Developments in Cancer Chemotherapy

Editor

Robert I. Glazer, Ph.D.

Chief
Applied Pharmacology Section
Laboratory of Medicinal
Chemistry and Pharmacology
National Cancer Institute
Bethesda, Maryland

C5
D53
1984

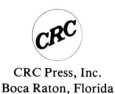

CRC Press, Inc.
Boca Raton, Florida

Library of Congress Cataloging in Publication Data
Main entry under title:

Developments in cancer chemotherapy.

    Bibliography: p.
    Includes index.
    1. Cancer—Chemotherapy. 2. Antineoplastic agents.
I. Glazer, Robert I. [DNLM: 1. Neoplasms—Drug
therapy. QZ 267 D4886]
RC271.C5D53 1984   616.99'4061   83-24034
ISBN 0-8493-5778-0

Direct all inquiries to CRC Press, Inc., 2000 Corporate Blvd., N.W., Boca Raton, Florida, 33431.

© 1984 by CRC Press, Inc.

International Standard Book Number 0-8493-5778-0

Library of Congress Card Number 83-24034
Printed in the United States

PREFACE

The field of cancer chemotherapy today is a rapidly expanding science which has now encompassed not only the more traditional areas of antimetabolite, antimitotic and intercalating agents, but also the fields of immunology and virology. Recent developments in these areas have involved new concepts in drug design, rational approaches for enhancing the synergism of combinations of drugs, detailed biochemical and molecular investigations into the nucleic acid and protein interactions of antimitotics and intercalators, mechanistic and clinical studies of old and new analogs as well as modification of the transformation and differentiation of cells by biological response modifiers such as the retinoids and interferons. The latter class of drug, in particular, has served as an impetus for the development of new pharmacological agents with interferon-like activity. The broad scope of this book was intentionally designed as such to emphasize the enormous complexity, as well as the number of biological processes which can be exploited to derive new approaches for the treatment of cancer. The tremendous effort of the contributing authors as well as the secretarial staff in the preparation of this book is gratefully acknowledged.

Robert I. Glazer

THE EDITOR

Robert I. Glazer, Ph.D., Chief, Applied Pharmacology Section, Laboratory of Medicinal Chemistry and Pharmacology, National Cancer Institute, National Institutes of Health, Bethesda, Maryland.

Dr. Glazer received his B.Sc. and M.S. from Columbia University and his Ph.D. in pharmacology from Indiana University in 1970. He was a recipient of a postdoctoral fellowship from the National Institutes of Health during his tenure in the Department of Pharmacology, Yale University School of Medicine. From 1972 to 1976, he was an Assistant Professor in the Department of Pharmacology, Emory University School of Medicine, during which time he was one of the first recipients of a Faculty Development Award in Basic Pharmacology from the Pharmaceutical Manufacturer's Association Foundation. He assumed his present post in 1977.

Dr. Glazer is a member of the American Society for Pharmacology and Experimental Therapeutics, The American Association for Cancer Research and the American Society of Biological Chemists. He serves on the Editorial Boards of *Molecular Pharmacology* and *Biochemical Pharmacology*.

His current major research interests include the mechanism of action of pyrimidine and purine antimetabolites, anthracyclines and interferons with respect to the synthesis and processing of RNA and nuclear protein phosphorylation. He has authored 90 research papers in the areas of cancer chemotherapy, carcinogenesis and drug metabolism.

CONTRIBUTORS

Theodore R. Breitman, Ph.D.
Senior Investigator
Laboratory of Medicinal Chemistry and
 Biology
National Cancer Institute
Bethesda, Maryland

Edwin C. Cadman, M.D.
Director, Cancer Research Institute
Professor of Medicine
Chief of Oncology and Hematology
University of California
San Francisco, California

Mrunal S. Chapekar, Ph.D.
Visiting Fellow
Laboratory of Medicinal Chemistry
National Cancer Institute
Bethesda, Maryland

Ernest Hamel, M.D., Ph.D.
Laboratory of Medicinal Chemistry and
 Pharmacology
National Institutes of Health
Bethesda, Maryland

Hiromichi Hemmi, Ph.D.
Department of Bacteriology
Tohoku University School of Medicine
Sendai, Japan

Hiremagalur N. Jayaram, Ph.D.
Senior Investigator
Laboratory of Medicinal Chemistry and
 Pharmacology
National Cancer Institute
Bethesda, Maryland

David G. Johns, M.D., Ph.D.
Chief
Laboratory of Medicinal Pharmacology
National Institutes of Health
Bethesda, Maryland

James B. Johnston, Ph.D.
Postdoctoral Fellow
Laboratory of Medicinal Chemistry and
 Pharmacology
National Cancer Institute
Bethesda, Maryland

Donna Kerrigan
Chemist
Laboratory of Medicinal Pharmacology
National Cancer Institute
Bethesda, Maryland

Victor E. Marquez, Ph.D.
Visiting Scientist
Laboratory of Medicinal Chemistry and
 Biology
National Cancer Institute
Bethesda, Maryland

Michael R. Mattern, Ph.D.
Cancer Expert
Department of Molecular Pharmacology
National Institutes of Health
Bethesda, Maryland

Yves Pommier, M.D.
Visiting Fellow
Laboratory of Molecular Pharmacology
National Cancer Institute
Bethesda, Maryland

Paul S. Ritch, M.D.
Assistant Professor
Department of Medicine
The Medical College of Wisconsin
Milwaukee, Wisconsin

Johanna D. Stoeckler, Ph.D.
Assistant Professor of Medicinal Science
 (Research)
Division of Biology and Medicine
Brown University
Providence, Rhode Island

Robert J. Suhadolnik, Ph.D.
Professor
Department of Biochemistry
Temple University School of Medicine
Philadelphia, Pennsylvania

Leonard A. Zwelling, M.D.
Senior Investigator
Laboratory of Molecular Pharmacology
National Cancer Institute
Bethesda, Maryland

TABLE OF CONTENTS

Chapter 1

PYRROLO [2,3-d] PYRIMIDINE NUCLEOSIDES

Paul S. Ritch and Robert I. Glazer

TABLE OF CONTENTS

I. INTRODUCTION

The pyrrolopyrimidine nucleoside antibiotics are structural analogs of adenosine, in which the imidazole portion of the purine is replaced by a pyrrole moiety (Figure 1). The three principal members of this group of compounds are tubercidin, toyocamycin, and sangivamycin. The biosynthesis of the pyrrolopyrimidines has been elucidated and total chemical synthesis of these compounds and derivatives has been achieved. Extensive biochemical studies indicate that the pyrrolopyrimidine nucleosides and their phosphorylated products are mutually competitive substrate inhibitors with adenosine and adenine nucleotides in a variety of cellular reactions. Tubercidin, toyocamycin, and sangivamycin have significant cytotoxic activity against mammalian cells and preliminary clinical studies have demonstrated antineoplastic activity. Interest in "old" anticancer drugs that were inadequately tested has recently been rekindled, and the pyrrolopyrimidine nucleoside antibiotics are among those drugs being resurrected for clinical evaluation. New information has become available that may suggest strategies for more effective clinical usage. Therefore, a review of this group of drugs is timely.

II. ISOLATION AND ANTIMICROBIAL ACTIVITY

Tubercidin, toyocamycin and sangivamycin were all initially isolated from various strains of *Streptomyces*. At least 13 different *Streptomyces* strains have been reported to produce this group of compounds. As with many other antitumor antibiotics, the pyrrolopyrimidines were discovered while screening for new antimicrobial agents. Initial biological testing demonstrated cytotoxicity against mammalian cells and subsequent investigations have further defined their antineoplastic activity.

A. Tubercidin

Anzai et al.[1] originally obtained tubercidin, or 7-deazaadenosine, from the broth of *Streptomyces tubercidus* isolated from the soil of Chiba Prefecture in Japan. Tubercidin has also been isolated from additional strains of *Streptomyces*.[2] The compound was discovered during a search for new antibiotics against tubercle bacilli. Antimicrobial activity was observed against *Mycobacterium* tuberculosis BCG (minimum inhibitory concentration, MIC <1 μg/

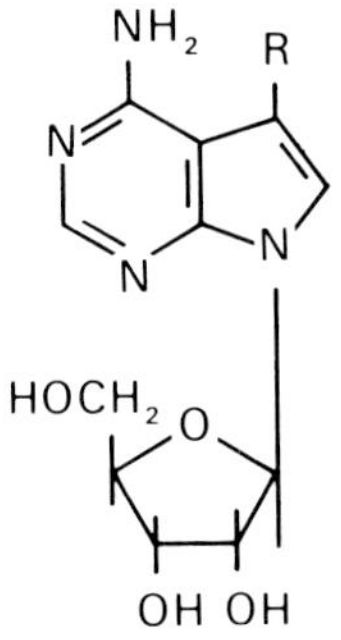

COMPOUND	R
Tubercidin	$-H$
Toyocamycin	$-C \equiv N$
Sangivamycin	$\overset{O}{\overset{\|}{-C-NH_2}}$
Thiosangivamycin	$\overset{S}{\overset{\|}{-C-NH_2}}$
Sargivamycin-amidine	$\overset{NH}{\overset{\|}{-C-NH_2}}$
Sangivamycin-amidoxime	$\overset{N-OH}{\overset{\|}{-C-NH_2}}$

FIGURE 1. The chemical structures of the pyrrolo-pyrimidine nucleosides.

mℓ) and *Candida albicans* (MIC 100 μg/mℓ), but not against a variety of Gram-positive and Gram-negative bacteria, other mycobacteria or *Candida* species, or against various fungi and yeast.[1] In subsequent studies, tubercidin was shown to inhibit the growth of *S. faecalis*[3] (IC$_{50}$ 2 × 10^{-8} M) and have activity against *Penicillium oxalicum*, *Glomerella* sp., and *Mycobacterium phlei*.[4] Several isolation procedures have been described.[2]

B. Toyocamycin

Toyocamycin was isolated from a culture of *Streptomyces tocoyaensis* by Nishimura et al.[5] using *Candida albicans* as test organism. The compound was extracted from both the culture filtrate and mycelium, although it was found to exist primarily in the fermentation medium. Numerous other strains of *Streptomyces* have been reported to produce toyocamycin.[2] Although the substance has been referred to by a variety of names including antibiotic 1037, antibiotic E-212, unamycin B, and vengicide, these antibiotics were subsequently shown to be identical to toyocamycin.[2,6-8] Additional isolation procedures have been described.[9]

Toyocamycin demonstrated antimicrobial activity against *Candida albicans* (MIC 1 μg/mℓ) and *Mycobacterium tuberculosis* var. *hominis* H37Rv (MIC 2 μg/mℓ), but little activity was seen against many Gram-positive and Gram-negative bacteria, fungi, or yeast.[5] Matsouka[10] reported that toyocamycin had growth inhibitory effects on *Candida tropicalis* (MIC 3 μg/mℓ), *Helminthosporium leptochloae* (MIC 3 μg/mℓ), and other microorganisms at higher drug concentrations.

C. Sangivamycin

Sangivamycin, initially designated BA-90912, was isolated by Rao and Renn[11] from the culture of a *Streptomyces* strain subsequently identified as *S. rimosus*.[12] Sangivamycin has only slight antibacterial or antifungal activity.[13] The fermentation conditions and isolation procedure have been described.[11] Suhadolnik has reported that the same organism is capable of producing both toyocamycin and sangivamycin.[2] At 30 hr after inoculation, similar concentrations of the two nucleosides were found in the culture filtrate. Toyocamycin production peaked at 42 hr, whereas sangivamycin concentration increased approximately sixfold over the subsequent 48 hr.

III. CHEMICAL STRUCTURE AND PROPERTIES

A. Tubercidin

Tubercidin is 6-amino-9-(β-D-ribofuranosyl)-7-deazapurine, or 4-amino-7-(β-D-ribofuranosyl)-pyrrolo[2,3-d]pyrimidine. The molecular formula is $C_{11}H_{14}N_4O_4$ and the molecular weight is 266. Suzuki and Marumo[14,15] elucidated the structure of tubercidin by chemical degradation. Mizuno and co-workers[16-18] provided proof of the structure and established the anomeric configuration as β. Tubercidin is a weakly basic, white crystalline compound. The pK_a of tubercidin is 5.3. The compound is readily soluble in acidic or alkaline solutions, slightly soluble is water, methanol, and ethanol, and insoluble in acetone, ethyl acetate, chloroform, benzene, and petroleum ether. Its UV and IR spectral characteristics and other physical and chemical properties have been described.[2,14,15,19,20] Total chemical synthesis of tubercidin was reported by Tolman et al.[21]

B. Toyocamycin

Toyocamycin is the 5-substituted cyano derivative of tubercidin: 4-amino-5-cyano-7-(β-D-ribofuranosyl)-pyrrolo[2,3-d]pyrimidine. Its molecular formula is $C_{12}H_{13}N_5O_4$ and the molecular weight is 291. The structure of toyocamycin was determined by Okhuma.[22,23] Toyocamycin is a colorless crystalline compound that is moderately soluble in methanol, ethanol, acetone, dioxane, and butanol, sparingly soluble in water and ether, and insoluble in ethyl acetate, chloroform, and petroleum ether. The UV absorption spectrum and other physical and chemical characteristics have been reported in detail.[5,8] Taylor and Hendress[24,25] synthesized the aglycone of toyocamycin, confirming its structure, and Tolman et al.[7,8] described the total chemical synthesis and established the β anomeric configuration of toyocamycin.

C. Sangivamycin

Sangivamycin is 4-amino-5-carboxamido-7-(β-D-ribofuranosyl)-pyrrolo[2,3-d]-pyrimidine. Its molecular formula is $C_{12}H_{25}N_5O_5$ and the molecular weight is 309. Rao[13] elucidated the structure of sangivamycin and described physical and chemical properties closely resembling those of toyocamycin. Sangivamycin is a weakly basic, colorless crystalline compound that is soluble in methanol, slightly soluble in water, and insoluble in acetone, ethyl acetate, chloroform, and ether. The UV, IR, and NMR spectral properties and chemical reactivity of sangivamycin are reported in detail.[13] The structural assignment of sangivamycin, as well as those of tubercidin and toyocamycin, was unequivocally established by total chemical synthesis.[7,8]

D. Pyrrolopyrimidine Derivatives

A number of additional pyrrolopyrimidine analogs have been synthesized. Gerster et al.[16] described the synthesis of various 4-substituted derivatives of tubercidin. The importance of the pyrrolopyrimidine 4-amino group was demonstrated by Saneyoshi and co-workers;[27]

a variety of 4-substituted compounds showed markedly diminished activity and toxicity (LD$_{50}$) in the NF mouse sarcoma model. Montgomery and Hewson[28] reported on the synthesis of 7-alkyl analogs of tubercidin, and additional pyrrolopyrimidine nucleosides similar to tubercidin were synthesized by Iwamura and Hashizume[29] and Pike et al.[30] Schram and Townsend[31] described the synthesis of fluorescent imidazo[1,2-c]pyrrolo[2,3-d]pyrimidine derivatives.

Gerster et al.[32] and Hinshaw et al.[33] discussed the preparation of new 4,5-disubstituted-7-(β-D-ribofuranosyl)-pyrrolo[2,3-d]pyrimidines by direct introduction of a functional group at position 5 via electrophilic substitution. Several 4-amino pyrrolopyrimidines with carboxamido-type groups at position 5 (i.e., sangivamycin derivatives) have been synthesized;[34] some of these have shown antitumor activity and may be of clinical interest.[35]

IV. BIOSYNTHESIS

A. Pyrrolopyrimidine Nucleoside Antibiotics

Suhadolnik and co-workers[2,9,36-39] have extensively studied the biosynthesis of pyrrolopyrimidine nucleoside antibiotics. Smulson and Suhadolnik[36] demonstrated that the pyrimidine ring of preformed purine (i.e., adenosine) is the direct precursor for the pyrimidine ring of tubercidin in *S. tubercidicus*; ^{14}C from adenine-2-^{14}C (but not adenine-8-^{14}C) was incorporated into the aglycone of the pyrrolopyrimidine nucleoside. When adenine-8-^{14}C was provided as the purine substrate, carbon-8 was lost as CO_2 in the conversion of the imidazole ring of the purine to the pyrrole ring of tubercidin. They also showed that ribose-1-^{14}C was incorporated into tubercidin, and that the label was equally distributed into the aglycone and ribose portions of the molecule, suggesting a metabolic conversion of C1 and 2 of D-ribose to the pyrrole carbons of the aglycone, analogous to the synthesis of the pteridine ring of folic acid and the indole ring of tryptophan.

Similar studies in *S. rimosus* showed that the pyrimido moiety of adenine-2-^{14}C served as the precursor for the pyrimido portion of toyocamycin.[9,37,38] Following isolation of the pyrrolopyrimidine, chemical degradation studies revealed that all of the ^{14}C was located in the pyrimidine ring and that it was found exclusively in the C-2 position of toyocamycin. As with tubercidin, C-8 of the imidazole ring of the purine (adenine-8-^{14}C) was lost during conversion to toyocamycin.

These findings can be explained by the loss of N-7 and C-8 during biosynthesis of the pyrrolo portion of the nucleoside.[2] The label from ribose-1-^3H was distributed equally to the aglycone and ribose portions of toyocamycin, whereas the tritium from ribose-3-^3H resided entirely in the ribose moiety. Further studies demonstrated that two ribose units attach to N-9 of the purine ring following removal of the ureido (C-8) carbon, and that C1 and 2 of both ribose units contribute equally to pyrrole ring formation.[38] Eistner and Suhadolnik[39] provided evidence that GTP (but not ATP or ITP) is the immediate precursor for the synthesis of the pyrrole ring of the pyrrolopyrimidine nucleosides. The ureido carbon is lost and replaced by a nitrogen via a reaction catalyzed by GTP-8-formylhydrolase.

The synthesis of sangivamycin is similar to that of the other pyrrolopyrimidine nucleoside antibiotics, and studies have shown that toyocamycin may serve as a direct precursor in the biosynthesis of sangivamycin.[2] Characteristics of the converting enzyme, nitrile hydrolase, are given by Suhdolnik.[2] Eistner and Suhadolnik[39] demonstrated that chloramphenicol interferes with the biosynthesis of sangivamycin in late-log phase *S. rimosus* by inhibiting GTP-8-formylhydrolase.

B. Nucleoside Q

In addition to those compounds that have been isolated from cultures of *Streptomyces*, other pyrrolopyrimidine nucleosides have been identified in prokaryotes and eukaryotes.

Nucleoside Q, a 7-deazaguanosine derivative bearing a C-7 cyclopentendiol side chain, has been demonstrated in tRNA from bacteria and a variety of plant and animal sources including mammalian tissues.[40,41] This nucleoside is present in the first portion of the anticodons of *Escherichia coli* tRNA[Tyr], tRNA[His], tRNA[Asn], and tRNA[Asp].[40] Nucleoside Q and Q*, which has a different side chain, have been identified in tRNA from starfish, lingula and hagfish, wheat germ, rat liver, ascites hepatoma (AH7974) and kidney, and rabbit liver.[41] A similar nucleoside has been detected in piperidine hydrolysates of tRNA from *Drosophila melanogaster*.[42]

Kuchino et al.[43] demonstrated that part of the carbon-nitrogen skeleton of the pyrrolo-pyrimidine aglycon of nucleoside Q is derived from a guanine residue. During the course of biosynthesis (G to Q), the C-8 carbon and N-7 nitrogen are expelled. Cheng et al.[44] also described a toyocamycin derivative that may serve as a precursor in the biosynthesis of nucleoside Q. Okada and co-workers[45,46] demonstrated that the incorporation of bases of Q precursors into the first portion of the anticodon of *E. coli* tRNA[Asn] and tRNA[Tyr] is catalyzed by the guanine insertion enzyme, tRNA transglycolase. This unique posttranscriptional modification involves cleavage of the N-C glycoside bond without breakage of the phosphodiester bond.

V. UPTAKE AND METABOLISM

Biochemical studies in numerous systems have shown that various analogs of adenosine, including the pyrrolopyrimidine nucleosides, are transported and anabolized to the corresponding nucleotides similar to the handling of adenosine itself. These data further indicate that the pyrrolopyrimidine nucleosides and adenosine are mutually competitive substrates for the same biochemical pathways.

A. Transport

Hakala et al.[47] studied the effects of tubercidin and toyocamycin on adenosine uptake in sarcoma 180 cells growing in monolayer. In this cell system, adenosine uptake is rapid and follows Michaelis-Menten kinetics (K_m 47 μM; V_{max} 300 nmol/min/g cells). After 15 min exposure to 3 to 30 μM labeled adenosine, 10 to 14% of cellular ^{14}C was in the form of ADP, 70 to 75% was found as ATP, and 5 to 7% was located in the acid-insoluble pool. When cells were simultaneously exposed to pyrrolopyrimidine nucleosides, uptake of adenosine (3 μM) was inhibited. Toyocamycin was a more potent inhibitor than tubercidin (IC_{50} ≤3 μM and 18 to 23 μM, respectively). Harley et al.[48] recently reported on the interaction between adenosine and tubercidin for transport into L5178Y cells. Replicate samples were exposed to tritiated nucleoside (adenosine, tubercidin) for graded brief intervals measured in seconds. Cellular uptake of the nucleosides was stopped by the addition of NBMPR (nitrobenzylthioinosine),[49,50] a potent nucleoside transport inhibitor, and the cells were immediately collected by centrifugation through silicone oil. Mutual inhibition studies demonstrated that adenosine and tubercidin are competitive permeants — i.e., substrates for the same transport mechanism. Iapalucci-Espinoza and co-workers[51] studied Ehrlich ascites cells under conditions of nutritional deprivation and demonstrated that toyocamycin uptake is unimpaired by amino acid starvation.

B. Phosphorylation

Following transport into the cell, major factors that determine whether the nucleoside (e.g., adenosine) will be salvaged for anabolism or degraded, in addition to allosteric regulation, are the relative K_m values for adenosine kinase and adenosine deaminase. In human erythrocytes, the K_m of adenosine with adenosine kinase is approximately 1.9 × $10^{-6} M$ (vs. sarcoma 180 K_m 5 × $10^{-7} M$), which is similar to that in Ehrlich ascites cells, H. Ep. 2 cells, and rat liver;[52] K_m for adenosine with adenosine deaminase is 1.2 × 10^{-4}

M, or 60-fold higher. Erythrocyte deaminase activity is considerably higher than adenosine kinase activity (0.15 vs. 0.027 μmol unit/mℓ cells). The concentration of the nucleoside will have an important influence on its disposition; at concentrations below $10^{-5}\,M$, adenosine would be preferentially salvaged by phosphorylation to AMP, whereas at levels exceeding $10^{-4}\,M$ adenosine would be primarily degraded by conversion to inosine and hypoxanthine.

Early studies demonstrated that tubercidin, toyocamycin, and sangivamycin are excellent substrates for adenosine kinase and that they are converted to the corresponding nucleoside monophosphate through 5′-position phosphorylation.[53] As with other adenosine analogs such as formycin,[54] these compounds are anabolized to mono-, di-, and triphosphate forms, although there may be differences in their relative contribution to the components of the nucleotide pool. Tubercidin is phophorylated to its nucleotide forms by human erythrocytes,[52,55] mouse fibroblasts,[56] mouse liver enzyme extracts,[57] mouse leukemia EL4 cells,[58] schistosomes,[59] and *S. faecalis*,[3] and serves as a substrate in cell-free systems for adenosine kinase from rat liver[60] and H. Ep. 2 human tumor cells.[61] Lindberg et al.[60] also demonstrated that toyocamycin is phosporylated by partially purified adenosine kinase from rat liver homogenates: K_m values for tubercidin, toyocamycin, and adenosine were $4.0 \times 10^{-5}\,M$, $8.0 \times 10^{-6}\,M$, and $1.6 \times 10^{-6}\,M$, respectively, and the corresponding V_{max} for each of these analogs was 2.7, 1.05, and 1.0 nmol 5′-MP per unit enzyme per min, respectively. Suhadolnik et al.[62] had previously demonstrated phosphorylation of toyocamycin to 5′-mono-, di-, and triphosphates by Ehrlich ascites tumor cells. Sangivamycin is similarly phosphorylated by adenosine kinase.[57] Glazer and Peale[63] reported that sangivamycin and thiosangivamycin reduced incorporation of ^{32}P into AMP to a much greater degree than GMP, CMP, and UMP in L1210 cells, and Bloch et al.[3] showed that tubercidin interfered with phosphorylation of adenosine and AMP — i.e., inhibited adenosine kinase and nucleoside diphosphokinase. Pyrrolopyrimidines may also participate in cyclic nucleotide formation. Zimmerman and co-workers[58] demonstrated metabolism of tubercidin to the corresponding 3,5′-monophosphate, and Blecher et al.[64] showed that cTuMP (cyclic 3′,5′ tubercidinyl monophosphate) had greater lipolytic activity in adipose tissue than cAMP.

The importance of phosphorylation as an essential initial step in cellular processing of the pyrrolopyrimidine nucleoside antibiotics has been readily demonstrated in kinase-deficient mutants. Resistance to tubercidin in *E. coli* deficient in adenosine kinase has been described,[53] and Gupta and Siminovitch[65] reported on adenosine kinase-deficient mutants of Chinese hamsters ovary cells resistant to tubercidin and toyocamycin. Bennett et al.[66] also described tubercidin resistance in an adenosine kinase-deficient subline of H. Ep. 2 cells.

C. Deaminase Resistance

In contrast to their anabolism according to the usual biochemical pathways for adenosine, pyrrolopyrimidine nucleosides are not disposed of via the mechanism primarily responsible for adenosine degradation. Bloch et al.[3] and Frederiksen[67] showed that tubercidin and toyocamycin are neither substrates nor inhibitors of calf intestine adenosine deaminase, and Agarwal et al.[68] demonstrated that these two nucleosides are devoid of both substrate and inhibitory activity with partially purified adenosine deaminase from human erythrocytes. Hardesty et al.[57] reported that sangivamycin is also resistant to mouse liver adenosine deaminase. Tubercidin is resistant to the effects of nucleoside phosphorylase, although it is a weak inhibitor of this enzyme.[3]

D. In Vivo Distribution and Disposition

There have been few studies on the distribution and disposition of pyrrolopyrimidine nucleosides administered to whole animals. Smith and co-workers[55] examined the in vivo handling of tubercidin, and Hardesty et al.[69] studied the tissue distribution and metabolism of sangivamycin in detail.

1. Tubercidin

Smith et al.[55] demonstrated that 80 to 98% of tubercidin (50 to 250 μg/mℓ) is absorbed by freshly drawn anticoagulated human blood, primarily in the erythrocytes. Tubercidin 5'-phosphate and 7-deazainosine, the deaminated analog of tubercidin, were absorbed to a considerably lesser degree. Uptake of tubercidin by RBCs occurred rapidly: 75% within 30 min and 95% absorption within 2 hr. Chromatographic analysis revealed that virtually all the absorbed drug had been phosphorylated to nucleotide form. Incorporation of tubercidin and toyocamycin into human erythrocyte nucleotide pools was also shown by Parks and Brown.[52]

When autologous erythrocytes were retransfused following incubation with tubercidin in vitro, the RBC half-life was not affected in either rabbits or dogs.[55] These data suggested that tubercidin does not significantly interfere with energy-providing reactions in the erythrocyte and are in contrast to findings in *S. faecais* in which tubercidin inhibited glucose utilization via interference by Tu 5'-TP (tubercidin 5'-triphosphate) with phosphofructokinase resulting in faulty regulation of the enzyme.[3,70] Smith et al.[55] suggested that the presence of Tu 5' TP per se does not necessarily result in cytotoxicity, and that lethality would be expressed only in those cells actively engaged in macromolecular synthesis.

In vivo studies in dogs revealed differences in the pattern of excretion depending on whether the tubercidin was injected directly into the vein or infused in autologous RBCs following in vitro incubation.[55] After rapid i.v. injection, 25% of the administered radioactivity was detected in the 24-hr urine, whereas only 0.29% of the biological activity was recovered as determined chromatographically. In contrast, when tubercidin-laden autologous erythrocytes were transfused, the drug was excreted more slowly; the 24-hr urine contained approximately 5% of the administered radioactivity and the excreted material exhibited the chromatographic mobility of tubercidin. Only after 21 days was approximately 18% recovery obtained. Smith and co-workers[55] suggested a two-component system for tubercidin following i.v. administration.

2. Sangivamycin

Hardesty et al.[69] studied the tissue distribution and metabolic fate of sangivamycin in mice following i.p. injection of radioactive nucleoside. As with tubercidin,[55] erythrocyte absorption was substantial; 90% of drug-derived radioactivity in the blood was in the RBC fraction, and at day 8 there was still 20% maximum activity in the red cells.[69] Sangivamycin half-life in whole blood following i.p. administration was 50 hr, similar to that observed for tubercidin.[55,69] Less than 1% of the acid-soluble fraction of sangivamycin in RBCs was free nucleoside; that is, >99% was phosphorylated. Sangivamycin was also taken up by liver, heart, brain, kidney, and spleen; however, the extent of drug phosphorylation varied among these tissues, and unmetabolized drug (free sangivamycin) comprised 1 to 5%, 8 to 12%, 12 to 15%, 50 to 60%, and 80% of the acid-soluble radioactivity in these tissues, respectively.

Maximum drug concentrations in all tissues were observed at 2 hr after injection, except for brain which reached peak concentration at 1 day. By day 12, brain tissue had also retained 12% of the maximum level of sangivamycin and SGM 5'-MP (sangivamycin 5'-monophosphate), whereas all other tissues had decreased sangivamycin concentrations to 1 to 5% of their maxima. The highest concentrations and most precipitous declines over the first 72 hr were seen in RBCs and liver. At day 3 there were still 50% maximum levels of SGM 5'-MP in kidney, spleen and brain, and by day 12 SGM 5'-MP was still detectable in all tissues. In RBCs SGM 5'-DP (sangivamycin 5'-diphosphate) concentration increased from 5.2% of the acid-soluble radioactivity at 1 hr to 21.6% at day 3; in other tissues the nucleoside diphosphate contributed only 0.1 to 2% to the acid-soluble fraction. SGM 5'-TP (sangivamycin 5'-triphosphate) was detected only in RBCs — 1.6% at 1 hr and 10% at day 3;

however, SGM 5'-TP conversion must have occurred in all tissues since the drug was incorporated into nucleic acids.

Incorporation of sangivamycin into RNA was observed within 30 min after drug administration. The most rapid initial rates of incorporation occurred in liver, heart, and spleen; maximum levels were reached at 24 hr. Less incorporation into RNA was seen in kidney, and there was no detectable increase in specific activity in brain tissue. By day 12, only 20% maximum levels persisted in liver, spleen, and kidney; in contrast, the heart had retained 65% of the incorporated radioactivity. There was a similar pattern of incorporation of sangivamycin into DNA, although to a lesser degree: approximately 25% of that for RNA in liver, spleen, heart, and kidney. No significant incorporation into DNA was observed in brain. By day 12 the levels had decreased to 20%, 10%, and 5% in kidney, spleen, and liver, respectively. As with free sangivamycin, SGM 5'-MP, and RNA, there was only a modest decline in DNA specific activity in heart; 50% maximum level persisted at day 12, probably reflecting the slow rate of turnover of cardiac cells.

The major excretory pathway for sangivamycin was the kidney,[69] and urinary excretion was slow. Only 8% of the drug-derived radioactivity was recovered in the first 24 hr. Approximately 40% of the administered material was accounted for by day 12.

Several similarities in the metabolism and disposition of tubercidin and sangivamycin are evident.[55,69] The half-life of sangivamycin following i.p. injection in mice (50 hr) is within the range of that observed for tubercidin administered i.v. to mice (43 hr) and rats (75 hr). Most of the drug-derived radioactivity is associated with the RBC fraction for both drugs. Also, the principal route of elimination for both tubercidin and sangivamycin is urinary excretion. The major apparent difference in the handling of these two drugs is in the degree of phosphorylation. The predominant species of tubercidin in erythrocytes is Tu 5'-TP. In contrast, sangivamycin is found primarily as the monophosphorylated derivative, SGM 5'-MP, although appreciable amounts of the di- and triphosphates are also detectable; at 72 hr the ratio of SGM 5'-MP:SGM 5'-DP: SGM 5'-TP in RBCs is 68:22:10. In this regard, sangivamycin more closely resembles toyocamycin; To 5'-MP (toyocamycin 5'-monophosphate) was found to be the predominant species in the acid-soluble nucleotide fraction in Ehrlich ascites cells.[62] It is possible that there are differences in the specificities of phosphorylating enzymes subsequent to monophosphate formation by adenosine kinase.

VI. INCORPORATION INTO NUCLEIC ACIDS

Incorporation of sangivamycin into DNA and RNA in erythrocytes[69] was referred to in the previous section. All three major pyrrolopyrimidines undergo phosphorylation and incorporation into nucleic acids. This has been studied in *S. faecalis*,[3] mouse fibroblasts,[56] Ehrlich ascites cells,[62] sarcoma 180 cells,[71] and human colon carcinoma HT29 cells,[72] and in cell-free systems with RNA polymerase and either DNA or deoxypolynucleotide templates.[73,74]

Acs et al.[56] demonstrated that tubercidin is rapidly incorporated into DNA and RNA in L cells. During exposure to 1 μg/mℓ tubercidin, 50% of the radiolabel was concentrated in the cells within 4 hr and, of this, 80 to 90% is in the acid-soluble fraction, entirely as ribonucleotides. In the acid-insoluble fraction, incorporation into RNA was threefold greater than DNA. Ritch and Glazer[71] observed a similar rapid incorporation of sangivamycin into DNA and RNA in cultured sarcoma 180 cells, and incorporation into RNA was tenfold higher than that for DNA in both log phase and plateau phase cells (Figure 2). Acs et al.[56] showed that only a small proportion of the tubercidin was incorporated into RNA as terminal-position nucleoside; 95% was incorporated as the ribonucleotide which was located throughout the polyribonucleotide chains. Suhadolnik et al.[62] demonstrated that toyocamycin is also incorporated into DNA and RNA, and that toyocamycin occupied both internal and terminal

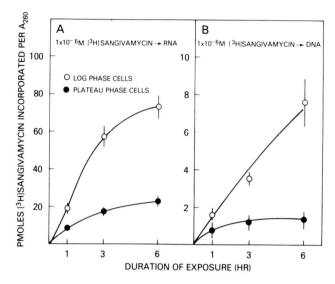

FIGURE 2.   Incorporation of [^{3}H]sangivamycin into RNA and DNA of sarcoma 180 cells.[71]

positions of RNA indicating that RNA synthesis continues for some time despite fraudulent incorporation of the pyrrolopyrimidine. The extent of incorporation of these analogs into DNA and RNA further suggested that the N-7 position of the purine is not a critical determinant of substrate specificity for those enzymes responsible for metabolizing adenine nucleosides. The demonstration that tubercidin[56] and toyocamycin[62] are incorporated into DNA as the 2'-deoxypyrrolopyrimidine nucleoside triphosphate also provided evidence that these compounds are substrates for ribonucleotide reductase.

The substrate specificity and allosteric regulation of pyrrolopyrimidines with ribonucleotide reductase from *E. coli* and *Lactobacillus leichmannii* have been studied extensively by Suhadolnik and co-workers.[75,76] Chassy and Suhadolnik[75] demonstrated that Tu 5'-DP (tubercidin 5'-diphosphate) and To 5'-DP (toyocamycin 5'-diphosphate) were enzymatically reduced to the corresponding 2'-deoxyribonucleotides by *E. coli* ribonucleotide reductase. SGM 5'-DP was not a substrate for the reaction, possibly due to the large 5-carboxamido group. Reduction of Tu 5'-TP and To 5'-TP (toyocamycin 5'-triphosphate), but not SGM 5'-TP, was stimulated by the prime effector, dGTP. However, SGM 5'-TP as well as Tu 5'-TP and To 5'-TP, inhibited the reduction of CDP and UDP, and inhibition of the reduction of ADP and GDP by 2'-dATP was potentiated by all three pyrrolopyrimidine nucleoside triphosphates.

In contrast to the substrate specificity observed with *E. coli* ribonucleotide reductase, Tu 5'-TP, To 5'-TP, and SGM 5'-TP were all substrates for ribonucleotide reductase from *L. leichmannii*, although the amount of Tu 5'-TP reduced was 36-fold greater than either To 5'-TP or SGM 5'-TP and, in the absence of Mg^{++}, Tu 5'-TP was a more effective substrate than ATP.[76] Both dGTP and 2'-dATP stimulated the reduction of Tu 5'-TP and To 5'-TP; reduction of SGM 5'-TP was stimulated by dGTP but not 2'-dATP. Without the prime effector, dGTP, Tu 5'-TP reduction was 75% that of ATP and 70% that of GTP; dGTP stimulated the reduction of ATP, Tu 5'-TP, To 5'-TP, and SGM 5'-TP by 18-fold, 20-fold, 472-fold, and 75-fold, respectively. Reduction of CTP and UTP by ribonucleotide reductase was stimulated by Tu 5'-TP and To 5'-TP, whereas these pyrrolopyrimidine nucleoside triphosphates inhibited GTP reduction and had no significant effect on the reduction of ATP. Comparing these results[76] with those reported by Chassy and Suhadolnik,[75] *E. coli* ribonucleotide reductase appears to have more rigid substrate specificity and less specific structural requirements for interaction at the allosteric site.[75,76]

Acs et al.[56] studied the effects of various inhibitors of nucleic acid synthesis on tubercidin handling in L cells. As might be expected, actinomycin D suppressed the incorporation of tubercidin into RNA. The DNA synthesis inhibitor, 5-fluorodeoxyuridine (FUDR), suppressed incorporation of tubercidin into DNA. After the removal of FUDR, however, a substantial amount of tubercidin was incorporated into DNA even in the presence of a tenfold excess of adenosine — i.e., during FUDR exposure a sufficiently large intracellular pool of tubercidin 5′-nucleotide derivatives accumulated to provide a source for 2′-deoxyribonucleotide conversion once DNA synthesis was permitted to resume. Radioactive 2′-deoxytubercidin was also incorporated into DNA but not RNA; however, the extent of incorporation into DNA was less than that observed when tubercidin served as the nucleoside precursor. Analysis of the intracellular acid-soluble fraction in cells exposed to 2′-deoxytubercidin revealed that there were no phosphorylated derivatives and that 2′-deoxytubercidin existed entirely as the free nucleoside. This is in marked contrast to the composition of the acid-soluble pool following exposure to tubercidin: 5 to 10% Tu 5′-MP (tubercidin 5′-monophosphate), 8 to 15% Tu 5′-DP, and 75 to 85% Tu 5′-TP.[56]

The work of Suhadolnik and co-workers[74] demonstrated that SGM 5′-TP competes with ATP, is a substrate for *Micrococcus lysodeikticus* RNA polymerase, and is incorporated into RNA with various DNA templates. With native calf thymus DNA primer, the initial rate of SGM 5′-TP incorporation over the first 20 min is only approximately half that for ATP incorporation; however, after 50 min SGM 5′-TP incorporation reaches 80% the efficiency of ATP. This is in contrast to the 26% incorporation efficiency of SGM 5′-TP using *E. coli* B RNA polymerase and denatured calf thymus DNA primer.[77] When poly d(A-T) primer was used with *M. lysodeikticus* RNA polymerase, SGM 5′-TP incorporation into the polymer was about 50% as efficient as ATP.[74] SGM 5′-MP and SGM 5′-DP were not incorporated, nor did these species inhibit ribonucleotide formation with poly d(A-T)-dependent incorporation of ATP and UTP into poly r(A,U), whereas SGM 5′-TP decreased ATP incorporation by 62%. Mixing experiments using RNA polymerase and poly d(A-T) primer, or calf thymus DNA primer in the presence of GTP, CTP, and UTP demonstrated that SGM 5′-TP is competitive with ATP for incorporation into RNA. Although little or no homopolymer formation occurred with SGM 5′-TP alone, SGM 5′-TP decreased ATP incorporation into homopolymer polyadenylate. Shigeura and Gordon[78] showed that 3′-deoxyATP inhibited the incorporation of both SGM 5′-TP and ATP into RNA. SGM 5′-TP incorporation into RNA is greater when Mn^{++} serves as the divalent metal ion, although incorporation does occur with Mg^{++}; SGM-5′-TP is incorporated into DNA with Mg^{++} as the divalent cation.[74]

Venkov et al.[79] demonstrated in *Saccharomyces cerevisiae* that after starvation for adenosine, toyocamycin is incorporated into pre-rRNA chains apparently replacing adenosine residues, and that the extent of replacement is dependent on toyocamycin concentration. Kapuler et al.[80,81] reported that Tu 5′-TP, To 5′-TP, and SGM 5′-TP can all replace ATP with mengovirus-induced RNA polymerase; relative efficiencies were 62, 41, and 81%, respectively. The 5′-triphosphates of tubercidin, toyocamycin, and sangivamycin were all capable of serving as ATP analogs for incorporation into alternating (A-U)-like ribonucleotide polymers with *E. coli* B RNA polymerase.[77] Suhadolnik et al.[74] demonstrated by alkaline hydrolysis or enzyme hydrolysis with bovine spleen phosphodiesterase that all of the ^{32}P in poly r(S-U) formed with RNA polymerase and poly d(A-T) primer was in SGM 2′(3′)-MP. Nearest neighbor studies by hydrolysis of susceptible phosphodiester bonds revealed SGM-3′-phosphate and adjacent uridine residues on both sides of sangivamycin. Apparently the N-7 of the imidazole ring of ATP is not essential for incorporation into RNA, and steric hindrance of the C-5 carboxamido group of sangivamycin is not a significant factor in polyribonucleotide formation.[74]

Incorporation of tubercidin into DNA alone results in loss of viability in L cells.[56] However, it is likely that incorporation into RNA is an important event in producing the lethal effects of pyrrolopyrimidines, and may be primarily responsible for cytotoxicity. Tubercidin inhibits the growth of double-stranded and single-stranded RNA-viruses as well as DNA-virus growth, and deoxytubercidin is less toxic to L cells than tubercidin itself.[56] Morphologic studies also demonstrated that actinomycin D prevents the development of cytological changes without suppressing tubercidin incorporation into DNA.[56] Tubercidin (1 μg/mℓ for 1 hr) produced cytoplasmic vacuolization and nuclear shrinkage, and caused the cells to detach from the culture dish. These changes did not occur in the presence of actinomycin D, suggesting than they may be related to ongoing RNA synthesis and drug incorporation. Desaminotubercidin was less toxic than the parent drug, and the aglycone of tubercidin was inactive even after prolonged exposures to high drug concentrations (10 μg/mℓ × 72 hr). Although 2′-deoxytubercidin was less toxic than tubercidin it did irreversibly inhibit growth at 1.9 μg/mℓ, but the cells remained attached to the culture dish. Cytological changes induced by 2′-deoxytubercidin were similar to those seen following irradiation or exposure to inhibitors of DNA synthesis, but cells did not develop the toxic appearance of tubercidin-treated cells.

Electron microscopic studies with toyocamycin revealed that low drug concentrations produced enlargement of the pars fibrosa of the nucleolus and high concentrations produced changes resembling those seen after exposure to actinomycin D.[82] Phillips and Phillips[83] reported on the time-dependence of ultrastructural alterations in the nucleolus during toyocamycin exposure. Treatment of Chinese hamster cells with toyocamycin (0.3 μg/mℓ) greatly inhibited accumulation of newly synthesized RNA in the cytoplasm without affecting the onset of nuclear or nucleolar RNA synthesis. Electron microscopic examination showed gradual disappearance of 150 Å granules from the particulate region of the nucleolus at 2 hr. At 4 hr the separate nucleolar regions could no longer be distinguished, and by 8 hr the ultrastructural alterations were more severe; the region that contains early rRNA became fibrillar. Effects of pyrrolopyrimidines on rRNA maturation will be discussed in a later section.

The function of tRNA that has incorporated pyrrolopyrimidine 5′-triphosphates has been studied. Ikehara and Ohtsuka[84] reported that triplets containing tubercidin at the 5′-end serve effectively as templates in the binding of tRNA to ribosomes, and that the incorporation of tubercidin does not interfere with the translation step of protein synthesis. However, tubercidin has effectively inhibited protein synthesis in a number of cell systems.[4,56,65,85] Uretsky et al.[86] demonstrated that all three pyrrolopyrimidine triphosphates are incorporated at the 3′-termini of tRNA from rat liver. Tubercidin-containing tRNA functioned satisfactorily in amino acid acceptor and transfer activities, and the coding properties of polysomes containing tubercidin were indistinguishable from those containing adenosine. In contrast to tubercidin-tRNA, which exhibited normal function in the esterification and transfer of amino acids into polysomes, tRNA containing toyocamycin or sangivamycin 3′-termini displayed greatly diminished acceptor activities. Although these nucleoside were incorporated normally, their presence did not permit normal function in the esterification of amino acids, possibly due to steric hindrance by the large cyano or carboxamido moieties. The effects of these drugs on protein synthesis have been discussed in detail.[2]

Ritch et al.[87] reported that log phase sarcoma 180 cells are more susceptible to the lethal effects of sangivamycin than early-plateau phase cells (Figure 3). Subsequent studies demonstrated that sangivamycin (1 × 10⁻⁶ *M*) is incorporated to a tenfold greater extent into RNA than DNA in both log phase and early-plateau phase cells,[71] and that incorporation into both nucleic acids occurs more rapidly and more extensively in log phase populations of both sarcoma 180 and human colon carcinoma HT29 cells.[71,72] The time- and concentration-dependent incorporation into DNA and RNA correlated with the effect of the drug on viability. Incorporation into poly(A)RNA was more pronounced in log phase cells, and an increased preferential incorporation into poly(A)RNA vs. nonpoly(A)RNA was observed in both log phase and early-plateau phase cell following prolonged exposure (Figure 4). As

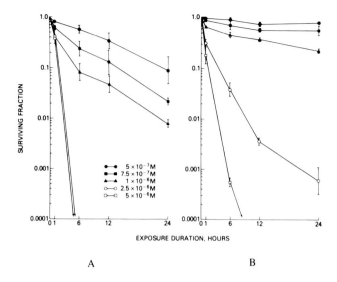

FIGURE 3. Time course of sangivamycin lethality in (A) log phase and (B) early plateau phase cultures. Surviving cell fractions at SGM concentrations of $5 \times 10^{-7} M$ (●), $7.5 \times 10^{-7} M$ (■), $1 \times 10^{-6} M$ (▲), 2.5 $\times 10^{-6} M$ (○), and $5 \times 10^{-6} M$ (□).[87]

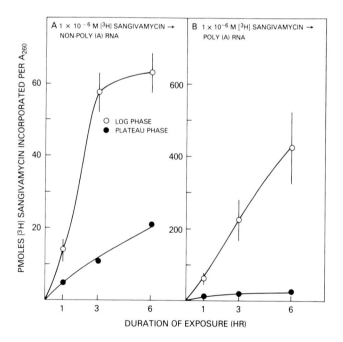

FIGURE 4. Incorporation of [³H]sangivamycin into nonpoly(A)- and poly(A)RNA of sarcoma 180 cells.[71]

the duration of drug exposure increased, progressively more sangivamycin was incorporated into poly(A)RNA in log phase cells than early-plateau phase cells: 6-, 11-, and 14-fold more at 1, 3, and 6 hr, respectively. There was a clear correlation between incorporation of sangivamycin into poly(A)RNA and cytotoxicity, and the increased proliferation rate-dependence of sangivamycin incorporation into poly(A)RNA closely reflected its lethality characteristics.[71,72,87]

VII. INHIBITION OF NUCLEIC ACID SYNTHESIS

Tubercidin produces a general inhibition of DNA, RNA, and protein synthesis.[4,56,85,88] Cass et al.[85] reported that tubercidin effected suppression of macromolecular synthesis at its IC$_{50}$ for L1210 cell growth; this was not observed for several nonpyrrolopyrimidine analogs of adenosine. Neither cytotoxicity nor inhibition of total RNA and DNA synthesis by tubercidin in L1210 cells was potentiated by 2′-deoxycoformycin.[85,89] Tavitian et al.[90] showed that the RNA-inhibitory concentration of tubercidin is also cytotoxic, but that DNA and protein synthesis continued for up to 6 hr; similar sequential inhibition has been described for actinomycin D, which inhibits RNA synthesis rapidly but permits DNA and protein synthesis to continue for much longer periods.[91] Gupta and Siminovitch[65] observed that tubercidin inhibited DNA and protein synthesis earlier than RNA synthesis in CHO cells, whereas toyocamycin inhibited RNA synthesis first, and DNA and protein synthesis subsequently. Ritch et al.[87] showed that the onset of inhibition of RNA synthesis in sarcoma 180 cells by sangivamycin preceded that for DNA synthesis, although neither was significantly suppressed at 1 hr, but DNA synthesis was more profoundly inhibited over the 3- to 24-hr observation period. This temporal pattern of inhibition for sangivamycin more closely resembled that seen with toyocamycin than tubercidin. At 24 hr, DNA synthesis was inhibited by 97% vs. 70% for RNA synthesis. Flow cytometry studies confirmed that the gradual suppression of ^{3}H-thymidine incorporation corresponded to delay in inhibition of DNA synthesis. During the first several hours there was continued progression of cells into and through early S. Inhibition of total RNA and DNA synthesis was dependent on drug concentration and duration of drug exposure. Flow cytometry showed a concentration- and time-dependent accumulation of cells in the late S-G$_2$ region of the DNA histogram. At prolonged exposure and at high drug concentrations there was a tenfold reduction in ^{3}H-thymidine incorporation, and there were no further changes in the DNA histogram.

Glazer and Hartman[72] reported that, after 2 hr of exposure, sangivamycin inhibited RNA synthesis by 40% in log phase HT29 cells with little effect on DNA synthesis; however, at 24 to 48 hr, DNA synthesis was significantly inhibited while there was little further suppression of RNA synthesis. In plateau phase cells, RNA synthesis was not suppressed even following prolonged exposure. Inhibition of both nonpoly(A)RNA and poly(A)RNA was seen in log phase cells, whereas neither RNA species was inhibited in plateau phase cells. Sangivamycin also inhibited synthesis of both nonpoly(A)RNA (IC$_{50}$ 5 × 10^{-5} M) and poly(A)RNA (IC$_{50}$ 2 × 10^{-5} M) in Ehrlich ascites cells.[92] Further separation of nonpoly(A)RNA into rRNA and tRNA showed that the inhibitory effects of sangivamycin were more pronounced on 28S than 18S rRNA (similar to xylosyladenine), but that 4S RNA synthesis was not inhibited (unlike xylosyladenine).

Kumar et al.[93] studied the effects of the nucleoside triphosphate of tubercidin on RNA chain elongation. Formation of the first phophodiester bond in RNA synthesis is accomplished by the liberation of a pyrophosphate from the complementary ribonucleoside triphosphate binding in the elongation site. Tu 5′-TP could effectively replace ATP as the chain-initiating nucleoside triphosphate, but was less effective in substituting for ATP as an RNA chain-elongating nucleotide.

The pyrrolopyrimidine nucleosides may also inhibit nucleic acid synthesis at other sites. Bennett and Smithers[94] and Henderson and Khoo[95] showed that tubercidin interfered with *de novo* purine synthesis. More recently, Bennett et al.[96] demonstrated that sangivamycin also interfered with formate utilization to a greater degree than hypoxanthine utilization in L1210 cells. However, the cytotoxic effects of sangivamycin were neither prevented nor reversed by providing 5-amino-4-imidazolecarboxamide (AIC), adenine, guanine, hypoxanthine, uridine, or uridine plus AIC. Thus, it is not likely that inhibition of *de novo* purine synthesis is a primary site of action for these compounds.

Table 1
THE EFFECT OF PYRROLOPYRIMIDINE ANALOGUES ON THE PHOSPHORYLATION OF HISTONE H1, HMG 14 AND 17, AND nRNA SYNTHESIS IN EHRLICH ASCITES CELLS[97]

| | ^{32}P incorporation | | | |
Drug	H1	HMG 14	HMG 17	nRNA
	(% control)			
Sangivamycin, 100 μM	48 ± 3	97 ± 3	99 ± 1	67 ± 1
Sangivamycin-amidine, 100 μM	56 ± 1	98 ± 6	104 ± 2	84 ± 1
Sangivamycin-admidoxime, 100 μM	53 ± 3	92 ± 11	96 ± 4	88 ± 1
Toyocamycin, 100 μM	45	98	94	64
Thiosangivamycin				
100 μM	10 ± 1	71 ± 4	69 ± 1	38 ± 1
10 μM	24 ± 1	96 ± 4	98 ± 4	60 ± 3
1 μM	93 ± 4	107 ± 5	102 ± 5	95 ± 4

Several new 5-substituted derivatives of sangivamycin have been synthesized.[34] Glazer and Peale[63] and Saffer and Glazer[97] identified important differences in the relative effectiveness of these analogs to serve as inhibitors of various cell functions. Thiosangivamycin was shown to be 50-fold more potent than sangivamycin as an inhibitor of nuclear RNA transcription.[63] At their respective IC_{50} concentrations for RNA synthesis, thiosangivamycin ($2 \times 10^{-7} M$) also inhibited DNA synthesis by 20 to 35%, while sangivamycin ($1 \times 10^{-5} M$) had no effect on DNA synthesis in L1210 cells. Both drugs suppressed the synthesis of nuclear rRNA, nonpoly(A)hnRNA, and poly(A)hnRNA by similar amounts, but sangivamycin was considerably less potent than the thio-derivative.

Saffer and Glazer[97] reported that sangivamycin inhibited histone H1 phosphorylation of Ehrlich ascites cells (IC_{50} 100 μM) whereas phosphorylation of high-mobility group (HMG) proteins, HMG 14 and 17,[98,99] was unaffected (Table 1). At all concentrations of sangivamycin, histone H1 phosphorylation was inhibited to a greater degree than nRNA synthesis (IC_{50} 400 μM). This is in contrast to actinomycin D, which inhibits nRNA synthesis but has no effect on histone H1 phosphorylation. Toyocamycin, sangivamycin-amidine, and sangivamycin-amidoxime were similar in potency to sangivamycin as inhibitors of histone H1 phosphorylation and nRNA synthesis, and also did not interfere with HMG 14 and 17 phosphorylation. Thiosangivamycin was 50-fold more potent than sangivamycin in inhibiting histone H1 phosphorylation and, in addition, demonstrated an inhibitory effect on HMG 14 and 17 phosphorylation. In cell-free assays with partially purified nuclear protein kinases, PK-I and PK-II, sangivamycin was a competitive inhibitor with either histone H1 or casein as substrate; K_i values with PK-I and PK-II were 200 and 100 μM, respectively. The IC_{50} for thiosangivamycin with PK-I was 40-fold less than that for sangivamycin, and closely paralleled the relative activities for inhibiting histone H1 phosphorylation in intact cells. The inhibition of nuclear protein kinase by sangivamycin and thiosangivamycin was a direct effect of the free nucleoside, since the enzyme preparations were devoid of nucleoside kinase activity. Other adenosine analogs such as cordycepin and xylosyladenine, when protected from deaminaton, also have an inhibitory effect on nuclear protein phosphorylation.[100,101] Tubercidin inhibited protein kinase from rat liver nuclei, and kinase NI was more sensitive than kinase NII (K_i $5 \times 10^{-5} M$ for NI; K_i $1 \times 10^{-4} M$ for NII); increasing the concentration of ATP reversed the inhibition.[102] Walter[103] and Walter and Ebert[104] reported on the stimulation of protein kinase from *Trypanosoma gambiense* and *T. cruzi* by tubercidin and adenosine.

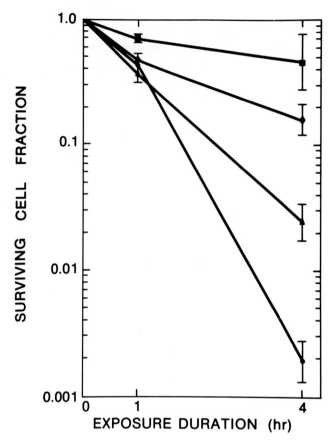

FIGURE 5.   Effects of 1-hr and 4-hr exposure to sangivamycin (●—●), thiosangivamycin (■—■), sangivamycin-amidoxime (▲—▲), and sangivamycin-amidine (♦—♦) at final drug concentrations of $5 \times 10^{-6} M$ on clonogenic cell survival.[35]

Ritch and Helmsworth[35] studied the relationship between RNA synthesis inhibition and drug lethality for several 5-substituted carboxamido-type pyrrolopyrimidine nucleoside derivatives in cultured sarcoma 180 cells (Figure 5). Comparable degrees of cell killing were produced by 1-hr exposures to $5 \times 10^{-6} M$ sangivamycin, sangivamycin-amidine, and sangivamycin-amidoxime; similar treatment with thiosangivamycin killed relatively few cells. After 4-hr drug exposures, significantly greater cell killing was observed for all analogs except thiosangivamycin, and sangivamycin was 12-fold, 85-fold, and 240-fold more cytotoxic than sangivamycin-amidoxime, sangivamycin-amidine, and thiosangivamycin, respectively. In contrast, the order of potency for inhibiting RNA synthesis was reversed; at 1 hr, RNA synthesis was inhibited 24, 57, and 73% by sangivamycin, sangivamycin-amidoxime, and thiosangivamycin, respectively. Log cell kill correlated inversely with early inhibition of RNA synthesis (r = −0.99), suggesting that fraudulent incorporation into RNA is a necessary first step in pyrrolopyrimidine lethality, and that early inhibition of RNA synthesis self-limits drug-related toxicity.

VIII. EFFECTS ON RNA PROCESSING

Tavitian et al.[90] studied the differential effects of toyocamycin on RNA transcription and maturation in mouse fibroblasts, HeLa S_3 cells, and Ehrlich ascites cells. At low drug concentration (0.1 μg/mℓ), toyocamycin completely inhibited synthesis of 28S and 18S

RNA, whereas synthesis of 45S RNA was unaffected; normally methylated 45S RNA continued to be synthesized for up to 6 hr and accumulate in the nucleolus. Analysis of the 45S RNA revealed that it contained toyocamycin, but otherwise the base composition was that of natural precursor 45S RNA. The inhibition of 45S RNA synthesis was reversible; following removal of toyocamycin, 45S RNA synthesis resumed. However, the 45S RNA that had been synthesized in the presence of toyocamycin was not converted to 28S and 18S RNA, even after removal of the drug. In contrast, normally pulse-labeled 45S RNA was converted to rRNA despite the presence of toyocamycin. Although the toyocamycin-containing RNA resembled RNA pulse-labeled with Me-^{3}H-methionine with respect to sedimentation coefficient, intracellular localization, and methyl acceptor activity, the substitution of toyocamycin for adenosine did not permit processing to rRNA. Gotoh et al.[105] demonstrated that 45S RNA which had incorporated toyocamycin was resistant to cleavage by ribonuclease III.

Tubercidin similarly caused accumulation of 45S RNA and completely inhibited rRNA synthesis; however, unlike toyocamycin. the effects of tubercidin were irreversible.[90] Although rRNA synthesis was totally abolished by toyocamycin and tubercidin, both drugs permitted 4S RNA (tRNA) synthesis to continue. Tavitian et al.[106] subsequently showed that, despite complete inhibition of rRNA synthesis, there was evidence of newly synthesized RNA bound to the polyribosomes. This *de novo* synthesized RNA was determined to have properties of mRNA.

Iapalucci-Espinoza et al.[51] examined the effects of toyocamycin on transcriptional and posttranscriptional processing of rRNA under conditions of amino acid starvation. Toyocamycin (2×10^{-6} M) reduced the transcription rate of rRNA in Ehrlich ascites cells in amino acid-rich medium; however, in amino acid-starved cells the decreased level of rRNA synthesis remained unaffected by the drug. In contrast, the processing of 45S pre-rRNA was markedly inhibited regardless of whether the cells were in complete or amino acid-deprived medium. The discordance between transcription and maturation indicated that drug uptake was not impaired by amino acid starvation. Since toyocamycin interfered with the activation of rRNA synthesis following refeeding of amino acid-starved cells without inhibiting the stimulation of protein synthesis accompanying refeeding, it was proposed that toyocamycin affected the mechanism regulating the rate of rRNA transcription.[51]

Radioautographic studies in CHO cells also demonstrated that toyocamycin interferes with rRNA processing. Exposure to 0.3 μg/mℓ of the drug inhibited the accumulation of newly synthesized RNA in the cytoplasm without affecting the onset of nuclear or nucleolar RNA synthesis.[83] Weiss and Pitot[107] showed that tubercidin and toyocamycin inhibited maturation of rRNA in Novikoff hepatoma cells in culture. Following drug exposure, processing of 45S RNA to 38S RNA continued, whereas formation of mature 28S and 18S RNA was significantly impaired; the labeling of 32S RNA intermediate precursors was affected to a lesser degree. They suggested that the drugs may prevent polyadenylation and/or methylation of adenosine residues.[107] Swart and Hodge[108] studied the effect of toyocamycin on adenovirus RNA processing and demonstrated that toyocamycin inhibited 3′ poly(A) additions without interfering with 5′ alterations (introduction of inverted dinucleotides) and internal methylations.

The effects of toyocamycin on processing of prelabeled pre-rRNA are concentration-dependent.[79] At low doses, there is a reduced rate of converting pre-rRNA into mature rRNA with accumulation of 27S and 20S pre-rRNA species; at higher doses, toyocamycin inhibits the last steps of pre-rRNA processing — conversion of 27S pre-rRNA to 25S rRNA and 20S pre-rRNA to 18S rRNA. Venkov et al.[79] concluded that the major site of action involves the last steps of rRNA processing, while transcription and early stages of rRNA processing are less affected.

Methylation reactions are crucial for maturation of nuclear rRNA, mRNA, and tRNA to their cytoplasmic counterparts.[109-111] The effects of pyrrolopyrimidine nucleosides on nRNA methylation have been studied extensively. Stern and Glazer[89] examined the effects of tubercidin in L1210 cells and demonstrated preferential inhibition of base methylation in mononucleotides, but not 2'-O-methylation in dinucleotides, similar to that seen with 8-azaadenosine and formycin, and in contrast to cordycepin and xylosyladenine which exhibited preferential inhibition of 2'-O-methylation in L1210 cells.[112] Sangivamycin had only a slight inhibitory effect on methylation of rRNA; thiosangivamycin was a more potent inhibitor of rRNA methylation, although methylation was inhibited to a lesser degree than nRNA synthesis,[63] and was similar in this respect to cordycepin and xylosyladenine.[112] Tubercidin also inhibited methylation of >18S nRNA to a greater extent than its synthesis at a concentration of $4 \times 10^{-6} M$. Increasing the concentration of tubercidin tenfold eliminated the preferential inhibition of methylation. Methylation of m^1A in 4S nRNA was relatively resistant to tubercidin, whereas methylation of m^2G, m^2_2G, m^7G, and m^1G was sensitive to the inhibitory effects of the drug.[89]

The uracil tRNA-methylating enzyme system which catalyzes the biosynthesis of ribothymidine in tRNA is relatively resistant to inhibition by a number of adenine derivatives that interfere with the activity of enzymes that catalyze the methylation of guanine in tRNA.[113] Adenosine preferentially inhibits guanine tRNA methylase as compared with uracil tRNA methylation in *E. coli*.[114,115] Wainfain et al.[116] demonstrated that tubercidin inhibits both guanine and uracil tRNA methylating enzymes. Although uracil tRNA methylase inhibition by tubercidin was decreased when the concentration of *S*-adenosylmethionine was raised, the relationship was felt to be more complex than simple competitive inhibition.[116] Lawrence et al.[117] reported that tubercidin is a competitive inhibitor of ATP for the ATP-PPi exchange reaction catalyzed by methyl-tRNA synthetase from *E. coli*. The K_i values for tubercidin and adenosine, which is also an inhibitor of the reaction, were 30 and 60 μM, respectively; the relative binding affinity of tubercidin with respect to adenosine was 200%.

Glazer et al.[92] demonstrated in Ehrlich ascites cells that sangivamycin did not affect methylation of nonpoly(A)RNA (unlike xylosyladenine) and was 20-fold less potent that xylosyladenine as an inhibitor of poly(A)RNA methylation. Xylosyladenine, but not sangivamycin, interfered with methylation of mono- and dinucleotide fractions arising from nonpoly(A)RNA, and sangivamycin was a considerably less potent inhibitor of methylation of mono-, di-, and oligonucleotide fractions of poly(A)RNA than xylosyladenine. Both sangivamycin and xylosyladenine exhibited slight preferential inhibition of base methylation over 2'-O-methylation. Transcription of rRNA, especially 28S rRNA (vs. 18S rRNA), and poly(A)RNA was preferentially inhibited by both drugs, while tRNA synthesis was unaffected by sangivamycin but sensitive to xylosyladenine. Since transcription proceeds toward the 3'-terminus, premature termination would result in preferential reduction of 28S synthesis. The greater sensitivity of 28S rRNA (than 18S rRNA) and the lack of inhibition of rRNA methylation by sangivamycin suggests the possibility of premature termination of ribosomal precursor RNA by some mechanism unrelated to hypomethylation.[92]

IX. METHYLASE INHIBITION BY *S*-TUBERCIDINYLHOMOCYSTEINE

The importance of *S*-adenosylmethionine as a principal donor in transmethylation reactions and in polyamine synthesis is well recognized. *S*-adenosylhomocysteine and the 7-deaza decarboxylated analog, *S*-tubercidinylhomocysteine (STH), both blocked methylation of tRNA in phytohemagglutinin-stimulated rat lymphocytes. *S*-adenosylhomocysteine also stimulated DNA synthesis via its degradation to yield adenosine, whereas STH inhibited DNA synthesis since its product of catabolism would be tubercidin.[118] Baxter and Byvoet[119] reported that tubercidin (0.1 $\mu g/m\ell$) inhibited rat liver histone arginine methyltransferase by 72%. STH is a potent inhibitor of mRNA methylases in vitro.[120,121] Kaehler et al.[122] demonstrated that STH inhibited 2'-O-methylation of cytoplasmic poly(A)RNA in Novikoff hepatoma cells. Inhibition of Newcastle disease virion mRNA (guanine-7)-methyltransferase by STH was reported by Pugh et al.[123] Chiang and Coward,[118] and Cass et al.[124] demonstrated inhibition of adenosylhomocysteinase by tubercidin. STH also acts as a potent inhibitor of spermidine synthase, as does the normal nucleoside substrate.[125] The biochemistry of reactions involving STH have been reviewed in detail by Suhadolnik.[77]

X. TUBERCIDIN ANALOG OF NAD$^+$

Bloch et al.[3] demonstrated that tubercidin served as a precursor for the biosynthesis of nicotinamide-7-deazaadenosine dinucleotide (NTuD$^+$) in *S. faecalis*. Lennon et al.[126] have studied the effects of changing the imidazole ring of NAD$^+$ to a pyrrole ring (NTuD$^+$) on various metabolic functions. In reactions involving dehydrogenases from several sources, replacement of the adenosine moiety by tubercidin had little effect on K_m and K_D, whereas V_{max} was markedly reduced. Substitution of tubercidin does not change the binding to the coenzyme domain of the dehydrogenase; however, there is a significant decrease in productive complex formation with the pyrrolopyrimidine analog.

Addition of NAD$^+$ to a cell-free synthesizing system derived from lysed rabbit reticulocytes replaces the requirement for an exogenously added energy-regenerating system. NAD$^+$ is effective at 5 μM and maximal stimulation is achieved above 25 μM NAD$^+$. NTuD$^+$ may effectively substitute for NAD$^+$ in this system and has 82% the activity of NAD$^+$ (vs. 27% for cordycepin and 18% for 2'-deoxyadenosine).[126]

NTuD$^+$ is also capable of serving as a substrate for the ADP ribosylation of elongation factor 2 by diphtheria toxin in lysed rabbit reticulocytes.[77] NTuD$^+$ is not an effective inhibitor of DNA synthesis in isolated rat nuclei. Toyocamydin and sangivamycin analogs of NAD$^+$ have not been studied.

XI. EFFECTS ON TRYPTOPHAN PYRROLASE INDUCTION

Tubercidin is a potent inhibitor of tryptophan pyrrolase induction by hydrocortisone in adrenalectomized rats when the drug is injected simultaneously with hydrocortisone.[4] The effect of tubercidin is dose-dependent (IC$_{50}$ 16 mg/kg). The methyl ester of tubercidin is a less potent inhibitor.

Injection of tubercidin 24 hr before hydrocortisone resulted in death for half the animals, and no enzyme activity could be detected in the survivors even after hydrocortisone injection. Tubercidin was ineffective as an inhibitor of substrate-induced stimulation of tryptophan pyrrolase by tryptophan.

Garren et al.[127] reported that actinomycin D given 4 hr after hydrocortisone produced a paradoxical transient increase in tryptophan pyrrolase activity; when tubercidin was administered 4 hr following hydrocortisone injection this paradoxical effect was not observed.[4] Puromycin produced a prompt reduction of tryptophan pyrrolase activity under these conditions.

XII. ANTISCHISTOSOMAL ACTIVITY

Protozoan and helminthic parasites have limited ability to synthesize the purine ring *de novo*; consequently, these organisms are dependent on salvage pathways using bases and nucleosides to satisfy requirements for purine nucleotides.[128] *Schistosoma mansoni* phosphoribosyl transferase activity is tenfold greater than that for adenosine kinase, and the principal pathway for conversion of adenosine to AMP is via adenosine deaminase and subsequent conversion of inosine to hypoxanthine. In this metabolic sequence, hypoxanthine phosphoribosylation is rate-limiting.[129] Earlier studies had indicated that tubercidin was active against various species of trypanosomes,[130,131] as was cordycepin.[132] Adenosine analogs would also be reasonable candidates to consider for chemotherapy against Shistosomes.

Tubercidin has multiple effects on schistosome nucleoside and nucleic acid metabolism, including inhibition of purine nucleoside phosphorylase — inosine accumulation exceeds that of hypoxanthine.[133] Of various adenosine analogs examined by Senft and Crabtree,[134] tubercidin was the most potent inhibitor of adenosine conversion to adenine nucleotides. Ross and Jaffe[135] demonstrated that the conversion of AMP to ADP and ATP was minimally affected by tubercidin and that Tu 5′-DP was not as good a substrate for schistosome adenylate kinase as ADP. In contrast, Tu 5′-DP was nearly as effective as ATP as substrate for rabbit muscle creatine phosphokinase, while Tu 5′-TP was a less effective substrate than ATP for Na^+, K^+-dependent ATPase in rabbit kidney.[135] Bloch et al.[3] had previously suggested that the toxicity of tubercidin in *S. faecalis* may be related to interference with glycolysis; however, Ross and Jaffe[135] showed that the adverse effects of tubercidin on *S. mansoni* could not be accounted for on the basis of inhibition of glucose uptake, glycolysis, or glycogen depletion. Studies by Miko and Drobnica[136] demonstrated that tubercidin only slightly inhibited rat liver mitochondrial respiration with both succinate as well as glutamate plus malate as substrates, and pigeon heart mitochondrial respiration, and did not inhibit endogenous respiration of Ehrlich-Lettre cells.

Stegman et al.[59] showed that tubercidin is converted to Tu 5′-TP by *S. mansoni* and interferes with the maintenance of normal ATP levels. At high concentrations of tubercidin (greatly exceeding those of adenine or adenosine), there was virtual shutdown of ATP synthesis. This could not be explained by interference with uptake since labeled adenine or adenosine was detectable; however, no label was incorporated into ATP. Cass et al.[85] similarly showed in L1210 cells that ATP levels were greatly reduced by tubercidin.

Exposure of schistosomes to tubercidin in vitro results in separation of copulating pairs, alteration of worm muscular activity pattern, and inhibition of egg-laying at drug concentrations as low as 10^{-7} M.[137] The onset of the tubercidin effects on *S. mansoni* were dose-related: at concentrations of 10^{-7}, 10^{-6}, and 10^{-5} M copulating worms were separated by 48, 24, and 6 hr, respectively. Both sexes are equally affected by the drug following in vitro exposure.[137]

Smith et al.[55] had demonstrated that tubercidin is rapidly absorbed into mammalian erythrocytes in vitro, and that 0.2 to 0.4 mg/mℓ whole blood can be sequestered without effect on longevity or function of RBCs when returned to the circulation. Since schistosomes feed on RBCs, it might be expected that the erythrocyte would be a good vehicle for drug delivery. Jaffe[128] showed in mice that the selective toxicity of tubercidin for the blood flukes of *S. mansoni* and *S. japonicum* in vivo can be increased when the drug is first incubated with a portion of the host's erythrocytes and the autologous drug-laden RBCs are transfused back into the infected animal. Lawrence[138] reported that intraerythrocytic tubercidin is more active against female worms since female schistosomes ingest erythrocytes ten times faster than male worms (330,000 vs. 39,000 cells per hr, respectively). Tubercidin has also been shown to be an effective antischistosomal agent in monkeys.[139]

XIII. ANTIVIRAL ACTIVITY

Tubercidin inhibits the growth of DNA-, double-stranded RNA-, and single-stranded RNA-viruses.[56] Brdar et al.[140] showed that the 5-bromo derivative of tubercidin reversibly inhibits the synthesis of hnRNA, rRNA, and mRNA, and interferes with SV-40 virus and Rous sarcoma virus proliferation. Several studies have shown that pyrrolopyrimidine nucleosides can inhibit the production of interferon and interfere with its antiviral effects.[141-143] De Clercq et al.[141] demonstrated that poly(Tu) inhibited interferon production in rabbit kidney cells challenged with vesicular stomatitis virus. Poly(Tu) appears to block interferon production by binding to a cellular receptor site.[142] Périès et al.[143] showed that toyocamycin inhibited the antiviral effects of interferon in encephalomyocarditis virus-infected cells.

XIV. ANTIPROLIFERATIVE EFFECTS

All the pyrrolopyrimidine nucleoside antibiotics have demonstrated inhibitory effects on the growth of mammalian cells. Tubercidin has been reported to have activity in vitro against NF mouse sarcoma,[1,27] mouse fibroblasts,[56,144] DON cells,[88] Ehrlich ascites cells,[144,145] CHO cells,[65] L1210 leukemia cells,[85] H. Ep. 2 cells,[66,144] HeLa cells,[13] and human epidermoid KB cells.[145-148] Acs et al.[56] demonstrated that exposure to 0.1 μg/mℓ tubercidin for 1 hr irreversibly inhibited colony-forming ability in L cells. Both desaminotubercidin and 2'-deoxytubercidin were less effective than the parent ribonucleoside, and the aglycone of tubercidin was inactive even at high concentrations and prolonged exposure. Cass et al.[85] also found that 2'-deoxytubercidin was less active than tubercidin in cultured L1210 leukemia cells, and Saneyoshi et al.[27] observed that 4-substitution (deamination) resulted in markedly reduced antiproliferative activity. Davoll also reported that the aglycone of tubercidin[149] was inactive.

Tubercidin is a potent inhibitor of KB cells in vitro (IC$_{50}$ 0.0075 μg/mℓ, or 3 × 10^{-8} M); at 0.15 μg/mℓ cell proliferation was completely suppressed.[145] Tubercidin was not cross-resistant with 6-mercaptopurine or its riboside; IC$_{50}$ was 0.006 μg/mℓ in the H. Ep. 2 parent cell line vs. 0.003 μg/mℓ in a 6-MP-resistant subline. Cass et al.[85] reported that tubercidin was highly cytotoxic to L1210 leukemia cells, and that tumorigenicity in mice was reduced greater than 5 orders of magnitude following exposure to 1 μM drug for 2 hr; xylotuberciden and aratubercidin were considerably less effective growth inhibitors. The activity of tubercidin was not potentiated by 2'-deoxycoformycin. Transport inhibition by NBMPR provided significant protection against the antiproliferative effects of tubercidin. Owen and Smith[145] demonstrated that tubercidin had significant in vivo activity against sarcoma 180 ascites tumor (1 mg/kg/day), Ehrlich ascites tumor (1 mg/kg/day), and Jensen sarcoma (0.5 mg/kg/day), and inhibited the growth of Dunning ascites leukemia. Tubercidin is also effective in vivo against NF mouse sarcoma[27] and L1210 leukemia.[13]

Toyocamycin has undergone less extensive testing than tubercidin. In vitro[13,27,65] and in vivo[27] activity has been seen against a variety of cell types, including L1210 leukemia, L cells, and HeLa cells.

Rao[13] reported that sangivamycin was cytotoxic to HeLa cells and had activity against L1210 leukemia in mice. More extensive studies on the antiproliferative effects of sangivamycin have been carried out in human colon carcinoma HT29 cells[72] and sarcoma 180 cells,[35,87] in vitro. Cell cloning studies have demonstrated that log phase cells are more susceptible to the lethal effects of sangivamycin than plateau phase cells.[72,87] The growth inhibitory effects of tubercidin and toyocamycin are also greater at lower cell densities.[65]

Ritch et al.[87] showed that drug exposure duration is a major determinant of sangivamycin lethality, and at prolonged exposures there is a steep dose-response relationship at drug concentrations above 5 × 10^{-7} M; as drug exposure was prolonged, small increments in drug concentration produced large increases in fractional cell kill. The preferential sensitivity of log phase vs. early-plateau phase cells also became more pronounced at longer durations of exposure to sangivamycin. Glazer and Hartman[72] also observed significantly increased cytotoxicity for both log phase and plateau phase HT29 cells as sangivamycin exposure was increased from 2 to 24 to 48 hr (Figure 6). They suggested that the time-dependency of sangivamycin lethality may relate to the requirement for the drug to be metabolized and incorporated into nucleic acids. This is supported by the slight to moderate inhibition of poly(A)RNA synthesis by sangivamycin, and the strong correlation between incorporation into poly(A)RNA (Figure 7) and drug lethality.[71,72,87] This effect is further substantiated by the inverse relationship between early inhibition of RNA synthesis and cell killing by various derivatives of sangivamycin.[35] Ritch et al.[87] suggested that pharmacological studies in man might provide information to optimize the schedule of administration; if "effective" plasma

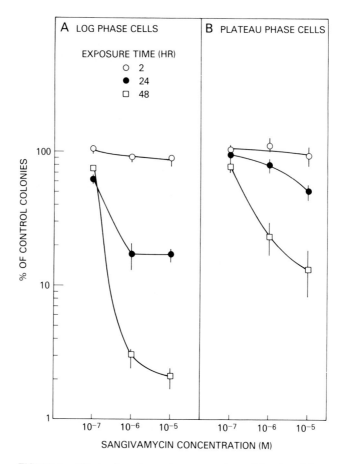

FIGURE 6.   Effects of sangivamycin concentration and duration of drug exposure on clonogenic cell survival of (A) log phase and (B) plateau phase human colon carcinoma cells in culture.[72]

levels are not sustained following intermittent pulse administration, prolonged i.v. infusion might be necessary to maintain cytotoxic drug concentrations.

Acs et al.[56] and Owen and Smith[145] reported that the growth inhibition of L cells and KB cells by tubercidin cannot be reversed by subsequent addition of various purines, pyrimidines, and nucleosides including adenosine, 2'-deoxyadenosine, and inosine. Recent studies by Ritch and Helmsworth[35] demonstrated that partial protection against sangivamycin toxicity in cultured sarcoma 180 cells can be provided by the simultaneous addition of adenosine plus 2'-deoxycoformycin, whereas neither adenosine nor 2'-deoxycoformycin alone had any effect on sangivamycin cytotoxicity (Figure 8). Adenosine could not be effectively replaced by 2'-deoxyadenosine in the combination with 2'-deoxycoformycin, and preliminary data indicate that 2'-deoxycoformycin plus adenosine (but not 2'-deoxyadenosine) interfere with the incorporation of sangivamycin into both nonpoly(A)- and poly(A)RNA.[150] When adenosine plus 2'-deoxycoformycin was added following exposure to sangivamycin, toxicity could not be reversed. These findings suggest that fraudulent incorporation into nonpoly(A)- and/or poly(A)RNA may be responsible for the lethal effects of pyrrolopyrimidines.

Relatively few other pyrrolopyrimidine analogs have been evaluated for antineoplastic activity. Both sangivamycin-amidine and sangivamycin-amidoxime inhibited colony formation in sarcoma 180 cells in vitro, but were less effective than sangivamycin, and thiosangivamycin had little activity in this cell system.[35] These derivatives were also active against L1210 leukemia, P388 leukemia, and colon carcinoma 26 in mice.[151] Kravchenko et al.[152]

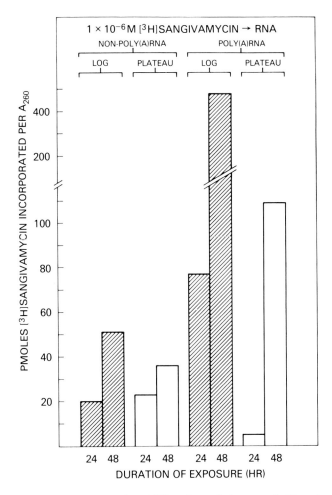

FIGURE 7. Incorporation of ^{3}H]sangivamycin into nonpoly(A)- and poly(A)RNA of log phase and plateau phase human colon carcinoma HT29 cells.[72]

reported that in vivo, sarcoma 180, sarcoma 45, and Jensen sarcoma were sensitive to additional pyrrolopyrimidine analogs.

Little information is available on the interaction between pyrrolopyrimidine nucleoside antibiotics and other cytotoxic drugs. Owen and Smith[145] studied the effects of tubercidin in combination with other antineoplastic agents against KB cells in vitro. No enhancement of tubercidin cytotoxicity was seen with methotrexate, 5-fluorouracil, 5-fluorodeoxyuridine, cytosine arabinoside, 6-mercaptopurine, streptozotocin, or uracil mustard.

XV. PRECLINICAL TOXICOLOGY

A. Tubercidin

The acute toxicity produced by a single dose of tubercidin was studied by Owen and Smith.[145] The LD_{50} according to route of administration was 35 mg/kg i.v., 32 mg/kg i.p., and 40 mg/kg p.o. in mice; 1.5 mg/kg i.v. and 20 mg/kg p.o. in rats; and >25 mg/kg i.v. in dogs. Following i.v. administration, toxicity was observed in lung tissue, pancreas, kidneys, liver, and gonads; hematological changes were insignificant. Anzai et al.[1] had observed an LD_{50} of 45 mg/kg in mice following i.v. administration.

Maximum tolerated dose for repeated injections in mice over 5 to 7 days was approximately

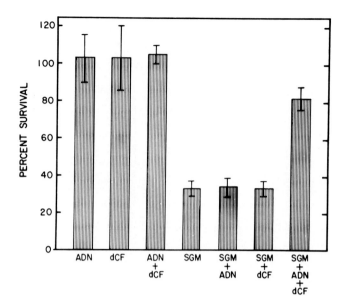

FIGURE 8.   Simultaneous exposure to 2'-deoxycoformycin plus adenosine provides partial protection against sangivamycin lethality in cultured sarcoma 180 cells.[35]

1 mg/kg in the studies reported by Owen and Smith.[145] More detailed evaluation of the
subacute toxicity following repeated injections in mice were reported by Smith et al.[4] Daily
injections were given either i.p. or p.o. for 5 days. There was a progressive increase in fatal
toxicity as the i.p. dose was escalated from 1 mg/kg to as high as 30 mg/kg. No deaths
occurred during the injection period at 1 mg/kg, although four of ten animals were dead at
day 11. At 3 mg/kg and 10 mg/kg, no animals survived beyond day 11 or day 5, respectively.
The 30 mg/kg dose was lethal to nine of the ten test animals by day 2. Considerably less
toxicity was observed after p.o. administration; all animals survived through day 11 at the
three lowest dose levels. At 30 mg/kg there were 1, 7, and 9 deaths by day 2, 5, and 11,
respectively.

Grage et al.[153] examined the chronic toxicity of tubercidin given repeatedly over more
prolonged periods. Maximum tolerated i.v. dose was <0.25 mg/kg/day × 19 days in rats,
<0.25 mg/kg/day × 31 days in dogs, and <1.0 mg/kg/day × 24 days in monkeys. The
only chemical alteration observed was an abnormal glucose tolerance curve. Postmortem
studies on dogs sacrificed at days 31 and 60 demonstrated fatty metamorphosis and necrosis
in the liver, and congestion and decreased size of the islets of Langerhans. Doses of 8 mg/
kg/day to monkeys was fatal after four injections. Autopsy examination revealed fatty
infiltration of the liver and disappearance of the islets of Langerhans. Prolonged dosing of
1 mg/kg/day was discontinued after 24 days because of venous access problems. Examination
of the sacrificed animals showed pancreatic acinar congestion.

B. Toyocamycin

Wilson[154] reported on preclinical toxicology of toyocamycin given in various dosage
schedules. Single i.p. injections in rats resulted in growth retardation and death on the 2nd
to 13th day. LD_{50} was 4 mg/kg in ICR Swiss mice and 5 mg/kg in BDF_1 mice. Single i.p.
injections in rats produced dose-dependent growth retardation and ascites; LD_{50} was 250
μg/kg. Dogs given a single i.v. dose of 100 to 500 μg/kg developed decreased appetite and
weight loss; at higher doses of 3.5 to 5 mg/kg the animals experienced vomiting, diarrhea,
lethargy and death within 2 to 5 days.

The LD_{50} for a series of 14 daily i.p. injections was 175 μg/kg/day in ICR Swiss mice and 250 μg/kg/day in BDF$_1$ mice. Growth retardation was observed in all animals. At the lower dose levels, animals died 1 to 9 days following completion of the series; at higher doses, all of the animals died during the injection period. Rats given 14 daily i.p. injections were asymptomatic at 25 μg/kg/day and showed evidence of growth retardation and ascites at 50 μg/kg/day. LD$_{50}$ for the 14-day series was 80 μg/kg/day. When the series of injections was extended to 24 days, slight reversible leucopenia was observed at 4.38 to 17.5 μg/kg/day and slight leucopenia and anemia was seen at 35 μg/kg/day. LD$_{50}$ for the extended series was 70 μg/kg/day.

Dogs given daily i.v. injections 6 days/week for up to 25 injections showed no clinical toxicity at 37.5 μg/kg/day, and only elevated fibrinogen was noted at 75 μg/kg/day. Dogs receiving 150-μg/kg doses developed anorexia, emesis, diarrhea, weight loss, and lethargy; none of the animals survived the injection period. Elevated levels of fibrinogen and nonprotein nitrogen were observed prior to death. Autopsy studies revealed pulmonary congestion, mucosal inflammation in the bladder and gastrointestinal tract, pancreatic hemorrhages and morphological changes in the liver and kidneys.

C. Sangivamycin

LD$_{50}$ for single doses of sangivamycin[155] was a 4 mg/kg i.p. in mice, 1.2 mg/kg i.p. in rats, and 2.5 mg/kg i.v. in dogs. The maximum tolerated dose for repeated injections in rats was 12.5 μg/kg/day × 25 days and the LD$_{50}$ was 25 to 50 μg/kg/day × 24 days. In dogs, the maximum tolerated dose on this schedule was 50 μg/kg/day. Toxicity in dogs included diarrhea, dehydration, lethargy, hematuria, lymphopenia, mild thrombocytopenia, azotemia, and electrolyte abnormalities including hyponatremia, hypokalemia, and hypochloremia. At higher doses hepatic and gallbladder toxicity were observed. LD$_{50}$ for repeated injections in dogs was 300 μg/kg/day. The maximum tolerated dose in monkeys was 400 μg/kg/day; toxicity included anemia and abnormal hepatic function. A dose of 1.6 mg/kg/day was lethal for two monkeys after 13 and 17 days, probably secondary to interstitial pneumonitis. Postmortem examination also revealed intestinal hemorrhages, hyperemia in the kidneys, and inflammatory muscle degeneration.

XVI. CLINICAL STUDIES

A. Tubercidin

Bisel et al.[156] reported on the initial Phase I clinical testing of tubercidin; 111 courses were given to 93 adult patients with a variety of solid tumors. Tubercidin was given i.v. daily × 10 days at an initial dose level of 25 μg/kg/day and escalated by increments to 300 μg/kg/day. Local venous irritation and venous thrombosis were observed in 12 patients; accidental subcutaneous extravasation resulted in local inflammation and ulceration. Mild anorexia, nausea, and vomiting were seen in ten patients. Hematological toxicity was mild and developed in only six patients; the lowest WBC recorded was 2900/mm^3 and there was no anemia or thrombocytopenia. Nephrotoxicity in the form of proteinuria and/or azotemia was noted in 18 patients; this seldom occurred at a dose less than 200 μg/kg/day and was observed in four of ten patients with renal cell carcinoma. There were no drug-related deaths. Tumor response was suggested in three patients and all of these had islet cell carcinoma of the pancreas.

Grage et al.[153] conducted a Phase I clinical trial in 45 patients in which tubercidin was given by intraerythrocytic administration to avoid local venous complications and extravasation necrosis. Tubercidin was incubated in vitro at 37°C with 500 mℓ autologous blood and transfused back into the patients. Doses ranged from 200 to 1500 μg/kg weekly for 2 weeks. Toxicity was mild and reversible. Minimal hematological toxicity developed in six patients, renal toxicity in five patients, hepatic toxicity in two patients, and severe gastrointestinal toxicity in one patient. Temporary carbohydrate intolerance was noted. Tumor regression was observed in four patients: three had islet cell carcinoma of the pancreas and one had carcinoid of the stomach.

Topically administered tubercidin 0.5% in a petrolatum base was given to eight patients with solitary nodular basal cell carcinoma (lesions 8 to 14 mm in diameter) and five patients with widespread actinic keratoses for 2 to 6 weeks.[157] Treatment produced complete regression of all eight basal cell carcinomas as defined by clinical disappearance, healing at the treatment site, rebiopsy 4 weeks later, and follow-up at $1^1/_2$ years with no recurrences. The sequence of changes at the treatment site was, in order of appearance: moist erythema; edema, oozing, and cyanosis; ulceration; escher formation; and reepithelialization. In contrast to the dramatic response rate seen in basal cell carcinoma, tubercidin treatment was unsuccessful in four of five patients with actinic keratoses.

Klein et al.[158] also reported on the use of topically applied tubercidin against a variety of cutaneous tumors. Tubercidin 1% produced more severe local reaction than appeared necessary for tumor eradication, and lowering the dose to 0.01 to 0.5% was effective with minimal side effects. No systemic toxicity was noted. Treatment was given locally to cutaneous lesions of mycosis fungoides, reticulum cell sarcoma, squamous cell carcinoma, and breast carcinoma. Antineoplastic activity was demonstrated in the majority of patients.

B. Toyocamycin

In a Phase I study of toyocamycin conducted by Wilson,[154] 35 courses of treatment were given to 23 patients over a dose range of 10 to 200 μg/kg/day × 5 days. No systemic toxicity was observed; however, there were severe local reactions with necrosis at the venipuncture site if the drug extravasated, and phlebitis proximal to the infusion. The trial was discontinued due to local toxicity.

C. Sangivamycin

Cavins et al.[159] reported a Phase I clinical trial of sangivamycin in which 40 evaluable patients received the drug by slow i.v. injection at doses of 10 to 120 μg/kg daily, 50 to 250 μg/kg thrice weekly, or 50 to 300 μg/kg weekly. Hypotension and flushing occurred if the drug was administered too rapidly and could be avoided by prolonging the infusion to 1 hr. Occasional mild nausea was observed. Leucopenia and thrombocytopenia developed in two patients and transient hypochloremia was seen in one patient. There were no drug-related abnormalities in liver function. No subjective or objective tumor responses were noted and the study did not establish a maximum tolerated dose.

Phase I studies in children raised a concern over possible cardiac toxicity.[160] Electrocardiographic abnormalities in children being treated with sangivamycin for acute leukemia included brief periods of sinus arrest, wandering atrial pacemaker, and atrioventricular block.[161] Sudden death occurred in one child with acute myelogenous leukemia who had achieved complete remission; post mortem examination showed no evident cause of death. Subsequent review of 75 adult patients who had received sangivamycin showed no clinical evidence of cardiac toxicity and EKG abnormalities, and primary and secondary AV block[161] were seen in only two patients.

XVII. CONCLUSION

The pyrrolopyrimidine nucleosides and their phosphorylated derivatives compete with adenosine and adenine nucleotides in a number of biochemical reactions and effectively serve as substrates or inhibitors in a variety of metabolic processes. Although a specific biochemical lesion that is directly responsible for cytotoxicity in mammalian cells has not been elucidated with certainty, recent studies have identified metabolic events that appear to be at least closely associated with the mechanisms that translate to lethality. Existing data suggest that drug incorporation into RNA, particularly poly(A)RNA, may be a prerequisite for the expression of the inhibitory effects on cell proliferation and viability. The relation between this and other biochemical effects, such as inhibition of DNA synthesis of rRNA maturation, remains to be determined.

Available data may be useful to suggest therapeutic strategies to be explored clinically. Initial clinical evaluation employed intermittent pulse administration according to various treatment schedules. However, if absorption by erythrocytes was rapid, it was likely that therapeutic plasma levels were sustained only transiently and drug delivery to the tumor may have been inadequate. If RBC absorption is saturable, prolonged i.v. infusion might be more effective in maintaining tumoricidal plasma concentrations. Since host toxicity may also be more severe at prolonged drug exposures, pharmacological monitoring would be useful to titrate drug delivery. If incorporation of the drug into poly(A)RNA is an essential step in effecting lethality, it may be possible to selectively enhance incorporation into this species in tumor cells with other agents (e.g., testosterone stimulates mRNA synthesis in prostate carcinoma cells) to potentiate the antineoplastic effects and improve the therapeutic index. Early Phase I studies suggested that certain endocrine tumors, such as pancreatic islet cell carcinomas and carcinoid tumors, are sensitive to pyrrolopyrimidines; activity against these neoplasms should be better defined in Phase II studies using more effective treatment schedules. In view of the potential cardiac toxicity of these compounds, close observation for conduction disturbances should be exercised during initial clinical studies with frequent EKGs and, if necessary, continuous Holter monitoring. Preliminary clinical trials examining some of these issues are currently in progress.

ACKNOWLEDGMENT

The authors gratefully acknowledge Melody K. Pringle for secretarial assistance in the preparation of this manuscript.

REFERENCES

1. **Anzai, K., Nakamura, G., and Suzuki, S.,** A new antibiotic, tubercidin, *J. Antibiot. (Tokyo),* 10A, 201, 1957.
2. **Suhadolnik, R. J.,** Pyrrolopyrimidine nucleosides, in *Nucleoside Antibiotics,* Suhadolnik, R. J., Ed., John Wiley & Sons, Inc., New York, 1970, chap. 8.
3. **Bloch, A., Leonard, R. J., and Nichol, C. A.,** On the mode of action of 7-deazaadenosine (tubercidin), *Biochim. Biophys. Acta,* 138, 10, 1967.
4. **Smith, C. G., Gray, G. D., Carlson, R. G., and Hanze, A. R.,** Biochemical and biological studies with tubercidin (7-deaza-adenosine), 7-deazainosine, and certain nucleotide derivatives of tubercidin, *Adv. Enzyme Regul.,* 5, 121, 1967.
5. **Nishimura, H., Katagiri, K., Sato, K., Mayama, M., and Shimaoka, N.,** Toyocamycin, a new anti-Candida antibiotic, *J. Antibiot. (Tokyo),* 9A, 60, 1956.
6. **Aszalos, A., Lemanski, P., Robison, R., Davis, S., and Berk, B.,** Identification of antibiotic 1037 as toyocamycin, *J. Antibiot. (Tokyo),* 19A, 285, 1966.
7. **Tolman, R. L., Robins, R. K., and Townsend, L. B.,** Pyrrolo[2,3-d]pyrimidine nucleoside antibiotics. Total synthesis and structure of toyocamycin, unamycin B, vengicide, antibiotic E-212, and sangivamycin (BA-90912), *J. Am. Chem. Soc.,* 90, 524, 1968.
8. **Tolman, L. R., Robins, R. K., and Townsend, L. B.,** Pyrrolopyrimidine nucleosides. III. The total synthesis of toyocamycin, sangivamycin, tubercidin, and related derivatives, *J. Am. Chem. Soc.,* 91, 2102, 1969.
9. **Uematsu, T. and Suhadolnik, R. J.,** Nucleoside antibiotics. VI. Biosynthesis of the pyrrolopyrimidine nucleoside antibiotic toyocamycin by *Streptomyces rimosus, Biochemistry,* 9, 1260, 1970.

10. **Matsouka, M.,** Biological studies on antifungal substances produced by *Streptomyces fungicidicus, J. Antibiot. (Tokyo),* 13A, 121, 1960.

11. **Rao, K. V. and Renn, D. W.,** BA-90912: an antitumor substance, *Antimicrob. Agents Chemother.,* 77, 1963.

12. **Rao, K. V., Marsh, W. S., and Renn. D. W.,** Sangivamycin and derivatives, *Chem. Abstr.,* 70, 191, 1979.

13. **Rao, K. V.,** Structure of sangivamycin, *J. Med. Chem.,* 11, 939, 1968.

14. **Suzuki, S. and Marumo, S.,** Chemical structure of tubercidin, *J. Antibiot. (Tokyo),* 13A, 360, 1960.

15. **Suzuki, S. and Marumo, S.,** Chemical structure of tubercidin, *J. Antibiot. (Tokyo),* 14A, 34, 1961.

16. **Mizuno, Y., Ikehara, M., Watanabe, K., Suzuki, S., and Itoh, T.,** Synthetic studies of potential antimetabolites. IX. The anomeric configuration of tubercidin, *J. Org. Chem.,* 28, 3329, 1963.

17. **Mizuno, Y., Ikehara, M., Watanabe, K., Suzuki, S., and Itoh, T.,** Synthetic studies of potential antimetabolites. X. Synthesis of 4-hydroxy-7-(β-D-ribofuranosyl)-7H-pyrrolo[2,3-d]pyrimidine, a tubercidin analog, *J. Org. Chem.,* 28, 3331, 1963.

18. **Mizuno, Y., Ikehara, M., Watanabe, K., and Suzuki, S.,** Structural elucidation of tubercidin, *Chem. Pharm. Bull.,* 11, 1091, 1963.

19. **Duvall, L. R.,** Tubercidin, *Cancer Chemother. Rep.,* 30, 61, 1963.

20. **Fox, J. J., Watanabe, K. A., and Bloch, A.,** Nucleoside antibiotics, *Prog. Nucleic Acid Res. Mol. Biol.,* 5, 251, 1966.

21. **Tolman, R. L., Robins, R. K., and Townsend, L. B.,** Pyrrolopyrimidine nucleosides. II. The total synthesis of 7-β-D-ribofuranosyl-pyrrolo[2,3-d]pyrimidines related to toyocamycin, *J. Heterocycl. Chem.,* 4, 230, 1967.

22. **Okhuma, K.,** Chemical structure of toyocamycin, *J. Antibiot. (Tokyo),* 13A, 361, 1960.

23. **Okhuma, K.,** Chemical structure of toyocamycin, *J. Antibiot. (Tokyo),* 14A, 343, 1961.

24. **Taylor, E. C. and Hendress, R. W.,** Synthesis of 4-amino-5-cyanopyrrolo[2,3-d]pyrimidine, the aglycone of toyocamycin, *J. Am. Chem. Soc.,* 86, 951, 1964.

25. **Taylor, E. C. and Hendress, R. W.,** Synthesis of pyrrolo[2,3-d]pyrimidines. The aglycone of toyocamycin, *J. Am. Chem. Soc.,* 87, 1995, 1965.

26. **Gerster, J. F., Carpenter, B., Robins, R. K., and Townsend, L. B.,** Pyrrolopyrimidine nucleosides. I. The synthesis of 4-substituted-7-(β-D-ribofuranosyl)pyrrolo[2,3-d]pyrimidines from tubercidin, *J. Med. Chem.,* 10, 326, 1967.

27. **Saneyoshi, M., Tokuzen, R., and Fukuoka, F.,** Antitumor activities and structural relationship of tubercidin, toyocamycin, and their derivatives, *Gann,* 56, 219, 1965.

28. **Montgomery, J. A. and Hewson, K.,** Analogs of tubercidin, *J. Med. Chem.,* 10, 665, 1967.

29. **Iwamura, H. and Hashizume, T.,** Synthesis in nucleoside antibiotics. III. Synthesis of 4-amino-5-cyano-6-methylmercaptopyrrolo[2,3-d]pyrimidine-7-β-D-ribosides (toyocamycin analogs), *Agric. Biol. Chem.,* 32, 1010, 1968.

30. **Pike, J. E., Slechta, L., and Wiley, P. F.,** Tubercidin and related compounds, *J. Heterocycl. Chem.,* 1, 159, 1964.

31. **Schram, K. H. and Townsend, L. B.,** Fluorescent nucleoside derivatives of imidazo [1,2-c]pyrrolo[2,3-d]pyrimidine. A new heterocyclic ring system, *Tetrahedron Lett.,* 14, 1345, 1974.

32. **Gerster, J. F., Hinshaw, B. C., Robins, R. K., and Townsend, L. B.,** A study of electrophilic substitution in the pyrrolo[2,3-d]pyrimidine ring, *J. Heterocycl. Chem.,* 6, 207, 1969.

33. **Hinshaw, B. C., Gerster, J. F., Robins, R. K., and Townsend, L. B.,** Pyrrolopyrimidine nucleosides. IV. The synthesis of certain 4,5-disubstituted-7-(β-D-ribofuranosyl)pyrrolo[2,3-d]pyrimidines related to the pyrrolo[2,3-d]pyrimidine nucleoside antibiotics, *J. Heterocycl. Chem.,* 6, 215, 1969.

34. **Hinshaw, B. C., Gerster, J. F., Robins, R. K., and Townsend, L. B.,** Pyrrolopyrimidine nucleosides. V. A study on the relative chemical reactivity of the 5-cyano group of the nucleoside antibiotic toyocamycin and desaminotoyocamycin. The synthesis of analogs of sangivamycin, *J. Org. Chem.,* 35, 236, 1970.

35. **Ritch, P. S. and Helmsworth, M.,** Pyrrolopyrimidine lethality in relation to ribonucleic acid synthesis in sarcoma 180 cells *in vitro, Biochem. Pharmacol.,* 31, 2686, 1982.

36. **Smulson, M. E. and Suhadolnik, R. J.,** The biosynthesis of 7-deazaadenine ribonucleoside, tubercidin, by *Streptomyces tubercidicus, J. Biol. Chem.,* 242, 2872, 1967.

37. **Suhadolnik, R. J. and Uematsu, T.,** On the biosynthesis of cyano-7-deazaadenine ribonucleoside, toyocamycin, *Fed. Proc.,* 26, 855, 1967.

38. **Suhadolnik, R. J. and Uematsu, T.,** Biosynthesis of the pyrrolopyrimidine nucleoside antibiotic, toyocamycin. VII. Origin of the pyrrole carbons and the cyano carbon, *J. Biol. Chem.,* 245, 4365, 1970.

39. **Eistner, E. F. and Suhadolnik, R. J.,** The biosynthesis of the nucleoside antibiotics. IX. Purification and properties of guanosine triphosphate 8-formylhydrolase that catalyzes production of formic acid from the ureido carbon of guanosine triphosphate, *J. Biol. Chem.,* 246, 6973, 1971.

40. **Kasai, H., Ohashi, Z., Harada, F., Nishimura, S., Oppenheimer, N. J., Crain, P. F., Liehr, J. G., von Minden, D. L., and McCloskey, J. A.,** Structure of the modified nucleoside Q isolated from *Escherichia coli* transfer ribonucleic acid, 7-(4,5-*cis*-dihydroxy-1-cyclopenten-3-ylaminomethyl)-7-deazaguanosine, *Biochemistry,* 14, 4198, 1975.

41. **Kasai, H., Kuchino, Y., Nihei, K., and Nishimura, S.,** Distribution of the modified nucleoside Q and its derivatives in animal and plant transfer RNAs, *Nucl. Acids Res.,* 2, 1931, 1975.

42. **White, B. N., Tener, G. M., Holden, J., and Suzuki, D. T.,** Activity of a transfer RNA modifying enzyme during the development of *Drosophila* and its relationship to the su(s) locus, *J. Mol. Biol.,* 74, 635, 1974.

43. **Kuchino, Y., Kasai, H., Nihei, K., and Nishimura, S.,** Biosynthesis of the modified nucleoside Q in transfer RNA, *Nucl. Acids Res.,* 3, 393, 1976.

44. **Cheng, C. S., Hinshaw, B. C., Panzica, R. P., and Townsend, L. B.,** Synthesis of 2-amino-5-cyano-7(β-D-ribofuranosyl)-pyrrolo[2,3-d]pyrimidin-4-one. An important precursor for the synthesis of nucleoside Q and Q*, *J. Am. Chem. Soc.,* 98, 2870, 1976.

45. **Okada, N. and Nishimura, S.,** Isolation and characterization of a guanine insertion enzyme, a specific tRNA transglycosylase, from *Escherichia coli, J. Biol. Chem.,* 254, 3061, 1979.

46. **Okada, N., Noguchi, S., Kasai, H., Shindo-Okada, N., Ohgi, T., Goto, T., and Nishimura, S.,** Novel mechanism of post-transcriptional modification of tRNA. Insertion of basis of Q precursor into tRNA by a specific tRNA transglycosylase reaction, *J. Biol. Chem.,* 254, 3067, 1979.

47. **Hakala, M. T., Kenny, L. N., and Slocum, H. K.,** Inhibition of adenosine (AR) uptake by N^6-Δ^2-isopentenyladenosine (IPA) and kenetin riboside (KR), *Fed. Proc.,* 30, 679, 1971.

48. **Harley, E. R., Paterson, A. R. P., and Cass, C. E.,** Initial rate kinetics of the transport of adenosine and 4-amino-7-(β-D-ribofuranosyl)pyrrolo[2,3-d]pyrimidine (tubercidin) in cultured cells, *Cancer Res.,* 42, 1289, 1982.

49. **Paterson, A. R. P., Babb, L. R., Paran, J. H., and Cass, C. E.,** Inhibition by nitrobenzylthioinosine of adenosine uptake by asynchronous HeLa cells, *Mol. Pharmacol.,* 13, 1147, 1977.

50. **Paterson, A. R. P., Yang, S.-E., Lan, E. Y., and Cass, C. E.,** Low specificity of the nucleoside transport mechanism of RPMI 6410 cells, *Mol. Pharmacol.,* 16, 900, 1979.

51. **Iapalucci-Espinoza, S., Cereghini, S., and Franze-Fernandez, M. T.,** Regulation of ribosomal RNA synthesis in mammalian cells: effect of toyocamycin, *Biochemistry,* 16, 2885, 1977.

52. **Parks, R. E., Jr. and Brown, P. R.,** Incorporation of nucleosides into the nucleotide pools of human erythrocytes. Adenosine and its analogs, *Biochemistry,* 12, 3294, 1973.

53. **Acs, G. and Reich, E.,** Tubercidin and related pyrrolopyrimidine antibiotics, in *Antibiotics I. Mechanism of Action,* Gottlieb, D. and Shaw, P. D., Eds., Springer-Verlag, New York, 1967, 494.

54. **Umezawa, H., Sawa, T., Fukagawa, Y., Homma, I., Ishizuka, M., and Takeuchi, T.,** Studies on formycin and formycin B in cells of Ehrlich carcinoma and *E. coli, J. Antibiot. (Tokyo),* 20A, 308, 1967.

55. **Smith, C. G., Reineke, L. M., Burch, M. R., Shefner, A. M., and Muirhead, E. E.,** Studies on the uptake of tubercidin (7-deazaadenosine) by blood cells and its distribution in whole animals, *Cancer Res.,* 30, 69, 1970.

56. **Acs, G., Reich, E., and Mori, M.,** Biological and biochemical properties of the analogue antibiotic tubercidin, *Proc. Natl. Acad. Sci.,* 52, 493, 1964.

57. **Hardesty, C. T., Chaney, N. A., Waravdekar, V. S., and Mead, J. A. R.,** Enzymatic phosphorylation of sangivamycin, *Biochim. Biophys. Acta,* 195, 581, 1969.

58. **Zimmerman, T. P., Wolberg, G., and Duncan, G. S.,** Metabolism of tubercidin and formycin to their 3′:5′-cyclic nucleotides in mammalian cells, *J. Biol. Chem.,* 253, 8792, 1978.

59. **Stegman, R. J., Senft, A. W., Brown, P. R., and Parks, R. E., Jr.,** Pathways of nucleotide metabolism in *Schistosoma mansoni*. IV. Incorporation of adenosine analogs *in vitro, Biochem. Pharmacol.,* 22, 459, 1973.

60. **Lindberg, B., Klenow, H., and Hansen, K.,** Some properties of partially purified mammalian adenosine kinase, *J. Biol. Chem.,* 242, 350, 1967.

61. **Schnebli, H. P., Hill, D. L., and Bennett, L. L., Jr.,** Purification and properties of adenosine kinase from human tumor cells of type H. Ep. No. 2, *J. Biol. Chem.,* 252, 1997, 1967.

62. **Suhadolnik, R. J., Uematsu, T., and Uematsu, H.,** Toyocamycin: phosphorylation and incorporation into RNA and DNA and the biochemical properties of the triphosphate, *Biochim. Biophys. Acta,* 149, 41, 1967.

63. **Glazer, R. I. and Peale, A. L.,** Comparison between the inhibitory activities of sangivamycin and thiosangivamycin on nuclear ribonucleic acid synthesis in L1210 cells *in vitro, Biochem. Pharmacol.,* 29, 305, 1980.

64. **Blecher, M., Ro'Ane, J. T., and Flynn, P. D.,** Biochemical acivities of tubercidin 3′,5′-cyclic monophosphate in rat epidymal adipose tissue, *Biochem. Pharmacol.,* 20, 249, 1971.

65. **Gupta, R. S. and Siminovitch, L.,** Genetic and biochemical studies with the adenosine analogs toyocamycin and tubercidin: mutation at the adenosine kinase locus in Chinese hamster cells, *Somat. Cell Genet.,* 4, 715, 1978.

66. **Bennett, L. L., Jr., Schnebli, H. P., Vail, M. H., Allan, P. W., and Montgomery, J. A.,** Purine ribonucleoside kinase activity and resistance to some analogs of adenosine, *Mol. Pharmacol.,* 2, 432, 1966.

67. **Frederiksen, S.,** Specificity of adenosine deaminase toward adenosine and 2′-deoxyadenosine analogues, *Arch. Biochem. Biophys.,* 13, 383, 1966.

68. **Agarwal, R. P., Sagar, S. M., and Parks, R. E., Jr.,** Adenosine deaminase from human erythrocytes: purification and effects of adenosine analogs, *Biochem. Pharmacol.,* 24, 693, 1975.

69. **Hardesty, C. T., Chaney, N. A., Waravdekar, V. S., and Mead, J. A. R.,** The disposition of the antitumor agent, sangivamycin, in mice, *Cancer Res.,* 34, 1005, 1974.

70. **Bloch, A.,** The structure of nucleosides in relation to their biological and biochemical activity: a summary, *Ann. N.Y. Acad. Sci.,* 255, 576, 1975.

71. **Ritch, P. S. and Glazer, R. I.,** Preferential incorporation of sangivamycin into ribonucleic acid in sarcoma 180 cells *in vitro, Biochem. Pharmacol.,* 31, 259, 1982.

72. **Glazer, R. I. and Hartman, K. D.,** Cytokinetic and biochemical effects of sangivamycin in human colon carcinoma cells in culture, *Mol. Pharmacol.,* 20, 657, 1981.

73. **Nishimura, S., Harada, F., and Ikehara, M.,** The selective utilization of tubercidin triphosphate as an ATP analog in the DNA-dependent RNA polymerase system, *Biochim. Biophys. Acta,* 129, 301, 1966.

74. **Suhadolnik, R. J., Uematsu, T., Uematsu, H., and Wilson, R. G.,** The incorporation of sangivamycin 5′-triphosphate into polyribonucleotide acid polymerase from *Micrococcus lysodeikticus, J. Biol. Chem.,* 243, 2761, 1968.

75. **Chassy, B. M. and Suhadolnik, R. J.,** Nucleoside Antibiotics. II. Biochemical tools for studying the structural requirements for interaction at the catalytic and regulatory sites of ribonucleotide reductase from *Escherieshea coli, J. Biol. Chem.,* 243, 3538, 1968.

76. **Suhadolnik, R. J., Finkel, S. I., and Chassy, B. M.,** Nucleoside antibiotics. I. Biochemical tools for studying the structural requirements for interaction at the catalytic and regulatory sites of ribonucleotide reductase from *Lactobacillus leichmannii, J. Biol. Chem.,* 243, 3532, 1968.

77. **Suhadolnik, R. J.,** Pyrrolopyrimidine nucleoside analogs, in *Nucleosides as Biological Probes,* Suhadolnik, R. J., Ed., John Wiley & Sons, New York, 1979, 158.

78. **Shigeura, H. T. and Gordon, C. N.,** The effects of 3′-deoxyadenosine on the synthesis of ribonucleic acid, *J. Biol. Chem.,* 240, 806, 1965.

79. **Venkov, P. V., Stateva, L. I., and Hadjiolov, A. A.,** Toyocamycin inhibition of ribosomal ribonucleic acid processing in an osmotic-sensitive adenosine-utilizing *Sarcharomyces cerevisiae* mutant, *Biochim. Biophys. Acta,* 474, 245, 1977.

80. **Kapuler, A. M., Ward, D. C., Mendelsohn, N., Klett, H., Acs, G., and Spiegelman, S.,** Steric requirements for base selection by template directed RNA synthetases, *Fed. Proc.,* 28, 731, 1969.

81. **Kapuler, A. M., Ward, D. C., Mendelsohn, N., Klett, H., and Acs, G.,** Utilization of substrate analogs by Mengovirus induced RNA polymerase, *Virology,* 37, 701, 1969.

82. **Heine, U.,** Electron microscopic studies on HeLa cells exposed to the antibiotic toyocamycin, *Cancer Res.,* 29, 1875, 1969.

83. **Phillips, S. G. and Phillips, D. M.,** Nucleoli of diploid cell strains. Their normal ultrastructure and the effects of toyocamycin and actinomycin D, *J. Cell Biol.,* 49, 784, 1971.

84. **Ikehara, M. and Ohtsuka, E.,** Stimulation of the binding of aminoacyl-sRNA to ribosomes by tubercidin (7-deazaadenosine) and N⁶-dimethyladenosine containing trinucleoside diphosphate analogs, *Biochem. Biophys. Res. Commun.,* 21, 257, 1965.

85. **Cass, C. E., Selner, M., Tan, T. H., Muhs, W. H., and Robins, M. J.,** Comparison of the effects on cultured L1210 leukemia cells of the ribosyl, 2′-deoxyribosyl, and xylosyl homologs of tubercidin and adenosine alone or in combination with 2′-deoxycoformycin, *Cancer Treat. Rep.,* 66, 317, 1982.

86. **Uretsky, S. C., Acs, G., Reich, E., Mori, M., and Altwerger, L.,** Pyrrolopyrimidine nucleotides and protein synthesis, *J. Biol. Chem.,* 243, 306, 1968.

87. **Ritch, P. S., Glazer, R. I., Cunningham, R. E., and Shackney, S. E.,** Kinetic effects of sangivamycin in sarcoma 180 *in vitro, Cancer Res.,* 41, 1784, 1981.

88. **Bhuyan, B. K., Scheidt, L. G., and Fraser, T. J.,** Cell cycle specificity of antitumor agents, *Cancer Res.,* 32, 398, 1972.

89. **Stern, H. J. and Glazer, R. I.,** Inhibition of methylation of nuclear ribonucleic acid in L1210 cells by tubercidin, 8-azaadenosine and formycin, *Biochem. Pharmacol.,* 29, 1459, 1980.

90. **Tavitian, A., Uretsky, S. C. and Acs, G.,** Selective inhibition of ribosomal RNA synthesis in mammalian cells, *Biochim. Biophys. Acta,* 157, 33, 1968.

91. **Reich, E., Franklin, R. M., Shatkin, A. J., and Tatum, E. L.,** Action of actinomycin D on animal cells and viruses, *Proc. Natl. Acad. Sci.,* 48, 1238, 1962.

92. **Glazer, R. I., Hartman, K. D., and Cohen, O. J.,** Effects of sangivamycin and xylosyladenine on the synthesis and methylation of polysomal ribonucleic acid in Ehrlich ascites cells *in vitro, Biochem. Pharmacol.,* 30, 2697, 1981.

93. **Kumar, S. A., Krakow, J. S., and Ward, D. C.,** ATP analogues as initiation and elongation nucleosides for bacterial DNA-dependent RNA polymerase, *Biochim. Biophys. Acta,* 477, 112, 1977.

94. **Bennett, L. L., Jr. and Smithers, D.,** Feedback inhibition of purine biosynthesis in H. Ep. #2 cells by adenosine analogs, *Biochem. Pharmacol.,* 13, 1331, 1964.

95. **Henderson, J. F. and Khoo, M. K. V.,** Synthesis of 5'-phosphoribosyl 1-pyrophosphate from glucose in Ehrlich ascites tumor cells *in vitro, J. Biol. Chem.,* 240, 2348, 1965.

96. **Bennett, L. L., Jr., Smithers, D., Hill, D. L., Rose, L. M., and Alexander, J. A.,** Biochemical properties of the nucleoside of 3-amino-1,5-dihydro-5-methyl-1,4,5,6,8 pentaazaacenaphthylene (NSC-154020), *Biochem. Pharmacol.,* 27, 233, 1978.

97. **Saffer, J. D. and Glazer, R. I.,** Inhibition of histone H1 phosphorylation by sangivamycin and other pyrrolopyrimidine analogues, *Mol. Pharmacol.,* 20, 211, 1981.

98. **Saffer, J. D. and Glazer, R. I.,** The phosphorylation of high mobility group proteins 14 and 17 from Ehrlich ascites and L1210 *in vitro, Biochem. Biophys. Res. Commun.,* 93, 1280, 1980.

99. **Saffer, J. D. and Glazer, R. I.,** The phosphorylation of high mobility group proteins 14 and 17 and their distribution in chromatin, *J. Biol. Chem.,* 257, 4655, 1982.

100. **Legraverend, M. and Glazer, R. I.,** Inhibition of the phosphorylation of nonhistone chromosomal proteins by cordycepin and xylosyladenine in L1210 cells *in vitro, Mol. Pharmacol.,* 14, 1130, 1978.

101. **Legraverend, M. and Glazer, R. I.,** Inhibition of the phosphorylation of nonhistone chromosomal proteins of rat liver by cordycepin and cordycepin triphosphates, *Cancer Res.,* 38, 1142, 1978.

102. **Hirsch, J. and Martelo, O. J.,** Inhibition of nuclear protein kinase by adenosine analogues, *Life Sci.,* 19, 85, 1976.

103. **Walter, R. D.,** Nucleoside-dependent protein kinase from *Trypanosoma gambiense, Biochim. Biophys. Acta,* 429, 137, 1976.

104. **Walter, R. D. and Ebert, F.,** Inhibition of protein kinase activity from *Trypanosoma cruzi* and *Trypanosoma gambiense* by 3'-deoxyadenosine, *Hoppe-Seyler's Z. Physiol. Chem.,* 358, 23, 1977.

105. **Gotoh, S., Nikolaev, N., Battaner, E., Birge, C. H., and Schlessinger, D.,** *Escherichia coli* RNase III cleaves HeLa cell nuclear RNA, *Biochem. Biophys. Res. Commun.,* 59, 972, 1974.

106. **Tavitian, A., Uretsky, S. C., and Acs, G.,** The effect of toyocamycin on cellular RNA synthesis, *Biochim. Biophys. Acta,* 179, 50, 1969.

107. **Weiss, J. W. and Pitot, H. C.,** Inhibition of ribosomal RNA maturation in Novikoff hepatoma cells by toyocamycin, tubercidin, and 6-thioguanine, *Cancer Res.,* 34, 581, 1974.

108. **Swart, C. and Hodge, L. D.,** Characterization of adenovirus RNA synthesized in the presence of an adenosine analog: failure of poly (A) addition, *Virology,* 84, 374, 1978.

109. **Almaric, F., Bachellerie, J.-P., and Caboche, M.,** RNA methylation and control of eukaryotic RNA biosynthesis: processing and utilization of undermethylated tRNAs in CHO cells, *Nucl. Acids Res.,* 4, 4357, 1977.

110. **Furuichi, Y., LaFiandra, A., and Shatkin, A. J.,** 5'-Terminal structure and mRNA stability, *Nature (London),* 266, 235, 1977.

111. **Caboche, M. and Bachellerie, J.-P.,** RNA methylation and control of eukaryotic RNA biosynthesis. Effects of cycloleucine, a specific inhibitor of methylation, on ribosomal RNA maturation, *Eur. J. Biochem.,* 74, 19, 1977.

112. **Glazer, R. I. and Peale, A. L.,** Cordycepin and xylosyladenine: inhibitors of methylation of nuclear RNA, *Biochem. Biophys. Res. Commun.,* 81, 521, 1978.

113. **Wainfain, E. and Landsberg, B.,** Inhibition of transfer ribonucleic acid methylating enzymes by cytotoxic analogs of adenosine, *Biochem. Pharmacol.,* 22, 493, 1973.

114. **Hurwitz, J., Gold, M., and Anders, M.,** The enzymatic methylation of ribonucleic acid and deoxyribonucleic acid. IV. The properties of the soluble ribonucleic acid-methylating enzymes, *J. Biol. Chem.,* 239, 3474, 1964.

115. **Wainfain, E. and Borek, E.,** Differential inhibitors of tRNA methylases, *Mol. Pharmacol.,* 3, 595, 1967.

116. **Wainfain, E., Chu, J., and Chheda, G. B.,** Tubercidin and isopropylureidopurine — inhibitors of ribothymidine synthesis *in vitro, Biochem. Pharmacol.,* 24, 83, 1975.

117. **Lawrence, F., Shire, D. J., and Walter, J.-P.,** The effect of adenosine analogs on the ATP-pyrophosphate exchange reaction catalysed by methionyl-tRNA synthetase, *Eur. J. Biochem.,* 41 73, 1974.

118. **Chiang, C.-D. and Coward, J. K.,** Effect of *S*-adenosylhomocysteine and *S*-tubercidinylhomocysteine on transfer ribonucleic acid methylation in phytohemagglutinin-stimulated lymphocytes, *Mol. Pharmacol.,* 11, 701, 1975.

119. **Baxter, C. S. and Byvoet, P.,** Effects of carcinogens and other agents on histone methylation by a histone arginine methyltransferase purified from rat liver cytoplasm, *Cancer Res.,* 34, 1418, 1974.

120. **Both, G. W., Banerjee, A. K., and Shatkin, A. J.,** Methylation-dependent translation of viral messenger RNAs *in vitro, Proc. Natl. Acad. Sci.,* 72, 1189, 1975.
121. **Toneguzzo, F. and Ghosh, H. P.,** Characterization and translation of methylated and unmethylated vesicular stomatitis virus mRNA synthesized *in vitro* by ribonucleoprotein particles from vesicular stomatitis virus-infected L cells, *J. Virol.,* 17, 477, 1976.
122. **Kaehler, M., Coward, J., and Rotman, F.,** *In vivo* inhibition of Novikoff cytoplasmic messenger RNA methylation by *S*-tubercidinylhomocysteine, *Biochemistry,* 16, 5770, 1977.
123. **Pugh, C. S. G., Borchadt, R. T., and Stone, O. H.,** Inhibition of Newcastle disease virion messenger RNA (guanine-7-)-methyltransferase by analogues of *S*-adenosylhomocysteine, *Biochemistry,* 16, 3928, 1977.
124. **Cass, C. E., Selner, M., Ferguson, P. J., and Phillips, J. R.,** Effects of 2′-deoxyadenosine, 9-β-D-arabinofuranosyladenine, and related compounds of *S*-adenosyl-L-homocysteine hydrolase activity in synchronous and asynchronous cultured cells, *Cancer Res.,* 42, 4991, 1982.
125. **Coward, J. K., Motola, N. C., and Moyer, J. D.,** Polyamine biosynthesis in rat prostate. Substrate and inhibitor properties of 7-deaza analogues of decarboxylated *S*-adeosylmethionine and 5′-methylthioadenine, *J. Med. Chem.,* 20, 500, 1977.
126. **Lennon, M. B., Wu, J., and Suhadolnik, R. J.,** The effect of NAD$^+$ and NAD$^+$ analogs on protein synthesis in rabbit reticulocytes: replacement of the energy regenerating system, *Biochem. Biophys. Res. Commun.,* 72, 530, 1976.
127. **Garren, L. D., Howell, R. R., Tomkins, G. M., and Crocco, R. M.,** A paradoxical effect of actinomycin D: the mechanism of regulation enzyme synthesis by hydrocortisone, *Proc. Natl. Acad. Sci.,* 52, 1121, 1964.
128. **Jaffe, J. J.,** Nucleoside analogs of antiparasitic agents, *Ann. N.Y. Acad. Sci.,* 255, 306, 1975.
129. **Senft, A. W., Crabtree, G. W., Agrawal, K. C., Scholar, E. M., Agrawal, R. P., and Parks, R. E., Jr.,** Pathways of nucleotide metabolism in *Schistosoma mansoni.* III. Identification of enzymes in cell-free abstracts, *Biochem. Pharmacol.,* 22, 449, 1973.
130. **Williamson, J.,** Nucleoside trypanocides, *Parasitology,* 59, 9P, 1969.
131. **Williamson, J.,** The activity of drugs on *Trypanosoma congolense in vitro, Trans. R. Soc. Trop. Med. Hyg.,* 3, 422, 1969.
132. **Williamson, J.,** Cordycepin, an antitumor antibiotic with trypanocidal properties, *Trans. R. Soc. Trop. Med. Hyg.,* 60, 8, 1966.
133. **Meich, R. P., Senft, A. W., and Senft, D. G.,** Pathways of nucleotide metabolism in *Schistosoma mansoni.* VI. Adenosine phosphorylase, *Biochem. Pharmacol.,* 24, 407, 1975.
134. **Senft, A. W. and Crabtree G. W.,** Pathways of nucleotide metabolism in *Schistosoma mansoni.* VIII. Inhibition of adenine and guanine nucleotide synthesis by purine analogs in intact worms, *Biochem. Pharmacol.,* 26, 1847, 1977.
135. **Ross, A. F. and Jaffe, J. J.,** Effects of tubercidin and its ribonucleotides on various metabolic pathways in *Schistosoma mansoni, Biochem. Pharmacol.,* 21, 3059, 1972.
136. **Miko, M. and Drobnica, Ľ.,** Effects of antibiotics nogalamycin, cirolemycin and tubercidin on endogenous respiration of tumor cells and oxidative phosphorylation of mammalian mitochondria, *Experientia,* 31, 832, 1975.
137. **Jaffe, J. J., Meymarian, E., and Doremus, H. M.,** Antischistosomal action of tubercidin administered after absorption into red cells, *Nature (London),* 230, 408, 1971.
138. **Lawrence, J. D.,** The ingestion of red blood cells by *Schistosoma mansoni, J. Parasitol.,* 59, 60, 1973.
139. **Jaffe, J. J., Doremus, H. M., Dunsford, H. A., Kammerer, W. S., and Meymarian, E.,** Antischistosomal activity of tubercidin in monkeys, *Am. J. Trop. Med. Hyg.,* 22, 62, 1973.
140. **Brdar, B., Rifkin, D. B., and Reich, E.,** Studies of Rous sarcoma virus. Effects of nucleoside analogues on virus syntheses, *J. Biol. Chem.,* 248, 2397, 1973.
141. **De Clercq, E., Torrence, P. F., and Witkop, B.,** Interferon induction by synthetic polynucleotides: importance of purine N-7 and strandwise rearrangement, *Proc. Natl. Acad. Sci.,* 71, 182, 1974.
142. **Torrence, P. F., De Clercq, E., Waters, J. A., and Witkop, B.,** A potent interferon inducer derived from poly(7-deazainosinic acid), *Biochemistry,* 13, 4400, 1974.
143. **Périès, J., Canivet, M., Olivie, M., and Tavitian, A.,** Effet d'un inhibiteur selectif des syntheses des RNAs ribosomiques sur l'action antivirale de l'interferon, *C.R. Acad. Sci. Ser. D.,* 278, 2079, 1974.
144. **Brindle, S. A., Guiffre, N. A., Amrein, B. J., Millonig, R. C., and Perlman, D.,** Antibiotic sensitivity of Ehrlich ascites cells grown in tissue culture, *Antimicrob. Agents Chemother.,* p. 159, 1961.
145. **Owen, S. P. and Smith, C. G.,** Cytotoxicity and antitumor properties of the abnormal nucleoside tubercidin (NSC-56408), *Cancer Chemother. Rep.,* 36, 19, 1964.
146. **Smith, C. G., Lummis, W. L., and Grady, J. E.,** An improved tissue culture assay. II. Cytotoxicity studies with antibiotics, chemicals, and solvents, *Cancer Res.,* 19, 847, 1959.
147. **Bhuyan, B. K., Renis, H. E., and Smith, C. G.,** A collagen plate assay for cytotoxic studies. II. Biological studies, *Cancer Res.,* 22, 1131, 1962.

148. **Renis, H. E., Johnson, H. G., and Bhuyan, B. K.,** A collagen plate assay for cytotoxic drugs. I. Methods, *Cancer Res.,* 22, 1126, 1962.

149. **Davoll, J.,** Pyrrolo[2,3-d]pyrimidines, *J. Chem. Soc.,* p. 131, 1960.

150. **Ritch, P. S. and Glazer, R. I.,** unpublished data, 1982.

151. NCI, Screening data summary, Dev. Ther. Prog. Div. Cancer Treat., National Cancer Institute, National Institutes of Health, Bethesda, Md., 1978.

152. **Kravchenko, A. I., Chernov, V. A., Shcherbakova, L. I., Filitis, L. N., Pershin, G. N., and Sokolova, V. N.,** Pyrrolo-(3,2-d)-pyrimidines as potential antitumor drugs, *Farmakol. Toksikol.,* 42, 659, 1979.

153. **Grage, T. B., Rochlin, D. B., Weiss, A. J., and Wilson, W. L.,** Clinical studies with tubercidin administered after absorption into human erythrocytes, *Cancer Res.,* 30, 79, 1970.

154. **Wilson, W. L.,** Phase I study with toyocamycin (NSC-63701), *Cancer Chemother. Rep.,* 52, 301, 1968.

155. NCI, Invest. Drug Branch, Cancer Ther. Evaluation Program, Div. of Cancer Treat., National Cancer Institute, National Institutes of Health, Bethesda, Md., 1965.

156. **Bisel, H. F., Ansfield, F. J., Mason, J. H., and Wilson, W. L.,** Clinical studies with tubercidin administered by direct intravenous injection, *Cancer Res.,* 30, 76, 1970.

157. **Burgess, G. H., Bloch, A., Stoll, H., Milgrom, H., Helm, F., and Klein, E.,** Effect of topical tubercidin on basal cell carcinomas and actinic keratoses, *Cancer,* 34, 250, 1974.

158. **Klein, E., Burgess, G. H., Bloch, A., Milgrom, H., and Holtermann, O. A.,** The effects of nucleoside analogs on cutaneous neoplasms, *Ann. N.Y. Acad. Sci.,* 255, 216, 1975.

159. **Cavins, J. A., Hall, T. C., Olson, K. B., Khung, C. L., Horton, J., Colsky, J., and Shadduck, R. K.,** Initial toxicity study of sangivamycin (NSC-65346), *Cancer Chemother. Rep.,* 51, 197, 1967.

160. **Morrison, R. K., Brown, D. E., Timmens, E. K., Nieglos, M. A., and Tassini, R.,** Cardiotoxicity studies with sangivamycin (BA-90912, NSC-63546), *Chem. Abstr.,* 74, 226, 1971.

161. NIH Summary Data, IND 964, National Institutes of Health, Bethesda, Md., 1965.

Chapter 2

PURINE NUCLEOSIDE PHOSPHORYLASE: A TARGET FOR CHEMOTHERAPY

Johanna D. Stoeckler

TABLE OF CONTENTS

I. INTRODUCTION

Mammalian purine nucleoside phosphorylase (PNP; nucleoside phosphorylase; purine nucleoside: orthophosphate ribosyltransferase; EC 2.4.2.1) catalyzes the reversible phosphorolytic reaction that cleaves the ribo- and 2'-deoxyribonucleosides of guanine and hypoxanthine, as well as many related analog nucleosides:

$$\beta\text{-nucleoside} + P_i \rightleftharpoons \text{base} + \alpha\text{-sugar } 1-P$$

The relatively recent appreciation of the importance of PNP in immunodevelopment and purine nucleoside analog metabolism (Section II.A and B) has encouraged detailed structural and kinetic studies (Section III.) and has generated strong interest in developing PNP inhibitors (Section IV.) as well as nucleoside substrate analogs that are resistant to cleavage (Section V.). The rationale and ultimate success of these efforts hinge on the role of PNP in purine metabolism and the levels of enzymic activity found in human and laboratory animal tissues.

Although in man[1] and other species[2-4] the synthesis of nucleosides is greatly favored under equilibrium conditions, PNP acts chiefly in the phosphorolytic direction in intact cells. As shown in Figure 1, PNP functions as a catabolic enzyme when it is coupled to guanase and/or xanthine oxidase in some tissues and as a salvage enzyme by providing substrates for hypoxanthine-guanine phosphoribosyltransferase (HGPRT). The liberated sugar phosphates may enter the pathway of carbohydrate metabolism or may participate in PNP or pyrimidine phosphorylase-mediated nucleoside exchange reactions, as was noted in an earlier review.[5] Ribose 1-P (R-1-P), via its conversion to ribose 5-P (R-5-P), is also an important precursor of 5-phosphoribosyl-1-pyrophosphate (PRPP). It has been shown that guanosine, a R-1-P donor, is incorporated much more rapidly into the nucleotide pools of human erythrocytes than guanine.[6] It is especially important to note that both ribo- and deoxyribonucleosides are salvaged by the PNP pathway to form only ribonucleotides. Thus PNP, in conjunction with adenosine deaminase (ADA), may represent a mechanism for limiting the production of deoxyribonucleotides to their synthesis by ribonucleoside diphosphate reductase, a highly regulated enzyme.[7]

PNP shows little regulation but is present in very high activities in man. Carson et al.[8] reported that its activity exceeds that of ADA in all human tissues examined except thymus and the highest activities per milligram of protein are found in extracts of kidney, peripheral lymphocytes, and granulocytes. Erythrocytes have about $1/_3$ as much activity as lymphocytes on the basis of protein in the supernates of cell lysates,[9] but when calculations are based on cell volumes red cells have about the same activity per milliliter of packed cells as peripheral lymphocytes.[6] Thus human erythrocytes, which are deficient in purine biosynthesis *de novo* and depend on salvage to meet their purine requirements, are the richest source of PNP. Furthermore, it may be significant that reticulocytes have almost seven times as much PNP activity as mature erythrocytes.[10] In contrast to lymphocytes,[11,12] erythrocytes transport nucleosides into the cell as rapidly as they can be split by PNP.[12] An activity of about 13 μmol inosine cleaved per minute per milliliter of packed cells at 30°C permits estimation of a rate in excess of 500 g/hr/2.5ℓ of erythrocytes (the approximate volume in an adult human).[6] This hypothetical rate illustrates the formidable phosphorolytic capacity of blood in man. An important consideration in extrapolating from laboratory animals to man is that PNP activity in erythrocytes is about 4- to 5-fold lower in mice,[13] 15-fold lower in rats,[14] and extremely low or nil in dogs and cats.[5]

II. THE SIGNIFICANCE OF PURINE NUCLEOSIDE PHOSPHORYLASE IN CHEMOTHERAPY

A. Relationship of PNP to Immunodeficiency

PNP became a primary target for chemotherapeutic intervention with the report by Giblett

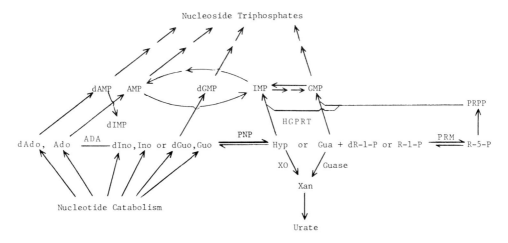

FIGURE 1. Central role of purine nucleoside phosphorylase (PNP) in purine salvage and catabolism. Inosine and guanosine are not phosphorylated. Radiolabeled deoxyinosine has been recovered as dIMP but not in di- or triphosphate deoxyribonucleosides.[8] Abbreviations: ADA, adenosine deaminase; Guase, guanase; HGPRT, hypoxanthine-guanine phosphoribosyltransferase; PRPP, 5-phosphoribosyl-1-pyrophosphate; PRM, phosphoribomutase; XO, xanthine oxidase.

and colleagues[15] in 1975 that a child exhibiting lymphopenia and severe deficiency of cellular immunity completely lacked this enzyme activity. The clinical manifestations of the immunodeficiency in a number of patients have been detailed by Ammann.[16] Investigations by Gelfand et al.[17] on incompletely deficient patients have indicated that proliferation-dependent T-suppressor cells are impaired while proliferation-independent T-helper cell functions are retained and may account for exaggerated humoral responses. This rare syndrome suggested a means of selectively suppressing cellular immunity for therapeutic purposes.[18-21] Since PNP deficiency is associated with T-cell lymphopenia, it has been proposed that a PNP inhibitor might be used to treat T-cell leukemias, to suppress the host-vs.-graft response,[19,21] or to counter autoimmune disease[20] without destroying the patient's humoral immunity. A caveat to these proposals is the finding that PNP-deficient patients have tended to develop neurological disorders, anemias, and autoantibodies.[16]

The PNP deficiency syndrome led to investigations of the roles of PNP substrates in cellular metabolism in attempts to determine the cause of selective immunosuppression. Deficient children have elevated levels of the PNP nucleoside substrates in blood and urine and show profound hypouricemia and hypouricosuria.[22,23] Considerable evidence, reviewed by Martin and Gelfand,[24] has accumulated indicating that dGTP generated from deoxyguanosine is the lymphocytotoxic agent. It was first noted by Cohen et al.,[25] and confirmed by other workers,[26,27] that dGTP accumulates to levels 100 times greater than normal in erythrocytes of enzyme-deficient individuals, with concomitant GTP depletion.[27] Improvement of cellular immune function by erythrocyte transfusion therapy also lowered dGTP concentrations to the normal range.[26] As reported by Chan[28] and Gudas et al.,[29] of all the PNP substrates, only deoxyguanosine inhibits the growth of the S49 mouse T-cell lymphoma line at 10^{-5} M concentrations. Mutant sublines isolated in Martin's laboratory demonstrate resistance to deoxyguanosine in cells that lack nucleoside transport or deoxycytidine kinase activity.[29,30] Cells are also resistant if they have a mutant ribonucleoside-diphosphate reductase[30] that is not subject to normal feedback control by dGTP.[7,31] Human lymphoma cell lines of T (but not B) cell origin have been shown by Mitchell et al.[32] and Gelfand et al.[33] to be significantly inhibited by deoxyguanosine concentrations in the 10^{-5} M range. Dosch et al.[34] have reported inhibition of the development of suppressor T cells in mice receiving intraperitoneal injections of deoxyguanosine. Deoxycytidine reverses the deoxyguanosine-induced growth inhibition of both human and murine cultured T-cell lymphoblasts.[28,29,32,33]

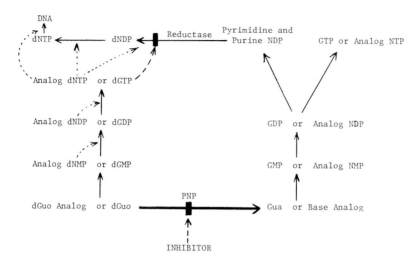

FIGURE 2. Rationale for the use of PNP inhibitors and deoxyguanosine analogs resistant to phosphorolysis:($\cdots\!>\blacksquare$) known sites of inhibition; ($\cdots\!>$) other potential sites. NMP, NDP, and NTP are nucleoside mono-, di-, and triphosphates.

Thus, the best-supported model for explaining the effects of PNP deficiency on the immune system is that depicted on Figure 2. In the absence of PNP activity (or in the presence of a potent PNP inhibitor) deoxyguanosine accumulates and is phosphorylated directly to form deoxyribonucleotides. dGTP, an allosteric inhibitor of ribonucleoside-diphosphate reductase, has the greatest effects on dCDP synthesis,[7,31] and DNA synthesis is blocked because of inadequate dCTP levels. The special sensitivity of T cells has been attributed by Carson et al. to the selective trapping of deoxyguanosine nucleotides because of the relative activities of phosphorylating and dephosphorylating enzymes in these cells.[8,35]

It is noteworthy that deoxyguanosine toxicity has been demonstrated in T-lymphoblast cells that possess normal PNP activity.[28,29,32,33] Ullman et al. have isolated a mutant of the S49 mouse T-cell lymphoma which has undetectable (less than 0.1% of the wild-type) PNP activity and yet is only slightly more sensitive to deoxyguanosine toxicity than wild-type cells.[29,30] In the absence of exogenous deoxyguanosine, the mutant cells have normal growth rates.[30] Thus, it appears that whole-body PNP must protect lymphocytes by maintaining low deoxyguanosine levels throughout the body. Studies of deoxyadenosine metabolism in mice by Smith and Henderson[36] suggest that the major source of deoxynucleotides accumulating in erythrocytes of deoxycoformycin-treated mice are normoblast nuclei extruded during erythropoiesis. A secondary source, which could become important during chemotherapy, is dying cells. Dietary purine nucleotides, overproduction of purine deoxyribonucleotides, and DNA repair appear to be only minor sources.[36] The extremely high PNP activity in erythrocytes (see above), which is not rate-limited by transport in these cells, may play a crucial role in removing circulating deoxyguanosine from the bloodstream.

While the above model is a reasonable explanation of the immunodeficiency associated with PNP deficiency, it does not explain all the clinical and experimental findings to date. In nine patients surveyed by Ammann, two had neurological abnormalities and four had anemias, of which only two were attributed to autoimmune disease.[16] The erythrocytes of PNP-deficient children may have depleted ATP and GTP and grossly elevated dGTP and NAD$^+$.[27] The partial replacement of erythrocytic ATP by dATP was found by Simmonds et al. in an ADA-deficient child[37] and by Siaw et al.[38] in a patient with lymphoproliferative disease who developed hemolytic anemia after clinical administration of the ADA inhibitor, deoxycoformycin. Hemolytic anemia and the accumulation of pyrimidine nucleotides have been reported in pyrimidine 5'-nucleotidase deficiency.[39] Thus there may be an association between hemolysis and perturbations of erythrocyte nucleotide levels. Inhibition of *S*-adenosylhomocysteine hydrolase occurs secondarily in ADA,[40] PNP, and HGPRT deficiencies.[41] Overproduction of purines *de novo* in the presence of elevated PRPP levels increases the serum inosine concentrations of PNP-deficient individuals to the 10^{-5} *M* range ($\sim$100-fold higher than normal).[22,23] An *S*-adenosyl homocysteine hydrolase activity only 7% of normal has been attributed by Hershfield to the irreversible inactivation of this enzyme by inosine.[41] The causes and/or importance of these and other clinical findings need further study since they may ultimately determine the clinical usefulness of PNP inhibitors as immunosuppressive agents. An understanding of the biochemical mechanisms involved may permit amelioration or prevention of the secondary effects of PNP deficiency or inhibition.

Finally, as illustrated in Figure 1, PNP is responsible for generating purine bases in the catabolic pathway. Xanthinuria and xanthine gout are occasionally observed and, as has been suggested elsewhere, might be ameliorated by a PNP inhibitor which would shift the purine excretion pattern to the more soluble nucleosides. A PNP inhibitor might also be useful in the treatment of secondary gout due to rapid cytolysis after irradiation or chemotherapy and might be given together with allopurinol.[19,21]

B. The Role of PNP in Purine Analog Metabolism

PNP also plays a significant role in purine analog metabolism by (1) cleaving both the ribo- and deoxyribonucleosides of many guanine and hypoxanthine analogs to release the bases, (2) catalyzing the synthesis of analog nucleosides from administered analog bases, and (3) synthesizing analog sugar phosphates from sugar-modified nucleosides.

It has long been noted in tests of antitumor activity that ribonucleosides of purine analogs are as effective as their free bases.[42] Parks et al.[6] have reported that 6-thioguanosine and 6-selenoguanosine, when incubated for 3 hr at 1 m*M* concentrations, are incorporated into the nucleotide pools of erythrocytes to a much greater extent than their free bases. 2'-Deoxy-6-selenoguanosine incorporation more resembled that of the base than of the nucleoside. These results are most readily explained by the rapid cleavage of the nucleosides by PNP and the generation of the PRPP precursor, R-1-P, from the ribonucleosides. From the viewpoints of solubility and potentiation of their own phosphoribosylation, ribonucleoside analogs of PNP substrates may have advantages over their bases. This may prove to be especially important if recent promising results showing differential protection of host and tumor tissues by transport inhibitors[43,44] receive further substantiation.

The rapid cleavage of the deoxynucleosides of guanine analogs by PNP raises the question of whether they might be directly phosphorylated (like deoxyguanosine) if their phosphorolysis were prevented. Studies by LePage et al., with mice, suggested that β-2'-deoxy-6-thioguanosine might be a more effective anticancer agent than 6-thioguanine.[45] Clinical tests did not demonstrate an advantage of the deoxynucleoside over the base; however, the high activity of PNP in human blood may have prevented significant doses of the nucleoside from reaching the target cells. Attempts to answer the question by (1) the use of PNP inhibitors, and (2) the use of deoxyguanosine analogs resistant to cleavage by PNP will be discussed in Section IV. and V.

Although PNP functions mainly as a phosphorolytic enzyme, the intracellular synthesis of analog nucleosides has been demonstrated. Krenitsky et al.[46] reported the synthesis of the nucleoside of allopurinol, 1-ribosylallopurinol, by human erythrocytic PNP and its identification in the urine of patients receiving this drug. Studies in mice show an extremely low rate of conversion of allopurinol to nucleotides in vivo[47] and although the nucleoside is a product of PNP catalysis, it is apparently unreactive or a poor substrate for PNP.[48] These factors would result in trapping the analog in its nucleoside form. Recently, the synthesis of 6-thioguanosine from 6-thioguanine in mouse Sarcoma 180 cells was reported by Lee and Sartorelli.[49] The rate of synthesis depended on the presence of glucose or R-1-P in the medium and was inhibited by a transport inhibitor which, presumably, prevented efflux of the 6-thioguanosine from the cells. These authors suggest that the PNP reaction may lower the potency of 6-thioguanine by making it unavailable for reaction with HGPRT. The flux of reactants through PNP and HGPRT must depend on their activities, on the relative affinities of the purine base for the two enzymes, and, perhaps most importantly, on the level of PRPP synthetase activity. This phenomenon may be worthy of further study to determine whether it is significant in other cell types and in whole animals.

Recent studies by Savarese et al. on the cytotoxicity of C(5′)-modified analogs of methylthioadenosine,[50,51] have indicated that C(5′)-substituted inosines are equally toxic in cells with high PNP activity. Certain substitutions at C(5′) result in very low substrate activity with PNP. As described in Section V., these poorly reactive nucleosides are still cleaved intracellularly to release the toxic analog sugar phosphates. Since tumor cell lines with low or absent methylthioadenosine phosphorylase activity have been identified,[50-52] the generation of toxic sugar phosphates by PNP may overcome their resistance.

III. CHARACTERIZATION OF PURINE NUCLEOSIDE PHOSPHORYLASE

A. Purification Methods

As interest in the function of PNP has risen, the enzyme has been purified from a wide variety of human and other mammalian tissues. Crystalline human erythrocytic PNP was isolated more than a dozen years ago in this laboratory[53,54] by modification of procedures described by Tsuboi and Hudson[55] and Abrams et al.,[56] using only the gentle techniques of ion-exchange chromatography, ammonium sulfate fractionation, and gel filtration. Similar techniques have been employed more recently to purify this enzyme from rabbit liver,[57] brain,[58] and erythrocytes;[59] from bovine liver[60] and brain;[61] and from Chinese hamster liver, kidney, and V79 tisse culture cells.[62] Chicken liver PNP was also purified to the crystalline state by like procedures.[63] A preparative electrophoresis step was added for purification of the enzyme from bovine thyroid;[64] isoelectric focusing was used as a last step in the isolation of PNP from human placenta.[65] Some of these purification schemes have also included heat treatment,[57,58,65] acid precipitation,[65] or extraction with organic solvents.[64]

Excellent purifications have been reported with two affinity chromatography procedures, both of which employ inosine for gentle ligand displacement. The first affinity ligand introduced was periodate-oxidized formycin B linked to iminobispropylamine-derivatized Sepharose® 4B.[66a,b] Formycin B affinity columns, following a single ion-exchange chromatography step, have been used to purify PNP from human erythrocytes,[66b,67] fibroblasts,[68] and granulocytes,[69] and from rat[66a] and chicken liver.[70] A second affinity ligand, 6-hydroxy-9-p-benzylaminopurine, coupled to trichloro-s-triazene-activated Sepharose® C1-6B, was used to purify human erythrocytic PNP by Osborne.[71] The latter affinity ligand was synthesized and tested in our laboratory[72] but we could not achieve the high binding capacity reported earlier.[71]

Affinity chromatographic purification was also used by Zannis et al.[68] for the microscale purification and subunit analysis of PNP from cultured human fibroblasts. The enzyme was radiolabeled by growing cells in [^{35}S]-methionine and enriched by the addition of unlabeled, purified human erythrocytic PNP prior to chromatography. The subunits of PNP were identified by autoradiography after denaturing polyacrylamide gel electrophoresis. Microscale analysis of PNP from crude extracts of human placenta and erythrocytes was achieved by Ghangas and Rheem[65] by forming immunoprecipitates of the enzyme with PNP-specific antibodies. The subunit composition of the enzymes was then studied by denaturing polyacrylamide gel electrophoresis.

Our laboratory has long been interested in the large-scale purification of human erythrocytic PNP.[73-75] A new technique, chromatofocusing, which was recently introduced commercially,[76] involves adsorption of proteins to an ion-exchange column at a pH above their isoelectric points and the step-wise elution at pH values slightly below their isoelectric

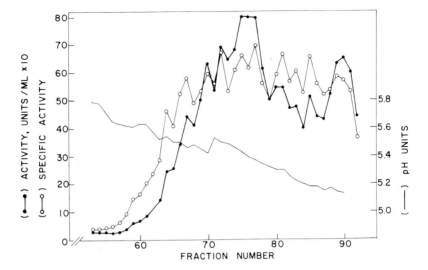

FIGURE 3. Chromatofocusing profile of human erythrocytic PNP. The activity and specific activity profiles suggest approximately ten variants. About 3700 units of partially purified PNP (spec. act. 6.7) were dialyzed against 0.025 M imidazole-HCl, pH 7.0, and applied to 1.5 × 62 cm column of polybuffer exchanger, PBE 94,[76] that had been equilibrated with the same buffer. The enzyme was eluted in 20-mℓ fractions with Polybuffer 74, 1[76] pH 5.0. The pooled fractions 64 to 91 contained 3163 units of PNP at spec. act. 69.

points. In trials conducted in this laboratory by Dowd and Chen,[134] this method has been highly effective in both small and large-scale purifications of PNP from human erythrocytes. Purifications of 5- to 20-fold have been obtained with negligible loss of activity. The fold purification has been inversely proportional to the purity of the applied enzyme. As much as 6000 units of PNP applied with ∼4 g of protein from a large-scale partial purification[74] have been purified tenfold on a 1.5 × 65 cm column. The elution pattern in Figure 3, illustrating the electrophoretic heterogeneity of PNP (see Section III.B.), demonstrates that this technique makes it possible to isolate quantitatively the different variants of PNP. Chromatofocusing has now replaced the DEAE-cellulose chromatographic step (which always resulted in significant loss of enzyme) in the standard procedure[75] for purification of PNP in this laboratory.

B. Physicochemical Properties

Studies of the structure of PNP have been spurred by its unusual subunit organization, the identification of genetic mutants with reduced or absent function, and the desire to elucidate the substrate binding site in order to design a potent inhibitor. Genetic studies of the human erythrocytic enzyme by Edwards et al.[77] indicated that PNP is the product of a single autosomal gene locus which was subsequently assigned by others to chromosome 14.[78,79]

Although trimeric enzyme structures are rare,[80] evidence from many sources indicates that human PNP has three subunits of equal size. Subunit molecular weights of about 30,000 to 33,000 have been determined by SDS gel electrophoresis for the enzyme from red cells,[66b,71,81,82] leukemic granylocytes,[69] and placenta.[65] The molecular weights determined by a variety of methods for these native enzymes range from 87,000 to 102,000. Suberimidate cross-linking confirms a trimeric structure.[65,82] The original crystalline human enzyme was shown to bind approximately three molecules of substrate per enzyme molecule.[54] Furthermore, the electrophoretic patterns of genetic variants[77] and of hybrids formed between the enzymes from human fetal liver and mouse liver,[77] and between those from human fetal liver and rabbit erythrocytes,[59] all suggest a protein composed of three subunits. Trimeric structures were also reported for the PNP from Chinese hamster tissues,[62] rabbit erythrocytes and liver,[59] and bovine spleen,[83] liver,[60] and thyroid.[64] The hamster enzyme was found to chromatograph as a mixture of trimers and dimers.[62] Reports of a monomeric rabbit liver PNP[57] and dimeric enzymes from human erythrocytes,[84] rabbit brain,[58] and bovine brain[61] are largely at variance with the findings of other laboratories.

Native human erythrocytic PNP shows considerable electrophoretic heterogeneity resulting from posttranslational modifications. Harris et al.[77] have shown by starch gel electrophoresis that human erythrocytic PNP from normal individuals migrates in at least seven bands, with the most activity found in the anodal forms; 10 to 15 variants were distinguishable in the patterns from individuals with rare mutant alleles. Normal PNP from other human tissues shows fewer electrophoretic bands with most of the activity present in the more alkaline forms. A correlation was found between the in vivo aging of erythrocytes and the progressive loss of alkaline variants and appearance of acidic variants.[85]

These posttranslational modifications could be mimicked in vitro with the generation of additional anodal bands when extracts of cultured human fibroblasts were incubated for up to 35 hr at 4°C. This process was not reversed or inhibited by sulfhydryl reducing agents.[77] Electrophoretic heterogeneity has also been detected by polyacrylamide gel isoelectric focusing of human PNP from placenta,[65] erythrocytes,[66b] brain and cultured fibroblasts,[68] leukemic granulocytes,[69] and by column isoelectric focusing in a sucrose gradient of the enzyme from erythrocytes.[14] Isoelectric points ranging from 5.0 to 6.1,[w6.5][66] 5.0 to 6.4,[68] 5.24 to 5.86,[65] and 5.85 to 5.25[14] have been reported for the erythrocytic variants.

Electrophoresis of the subunits of human erythrocytic PNP in 8.5 M urea has demonstrated the existence of four major components with isoelectric points between 6.20 and 6.63, and two minor ones.[66] PNP enzymes from fibroblasts and placenta, which show fewer electrophoretic bands under nondenaturing conditions, also have simpler subunit electrophoretic patterns.[65,68] McRoberts and Martin[67] have detected two additional alkaline subunits in the erythrocytic enzyme from the heterozygous parents of a PNP-deficient patient. Peptide mapping of these slightly larger mutant subunits indicated that the polypeptide chains were modified internally rather than at their termini.

On the basis of the isoelectric points of the four major subunits of normal erythrocytic PNP, Zannis et al.[66] suggested that the acidic subunits differed from the most alkaline one by two, three, and four negative charges and could be assembled into 20 different trimer combinations that reduce to just 12 possible variants with distinct charges. Electrophoresis of the native erythrocytic enzyme often gives diffuse patterns and has demonstrated a minimum of seven bands;[77] column isoelectric focusing over a narrow pH range produced six distinct peaks plus a broad shoulder on the acidic side.[14] Thin-layer isoelectric focusing of crystalline human erythrocytic PNP by the method of Radola,[86] with Sephadex® G-75 Superfine gel as the stabilizing support medium, has permitted the visualization of 11 distinct bands by protein staining. Alternative staining for enzymic activity yields a single broad band extending over the same region.[87] It is not certain whether this complex pattern represents the true PNP isozymes or is an artifact of the ampholyte gradient. However, this technique permits the immediate transfer of enzyme protein to a paper print and may minimize diffusion. The chromatofocusing profile in Figure 3 also suggests the presence of at least ten variants.

Determination of the complete structure of human erythrocytic PNP is in progress in a collaborative effort with the X-ray crystallography group of Bugg.[135] The enzyme was originally crystallized from ammonium sulfate in Tris buffer at pH 7.5.[54] The crystals appear as thin rods, individually or in bundles, unsuitable for X-ray analysis. However, as reported by Cook et al.,[88] at lower pH values a predominance of rhombohedral-shaped crystals is seen. Figure 4 shows a mixture of rod bundles and rhombohedral-shaped crystals observed at pH values between 5.3 and 5.9. Large rhombohedral-shaped crystals obtained at pH 5.3

43

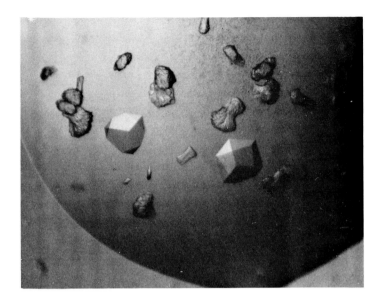

FIGURE 4. Rhombohedral-shaped crystals and bundles of rod-shaped crystals of human erythrocytic PNP. As previously reported,[54] only thin rod-shaped crystals grow at pH 7.5. The two crystal shapes are observed at pH 5.3 to 5.9.[88] The rhombohedral-shaped crystals are suitable for X-ray crystallographic analysis.

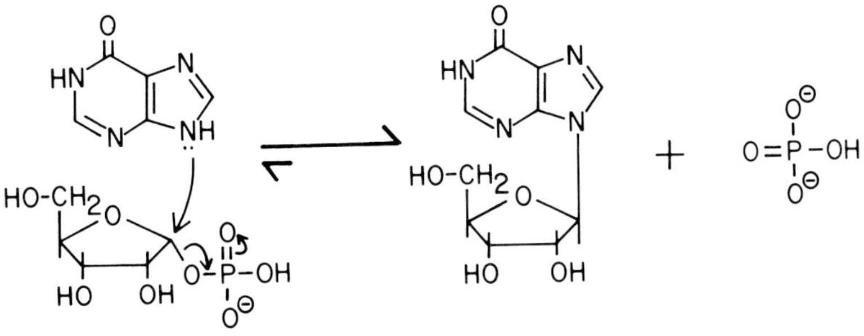

FIGURE 5. The reaction mechanism of PNP. At equilibrium, synthesis of inosine from hypoxanthine and R-1-P is favored.

to 5.4 in citrate buffer diffract to at least 3 Å resolution. Derivatives of PNP with iodinated substrate analogs and other heavy atoms are currently under study by Ealick and colleagues.[135] Preliminary results based on a 6Å electron density map indicate that PNP exists as a trimer with one subunit per assymetric unit.[1] Goddard et al.[136] have recently cloned human PNP.

C. Kinetic Behavior

The PNP reaction has an S_N2 catalytic mechanism which generates α-sugar phosphates from β-nucleosides, as shown in Figure 5. An ordered reaction mechanism has been proposed for the enzyme from human erythrocytes,[84,89] calf spleen,[90] bovine brain[61] and thyroid,[91a] and rabbit liver[57] on the basis of substrate binding, initial velocity, and product inhibition studies. The transribosylation reaction catalyzed by PNP requires the presence of inorganic phosphate and involves free R-1-P rather than a phosphorylated or ribosylated enzyme, as shown by kinetic[89,90,91b] and ^{31}P NMR studies.[92]

Perhaps the most interesting feature of the PNP reaction is activation by high substrate concentrations, which is characterized by a downward curvature of the line obtained from

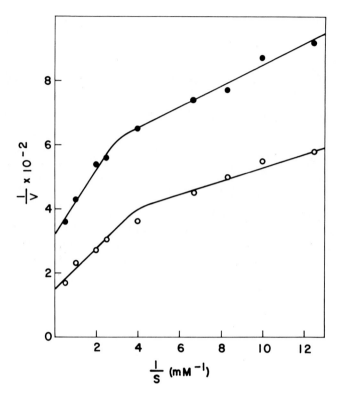

FIGURE 6.   Apparent substrate activation of human erythrocytic PNP by high phosphate concentrations occurring with either high or low fixed inosine concentrations. Double-reciprocal plots of the reaction of PNP with varying concentrations of inorganic phosphate (P_i) at two fixed concentrations, (●) 100 μM and (○) 500 μM, of inosine. K_m values for P_i at low and high concentration are 71 and 376 μM with 100 μM inosine, and 66 and 423 μM with 500 μM inosine. Inosine itself shows substrate activation at concentrations >200μM in the presence of saturating P_i concentrations (not shown).[54]

plots of 1/v vs. 1/S. This is the only evidence of possible cooperativity between the subunits of this trimeric enzyme. There is no known allosteric activation or inhibition of PNP by metabolites other than its substrates. All the normal purine and pyrimidine bases, nucleosides, and nucleotides have been tested as effectors of the human granulocytic enzyme[69] and purine nucleotides and phosphorylated sugars have been tested with the human erythrocytic enzyme.[87] Negative cooperativity at high substrate concentrations is seen with PNP from human erythrocytes,[14,53,85] calf spleen,[14,60,90] bovine thyroid and liver,[60] and rabbit erythrocytes;[59] it has been noted for both purine bases[21,90] and their nucleosides,[14,53,60,77,90] as well as for phosphate[54,60,91b] and arsenate.[60,91b] With human erythrocytic PNP, the deviation from linearity of the double-reciprocal plot is apparent at inosine concentrations greater than 200 μM.[53] Figure 6 presents a kinetic study by Choi et al.[1] which shows that activation at high inorganic phosphate concentrations can be observed in the presence of either low (100 μM) or high (500 μM) concentrations of inosine.

Turner et al.[85] discovered that substrate activation by inosine was a feature of the most acidic variants of human erythrocytic PNP. It was not observed with the most alkaline isozymes that were found in the youngest erythrocytes, or with PNP from fresh extracts of cultured human lymphocytoid cells. However, lengthy storage of the cell extracts at 4°C, which resulted in the generation of multiple electrophoretic bands, also gave rise to the apparent substrate activation. Agarwal et al.[14] isolated individual peaks after isoelectric focusing of the human red cell enzyme and also found the downward curvature of the double-reciprocal plot to be most pronounced with the most acidic variant. Thus, the substrate activation phenomenon appears to be the result of the progressive posttranslational modification of PNP. Umemura et al.[70] recently reported that chicken liver PNP, a trimer that in many respects resembles the mammalian enzyme, loses substrate activation when every subunit sustains a proteolytic nick near the -COOH terminus. This enzyme was isolated by affinity chromatography and has a native molecular weight of 90,000. Under denaturing conditions it dissociates into 24,000- and 6000-mol wt peptides. When chicken-liver PNP was isolated earlier by standard ion-exchange chromatographic procedures,[63] it also had a molecular weight of 90,000, but dissociated at a 1:2 ratio into large (30,000 to 32,000) and small (27,000 to 28,000) subunits.[93] This enzyme preparation did display substrate activation.[63] Agarwal and Parks[94] effected the loss of activation by high inosine concentrations by treatment of the human erythrocytic enzyme with the sulfhydryl reagent, 5,5′-dithiobis(2-nitrobenzoic acid) (DTNB). The reaction of approximately 3 mol of DTNB per mole of enzyme also caused a 60% loss of enzymic activity and a four- to fivefold increase in the K_m value for inosine. Guanine did not protect the enzyme from these kinetic changes, all of which were reversible by dithiothreitol. Similar behavior has been reported for PNP from rabbit erythrocytes.[59]

Participation of both cysteine (pK_a 8.2 to 8.5) and histidine (pK_a 5.5 to 6.4) in the catalytic mechanism of PNP has been indicated by the pH-dependence of the kinetic parameters.[54,57,58,61,64] Further evidence for the essentiality of a cysteine is provided by the complete inactivation of the enzyme by p-chloromercuribenzoate (PCMB),[57,58,61,64,94] which requires the reaction of only about 6 mol of PCMB per mole of human enzyme.[94] Formycin B,[64] but not guanine,[94] protects against PCMB inactivation. The pH-dependence of photoinactivation is indicative of the modification of histidine.[58,61,64] Partial protection against inactivation is provided by hypoxanthine[58] and the nucleoside analog, formycin B.[64] An essential lysine residue has been suggested by Carlson and Fischer[64] in PNP from bovine thyroid on the basis of pH-dependent inactivation by pyridoxal 5-phosphate, which could be partly blocked by inosine or high concentrations of phosphate. On the other hand, Jordan and Wu[95a] could not inactivate human erythrocytic PNP with maleic anhydride, a lysine-specific reagent. These authors identified an essential arginine residue in human and calf spleen PNP which was modified by reaction with 2,3-butanedione, but could be partially protected by R-1-P, phosphate, arsenate, or inosine. Modification of arginine was confirmed by amino acid analysis of inactivated homogeneous calf spleen PNP. Salmone and Jordan[95b] recently synthesized the first active site-directed irreversible PNP inhibitor, 9-(3,4-dioxyl)hypoxanthine which forms borate-stabilized adducts with arginine. Formycin B protected the enzyme against this inhibitor. Carlson and Fischer[64] have proposed a model for the catalytic mechanism of mammalian PNP in which histidine interacts with both N-1 and the hydroxyl at position 6, while a cysteinyl residue protonates N-7 of the base moiety of inosine. They depict the catalytic site as a pocket with the cysteine and histidine side-chains flanking the opening, and a lysyl residue that binds to phosphate at the bottom. This model reflects the reported finding that P_i is the first substrate to bind to bovine thyroid PNP and R-1-P is the last product released.[91a,b] In contrast, the calf spleen[90] and human erythrocytic[89] enzymes were found to bind purine base or nucleoside first and release it last. The exact nature of the interaction of essential amino acid side-chains with the substrates and of the orientation of the substrate molecules with respect to the enzyme surface must await clarification by X-ray crystallography.

IV. INHIBITORS OF PURINE NUCLEOSIDE PHOSPHORYLASE

A. Structure-Activity Relationship Studies

In recent years structure-activity relationship studies with PNP have focused on the iden-

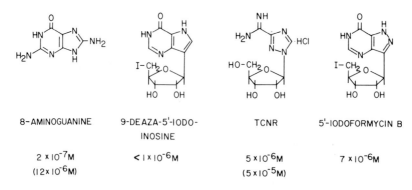

8-AMINOGUANINE   9-DEAZA-5'-IODO-   TCNR   5'-IODOFORMYCIN B
INOSINE

$2 \times 10^{-7}M$ $< 1 \times 10^{-6}M$ $5 \times 10^{-6}M$ $7 \times 10^{-6}M$
$(12 \times 10^{-6}M)$ $(5 \times 10^{-5}M)$

FIGURE 7.   Structures and K_i values of the most potent PNP inhibitors. The values in parentheses were determined at high inhibitor concentrations. TCNR is 1-β-D-ribofuranosyl-1,2,4-triazole-3-carboxamidine hydrochloride.

tification of a useful inhibitor. The compounds shown in Figure 7 are the best inhibitors identified to date, with K_i values ranging from 10^{-6} to 10^{-7} *M*. It is indicative of the awakening of interest in PNP that two of these, 8-aminoguanine (8-AG) and 1-β-D-ribofuranosyl-1,2,4-triazole-3-carboxamidine (TCNR), were synthesized earlier and only recently appraised as PNP inhibitors. The potencies of these PNP inhibitors do not approach those of the adenosine deaminase inhibitors, 2'-deoxycoformycin ($K_i = 2.5 \times 10^{-12}$ *M*) or *erythro*-9-(2-hydroxy-3-nonyl)adenine ($K_i = 1.6 \times 10^{-9}$ *M*),[96] which can simulate ADA deficiency in vivo.[36,38] However, as described below, 8-AG and TCNR have been shown to inhibit PNP in intact cells. Furthermore, these compounds exemplify the types of modifications that may lead to the synthesis of more potent inhibitors. The compounds in Figure 7 have diverse chemical structures and properties: 8-AG is an alternative substrate of PNP;[21] 9-deaza-5'-deoxy-5'-iodoinosine and 5'-deoxy-5'-iodoformycin B are C-nucleosides resistant to phosphorolysis; and TCNR, which is also not cleaved by PNP,[97] resembles the intermediate of purine biosynthesis *de novo*, 5-amino-4-imidazolecarboxamide ribonucleotide (AICAR).

The synthesis of 8-AG, which was obtained from the drug library of the National Cancer Institute,[98] was reported in 1950 by Cavalieri and Bendich.[99] The affinity of 8-AG for PNP was first reported 29 years later.[100] 8-AG is the best inhibitor of PNP characterized to date and has an apparent K_i value of 2×10^{-7} *M* for the human erythrocytic enzyme, whereas the natural substrate, guanine, has a K_i value of 5×10^{-6} *M*.[21] Like guanine[21] and hypoxanthine,[90] 8-AG causes apparent substrate activation so that plots of 1/v vs. inhibitor concentrations, and replots of the slopes of double-reciprocal plots at different fixed inhibitor concentrations are nonlinear. Therefore, K_i values of about 1.2×10^{-6} *M* are obtained for 8-AG when it is tested as an inhibitor of phosphorolysis at concentrations greater than 5×10^{-7} *M*.[21] 8-AG is an alternative substrate of PNP and 8-aminoguanosine (8-AGuo) can be synthesized enzymatically with R-1-P.[18,19,21] 8-AGuo, whose chemical synthesis was reported in 1965 by Holmes and Robins,[101] has a K_i value of 17×10^{-6} *M* for the synthetic PNP reaction.[21] This higher K_i value for the nucleoside parallels findings with the natural substrates that the nucleosides (K_m values from 30 to 83×10^{-6} *M*)[21,53,84,102,103] have lower affinity for human erythrocytic PNP than the purine bases (K_m values 20 and 19×10^{-6} *M*).[21,104] The substrate activity of 8-AGuo was noted earlier by Jordan and Wu,[103] but the extremely high K_m and K_i values of 3.2×10^{-2} *M* and 2.9×10^{-4} *M*, respectively, reported by these authors for the nucleoside did not lead to an appreciation of the affinity of 8-AG and 8-AGuo for PNP. Because it is an alternative substrate, 8-AGuo can serve as a pro-drug from which the less soluble base can be generated intracellularly. The absence of substrate or inhibitory activity of 8-AG with xanthine oxidase, hypoxanthine-guanine phosphoribosyl-

Table 1
INHIBITION OF HUMAN ERYTHROCYTIC PNP BY C(8)-
SUBSTITUTED PURINE ANALOGS[a]

	Purine ring substituent			Inhibition[b] (%)	K_i (μM)	Substrate activity[c]
	C(2)	C(6)	C(8)			
1.	NH_2	OH	NH_2	95	0.2	+
2.	H	OH	NH_2	57	10	+
3.	NH_2	OH	I	22	51	−
4.	NH_2	OH	SH	25	53	+
5.	H	SH	NH_2	26	79	+
6.	H	OH	S-(o-nitrobenzylthio)	22		−
7.	H	OH	S-(m-nitrobenzylthio)	20		−
8.	H	OH	$SONH_2$	18		−
9.	NH_2	SH	CH_3	18		−
10.	NH_2	OH	CH_3	17		+
11.	H	OH	S-(m-aminobenzylthio)	17		−
12.	H	OH	CHOH-phenyl	13		−
13.	H	OH	m-nitrophenyl	12		−
14.	NH_2	OH	SCH_3	12		−

[a]   All data from Reference 21; by purine numbering, guanine is 2-NH_2-6-OH-purine.
[b]   Percent inhibition of guanosine phosphorolysis was determined by spectrophotometric assays with guanosine and inhibitors both present at 30 μM concentration, which is approximately the K_m value for the substrate.
[c]   Substrate activities were determined by spectral shift assays with 50 to 75 μM analog concentrations, 300 μM R-1-P, and 0.1 to 0.6 units of PNP.

transferase, or guanase[21] eliminates metabolic depletion of the inhibitor and may prevent it from exerting secondary effects on purine metabolism.

Table 1 presents the results of a SAR study of substituents on C(8) of the purine ring.[21] Of all compounds tested, only 8-AG and 8-aminohypoxanthine bind better to human erythrocytic PNP than the normal substrates. The relative affinities of analogs 1, 2, and 5 parallel those of the parent compounds, since guanine, hypoxanthine, and 6-mercaptopurine have K_i values of 5 μM, 17 μM,[21] and 73 μM,[105] respectively. 8-Aminohypoxanthine was reported earlier to react with bovine thyroid PNP with K_m = 118 μM and V_{max} = 0.26% (relative to hypoxanthine).[90] The more favorable kinetic parameters seen with the human erythrocytic enzyme, K_m = 6 μM and V_{max} = 6% (relative to guanine),[21] might reflect differences in the binding sites of these enzymes (Section III.C.). In addition to the analogs listed in Table 1, bases with OH, SCH_3, propyl or phenyl groups substituted at C(8) show little or no inhibition of PNP when tested as described.[21] Jordan and Wu[103] have reported that $NHCH_3$ and $N(CH_3)_2$ groups at C(8) of guanosine cannot be accommodated by PNP. Although the nature of the inhibition by the analogs with bulky substituents at C(8) has not been determined, it is possible that these aglycones can bind to the active site. Although the data in Table 1 suggest that C(8) substituents other than NH_2 hinder binding to PNP, it is possible that some other group not yet tested, e.g., CH_2NH_2, may improve affinity, and further exploration of the 8-position may be worthwhile.

The newest addition to the list of PNP inhibitors is 9-deaza-5'-deoxy-5'-iodoinosine. This C-nucleoside was very recently synthesized by Klein et al. and preliminary testing with the human enzyme indicates that it is a competitive inhibitor with a K_i -value in the 10^{-7} M range.[106] A K_i value of 47 μM has been reported for 9-deazahypoxanthine with bovine thyroid PNP.[91a] This relatively high value may again reflect a species difference. However, it is likely that the enhanced binding of the nucleoside is due to the iodo substituent at C(5'). This is discussed in more detail below. Complete kinetic studies are needed to determine

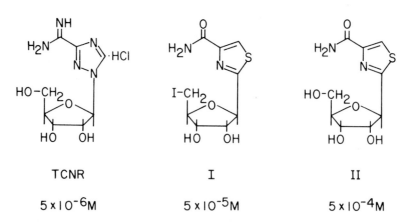

TCNR   I   II

$5 \times 10^{-6} M$ $5 \times 10^{-5} M$ $5 \times 10^{-4} M$

FIGURE 8.   Structures and K_i values of triazole and thiazole nucleoside inhibitors of PNP.
Abbreviations: TCNR, 1–β-D-ribofuranosyl-1,2,4-triazole-3-carboxamidine hydrochloride; I,
2-(5-deoxy-5-iodo-β-D-ribofuranosyl)thiazole-4-carboxamide; II, 2-β-D-ribofuranosylthia-
zole-4-carboxamide.

whether this compound is as potent as 8-AG, but it appears to be the tightest-binding
nucleoside tested to date.

TCNR is perhaps the least likely looking PNP inhibitor, since it has only one heterocyclic
ring. Its synthesis and testing as an antiviral agent was reported in 1973 by Witkowski et
al;[107] its high affinity for human PNP from lymphoblasts of B-cell origin was documented
in 1980 by Willis et al.[97] TCNR has a K_i value of $5 \times 10^{-6} M$ when tested at low inosine
concentrations. Like 8-AG, TCNR is affected by apparent substrate activation and a K_i value
of $5 \times 10^{-5} M$ is obtained when it is tested at higher inosine concentrations. TCNR is
resistant to phosphorolysis but it is not a "pure" PNP inhibitor because it undergoes adenosine kinase-dependent phosphorylation (Section IV.B.).[97] Figure 8 compares the structure
of TCNR to two other AICAR-like nucleosides. The C-nucleosides, 2-β-D-ribofuranosyl-
thiazole-4-carboxamide (II) and its 5'-deoxy-5'-iodo derivative (I) were also synthesized by
Robins et al.[108] and tested as inhibitors of human erythrocytic PNP.[109] Although these
compounds are not themselves good inhibitors, they illustrate the tenfold enhancement of
affinity by the halogen at the C(5') position. This suggests that substitution of iodine for
the 5'-OH of TCNR might improve its affinity for PNP as well as eliminate the possibility
of phosphorylation and secondary inhibitory effects.

5'-Deoxy-5'-iodoformycin also illustrates the enhancement of binding to PNP by iodination
at C(5'). The antibiotic, formycin B,[110] inhibits human erythrocytic PNP with $K_i = 1 \times 10^{-4} M$.[111] Affinity for PNP is improved more than tenfold by the iodine substituent.[21] The
data in Table 2 illustrate that although modifications at C(2') and C(3') drastically reduce
the ability of PNP to bind nucleosides, there is surprising flexibility at the 5' position. The
5'-hydroxyl has no apparent effect on affinity since 5'-deoxyinosine has the same Michaelis
constant as inosine, although the relative V_{max} is reduced by 55%. Enzymatically synthesized
5-deoxyribose 1-phosphate has been partially purified and used to demonstrate synthesis of
5'-deoxyguanosine by PNP.[102] It has been reported by others that 5'-deoxyinosine binds but
has no substrate activity with PNP from human erythrocytes[103] or bovine thyroid.[91a] The
reason for this discrepancy is not known; however, these workers obtained the compound
from a different source. The inosine analogs with a halogen or thioalkyl group at C(5'),
which have been synthesized by Chu et al.,[21] all display as good or better affinity than the
parent compounds, but extremely low substrate activity.[21] Only the 5'-fluoro substituent,
which has the approximate size of a hydrogen atom, permits a V_{max} greater than 1%. It is
interesting that α-L-lyxosylhypoxanthine, which resembles inosine with the 5'-hydroxy-
methyl group extended below the furanose ring, has moderately good affinity and reactivity.

Table 2
THE EFFECTS OF SUGAR MODIFICATION ON THE
BINDING AND ACTIVITY OF NUCLEOSIDE
ANALOGS WITH HUMAN ERYTHROCYTIC PNP[a]

Nucleoside	K_i (μM)	K_m (μM)	Rel. V_{max}
1. Inosine		30 — 46	100
2. 5'-Deoxyinosine		31	45
3. α-L-Lyxosylhypoxanthine		160	38
4. 5'-Methylthioinosine	22	15	0.7
5. 5'-Isobutylthioinosine	105	42	0.2
6. 5'-n-Butylthioinosine	63	32	0.6
7. 5'-Fluoroinosine		13	4
8. 5'-Chloroinosine	26	10	0.8
9. 5'-Bromoinosine	50	20	0.4
10. 5'-Iodoinosine	18	12	0.1
11. 5'-Benzylthioinosine	300		0
12. 5'-S-COOH-inosine			0
13. 5'-Aminoinosine			0
14. Formycin B	100		
15. 5'-Chloroformycin B	10		
16. 5'-Iodoformycin B	7		
17. 2'-Deoxyinosine		45	53
18. 2'-Deoxyguanosine		44	42
19. 2'-O-methylguanosine			0
20. 2'-Fluoroinosine		490	<0.2
21. 2'-Fluorarabinosylhypoxanthine			0
22. 2'-Azidoinosine (ara and ribo)			0
23. 2'-Bromoguanosine			0
24. 2'-Chloroguanosine			0
25. 2'-Iodoguanosine			0
26. 3'-Deoxyinosine		1100	2
27. 2',3'-Dideoxyinosine		440	1
28. 2',5'-Dideoxyinosine		120	53
29. Arabinosylhypoxanthine		>2000	<1
30. Xylosylhypoxanthine			0
31. 4'-Thioinosine		1900	<1
32. Carbocyclic inosine			0
33. Inosine dialdehyde			0

[a] All data are from References 21, 102, 111, 122, and 126. Except for the formycin series and 5'-benzylthioinosine, compounds that have no substrate activity also show no inhibition of PNP when tested at concentrations equimolar to the substrate concentration.

The bulkier benzylthio group and charged substituents are tolerated poorly, or not at all. Although the 5'-substituted inosines are very poor substrates, they are cleaved by PNP in intact cells (Section V.) and, of the compounds in Table 2, only formycin B and its analogs are true inhibitors, and the 5'-modified formycin Bs may also be "pure" PNP inhibitors since they cannot be phosphorylated.

With the exception of the 5'-halogenated C-nucleosides and some 8-azapurines, ring-modified bases and nucleosides examined to date bind poorly or are unreactive with human erythrocytic PNP. This is illustrated by the data in Table 3. Carlson and Fischer[91a] have reported high K_i values for 7-deaza- and 8-azahypoxanthine and a value of 47 μM for 9-deazahypoxanthine with bovine thyroid PNP. It is very interesting that although analogs 13 to 15 in Table 3 have less affinity for PNP than the natural substrates, 5'-iodoformycin B

Table 3

**THE EFFECTS OF RING MODIFICATIONS ON THE AFFINITY
OF PURINE ANALOGS FOR HUMAN ERYTHROCYTIC PNP**

	K_i (μM)	Inhibition[a] (%)	Substrate activity[b] or K_m (μM)	Ref.
1. Guanine	5		20	21
2. Hypoxanthine	17		19	21,104
3. 1-Deazaguanine		0	−	112
4. 3-Deazaguanine		12	+	112
5. 3-Deazaguanosine		42	233	112
6. 7-Deazaguanine		0	−	113
7. 7-Deazainosine	330			105
8. 1,7-Dideazahypoxanthine		0	−	114
9. 3,7-Dideazaguanine		0	−	115
10. 2-Aza-3-deazahypoxanthine		12	+	116
11. 8-Azaguanosine			42	117
12. 8-Aza-7-deazahypoxanthine (allopurinol)	970		+	46,105
13. 8-Aza-7-deazaguanine			52	113
14. 8-Aza-9-deazaguanine	41		−	113
15. 8-Aza-9-deazaguanosine	75		−	113
16. 8-Aza-9-deazainosine (formycin B)	100			111

[a]   Inhibition was tested with substrates (guanosine or inosine) at 30 or 50 μM concentration
       and equimolar analog concentrations.
[b]   The + or − denotes presence or absence of substrate activity, if tested.

and 9-deaza-5'-iodoinosine have lower K_i values than 5'-iodoinosine. Finally, SAR studies
by Krenitsky et al.[105] showed that all methyl or thio substitutions on the purine ring also
greatly reduce the affinity of base analogs for human erythrocytic PNP. A summary of some
of the results of SAR studies with this enzyme is presented in Figure 9.

B. Biological Effects

The major symptoms of PNP deficiency, abnormalities of the immune system, appear
between the ages of 3 to 18 months,[24] indicating that lack of PNP per se is not lethal to
most human tissues. PNP-deficient mutants of the S49 mouse T-cell lymphoma line have a
growth rate comparable to that of the parent line.[30] They show only slightly enhanced
sensitivity to deoxyguanosine toxicity relative to the parent line, with ID_{50} values of 19 and
26 μM respectively.[29,30] The sensitivity of the parent line[29] and the loss of T-suppressor cell
activity in normal mice following i.p. deoxyguanosine injections[34] suggest that intracellular
PNP cannot fully protect certain lymphoblasts from exogenous deoxyguanosine, but that
under normal conditions whole-body PNP may prevent plasma and tissue concentrations
from reaching toxic levels.

Thus, it is not surprising that "pure" PNP inhibitors are generally nontoxic in the absence
of exogenous nucleosides. The growth of human T-cell-derived CCRF-CEM cells and human
colon tumor lines is not inhibited by 100 μM 8-AGuo or 5'-chloroformycin B,[118] nor is
there growth inhibition of T– and B–lymphoblast MOLT-4 and MLG-8 cell lines by 100
μM 8-AGuo.[20] However, the blastogenesis of PHA- or LPS-stimulated mouse spleen cells
is inhibited by 8-AGuo, with an ID_{50} value of ~60 μM.[18]

In contrast, growth inhibition in the absence of exogenous deoxyguanosine is seen with
inhibitors that have additional sites of action. Formycin B is growth inhibitory to human
B[97] and T[119] cell lines, to mitogen-stimulated mouse spleen cells,[18,119] and PHA-stimulated

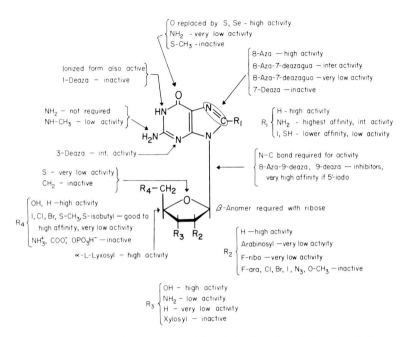

FIGURE 9. Summary of the structure-activity relationships of substrate analogs for human erythrocytic PNP. (Figure modified from Parks, R. E., Jr., et al.[19]).

human peripheral lymphocytes.[120,121] The effect on cell proliferation is associated with inhibition of DNA synthesis in peripheral lymphocytes and no synergy is observed with deoxyguanosine toxicity.[121] TCNR exerts growth inhibition related to inhibition of IMP dehydrogenase in cultured lymphoblasts of B-cell origin — effects that are absent in adenosine kinase and HGPRT-deficient double mutants that permit accumulation of the ribo- and deoxyribonucleoside PNP substrates in the medium.[97]

Allopurinol riboside has been reported to inhibit calf spleen PNP with a K_i value of 277 μM, to inhibit mitogen-stimulated blastogenesis of peripheral human lymphocytes (especially with PHA and Con A) at 2.5 to 10 mM concentrations, and to significantly suppress delayed-type hypersensitivity to sheep red blood cells in mice injected for 7 days with 1 mg/g body weight.[48] It is difficult to judge whether these effects can all be ascribed to ''pure'' PNP inhibition, since its intracellular cleavage is possible at these very high concentrations and allopurinol can be metabolized and exert secondary effects.[47]

The effectiveness of PNP inhibition by 8-AGuo and 8-AG has been examined in a number of cell types. In the T-lymphoblast MOLT-4 cells the ID_{50} of deoxyguanosine is dramatically lowered from 26 to 1.5 μM by 100 μM 8-AGuo, whereas the ID_{50} values with the B-lymphoblast MLG-8 cells are 85 and 45 μM, respectively. This concentration of inhibitor also blocks the cleavage of 200-μM inosine by 98% during a 1-hr incubation with MOLT-4 or MLG-8 cells, and 8-AGuo itself is not depleted from the medium.[20] In contrast, the toxicity of deoxyguanosine is not potentiated by 8-AGuo in CCRF-CEM cells;[118] the complete phosphorolysis of 200 μM guanosine or deoxyguanosine is delayed but not prevented by 100 μM 8-AG or 8-AGuo during a 1-hr incubation with human erythrocytes or murine L1210 cells, which have very high PNP activity.[21] In mouse Sarcoma 180 and L5178Y cells, which have lower PNP activity, 40 to 50% of the nucleoside is intact after 1 hr.[21] Also, 8-AGuo is itself cleaved during the incubations to form the more potent inhibitor, 8-AG.[21] It appears that both sensitivity to deoxyguanosine, as well as the response to a given PNP inhibitor, varies greatly among cell types. The transport of PNP inhibitors into cells has not yet been examined and may also differ among cell lines, as may the transport of deoxyguanosine. Since the inhibition of deoxyguanosine phosphorolysis in L5178Y and

L1210 cells by 8-AG is comparable to that caused by 8-AGuo,[21] transport of the inhibitor may not be a limiting factor in these cells. A striking difference seen between the erythrocytes and the mouse tumor cells is that GTP synthesis in the tumor cells keeps pace with the nucleoside phosphorolysis, whereas in the erythrocytes only 25% conversion to GTP is seen at a time (30 min) when 90% of the nucleoside has been cleaved.[21] This suggests that efficient phosphorolysis of nucleosides in red cells does not require metabolic removal of the base product.

V. ANALOGS OF 2′-DEOXYGUANOSINE AND 5′-MODIFIED NUCLEOSIDES

A. Structure-Activity Relationship Studies

Recent studies have also sought to delineate the structure-activity relationships of substrate analogs resistant to cleavage by human erythrocytic PNP.[19,21,22] The goal of these efforts has been to identify PNP-resistant analogs of 2′-deoxyguanosine that might be phosphorylated directly by a nonspecific deoxynucleoside kinase and form analogs of dGMP, dGDP, and dGTP as indicated in Figure 2. Two classes of analogs are fully resistant to phosphorolysis, those that bind to PNP but have a structure like TCNR or an unreactive C–C glycosidic bond, and those that have base or sugar modifications that prevent binding to PNP. Many substrate analogs fall midway between these two categories in that they bind poorly and react very slowly. The most interesting examples of this kind are allopurinol (4-hydroxy-pyrazolo[3,4-d]pyrimidine) and its 2-amino derivative — compounds 12 and 13 in Table 3. Both bases react with human erythrocytic PNP[46,113] to form nucleosides. However, the ribonucleosides of these compounds have extremely low substrate activities. In vitro phosphorolysis of allopurinol riboside by 1.25 units of calf spleen PNP is not detectable after 30 min,[48] and phosphorolysis or arsenolysis of the 2-amino derivative by human erythrocytic PNP occurs at $\leqslant$1% of the rate observed with inosine, whereas its synthesis has a V_{max} of ~8%.[123] Other substrate analogs that react slowly and bind poorly with human erythrocytic PNP include base-modified compounds like N^2-methylguanosine[87] or 3-deazaguanosine,[112] and sugar-modified compounds such as 3′-deoxy-, 2′,3′-dideoxy-, and 4′-thioinosine and arabinosylhypoxanthine (see Table 2);[102] and arabinosylguanine.[87]

Few deoxyguanosine analogs that bind to PNP but cannot undergo phosphorolysis have been available to date. The 2′-deoxy and arabinose derivatives of 8-aza-9-deaza-6-thioguanosine (2-amino-6-thiopyrazolo[4,3-d]pyrimidine),[54] which were recently provided by Acton et al.,[124] have much poorer affinity for PNP than 8-aza-9-deazaguanosine (compound 15, Table 3). It would be of interest to test the 2′-deoxynucleosides or arabinose derivatives of other C-nucleosides and of TCNR for binding to PNP and biological activity.

A group of cleavage-resistant, nonbinding deoxynucleoside substrate analogs of human erythrocytic PNP was recently identified in the 2′-halo- or 2′-azido-substituted 2′-deoxy-inosines and 2′-deoxyguanosines. The 2′-azido- (in either the *ribo* or *ara* configuration) and 2′-fluoro- (in the *ara* configuration) inosines are inert with PNP, although 2′-fluoroinosine (the *ribo* form) reacts very slowly, with $V_{max} < 0.2\%$ and $K_m = 4.90 \times 10^{-4}\ M$.[122] This surprising effect of the small fluorine atom may be due to an unusual ring-puckering of the fluorinated ribofuranose, which has been detected by X-ray crystallography.[125] Of the 2′-deoxy-2′-F, -Cl, -Br, and -I-substituted guanosines made available for testing by Ikehara et al.,[126] again only the 2′-fluoro analog shows barely detectable substrate activity with the isolated enzyme.

Another type of PNP substrate analog with potential chemotherapeutic applications is the group of 5′-deoxy-5′-substituted inosines and guanosines. These compounds cannot be phosphorylated, but serve instead as generators of cytotoxic analogs of R-1-P.[19,50,51] The data in Table 2 show that these compounds have very low substrate activity, but bind to PNP as well as, or better than, inosine. This is the only class of compounds known in which good affinity is coupled with low reactivity. The iodine atom enhances binding to the greatest extent.

B. Biological Effects

The chemotherapeutic potential of analogs of 2'-deoxyguanosine obviously does not depend only on their resistance to (or protection from) cleavage by PNP. Their capacity to be activated by nucleoside and nucleotide kinases, the biological activities of the analog nucleotides, and their susceptibility to inactivation by nucleotidases are all crucial factors whose net effects determine cytotoxicity. The S49 mouse T-cell lymphoblast line and its PNP-deficient mutant subline, NSU-1, which have ID_{50} values of 26 and 19 $\times$ 10^{-6} M, respectively, with deoxyguanosine,[29,30] have been provided by D. W. Martin, Jr., and colleagues for testing the biological activities of 2'-deoxyguanosine analogs, alone or in combination with PNP inhibitors. To date, tissue culture growth inhibition studies by Robison[137] have shown that the 2'-deoxynucleosides of 6-thioguanine and 6-selenoguanine are significantly more toxic to the parent line and, thus, appear to require activation by HGPRT. The low toxicity in the mutant subline of β-2'-deoxy-6-thioguanosine (ID_{50} ∼1 $\times$ 10^{-4} M) can be abolished by coincubation with 8-AGuo, indicating that very low residual PNP activity (undetectable, i.e., <0.1% of the wild-type activity, in cell extracts[30]) may be sufficient to cleave a small fraction of the nucleoside under favorable intracellular conditions.

No toxicity was found with 8-aza-7-deaza-2'-deoxyguanosine, which has low substrate activity with PNP and was tested against the mutant line. The PNP-resistant 2'-deoxy and *ara* analogs of 8-aza-9-deaza-6-thioguanosine were nontoxic with both cell lines. Only arabinosylguanine (ara-G) was found to have comparable cytotoxicities in the 10^{-6} M range with the parent and PNP-deficient cell lines. These results are only in partial agreement with SAR studies of calf thymus deoxycytidine kinase by Krenitsky et al.[127] Deoxyguanosine, 2'-deoxy-6-thioguanine (the β-anomer), and ara-G were reported to have 10, 5.8, and 3.1%, respectively, of the substrate efficiency (V'_{max}/K'_m) of deoxycytidine. Thus, unless the species difference in the kinase accounts for the absence of toxicity with 2'-deoxy-6-thioguanosine, factors other than substrate efficiency with deoxycytidine kinase must play a role in these cells. Brink and LePage[128] reported the incorporation of ara-G into the RNA of several murine tumor lines when mice bearing the ascites tumors were injected with either ara-G or arabinosyladenine. Elion et al.[129] determined significant antiviral activity in vivo, but very low antitumor activity (ID_{50} = 1 $\times$ 10^{-4} M), with ara-G in human Detroit 98 and murine L cells. They also found considerable phosphorolysis of radiolabeled ara-G in erythrocytes and in vivo in mice, and its excretion as uric acid. This illustrates the cleavage in vivo or in intact cells of analogs that show extremely low substrate activity with the isolated enzyme. The 2'-halogenated 2'-deoxyguanosines were not toxic at 10^{-4} M concentrations in CCRF-CEM cells.[118]

Recent studies by Savarese and co-workers have indicated the chemotherapeutic potential of analogs of methylthioadenosine.[19,50,51] The finding that 5'-iodoinosine is more toxic than 5'-iodoadenosine in L1210 cells which have high PNP but low MTA phosphorylase activity[21,51] points to 5-iodoribose 1-phosphate, which is generated from both nucleosides, as the toxic moiety. The mode of cytotoxic action of the sugar analog has not been defined, but it may interfere with the reported salvage of 5-methylthioribose 1-phosphate to methionine.[130] Studies in progress by Choi et al.[1] of this laboratory, have shown 5-iodoribose-1-phosphate to have inhibitory effects on purine metabolism. Kamatani et al.[131] have documented the PNP and MTA-phosphorylase-dependent interconversion of 5'-isobutylthioadenosine and 5'-isobutylthioinosine in several human cell lines. Although the 5'-modified nucleosides have very low substrate activity with the isolated enzyme, even when xanthine oxidase is used to remove the hypoxanthine product, significant intracellular cleavage is probably favored by their high affinities for PNP. The incubation of 200 μM 5'-iodoinosine with L1210 and L5178Y cells (5% v/v) results in 70 and 20% cleavage, respectively, within 60 min.[21]

VI. CONCLUSION

The selective cellular immunodeficiency associated with PNP deficiency has provided a good rationale for developing PNP inhibitors for the chemotherapy of T-cell-derived leukemias and to suppress the host-vs.-graft response without destroying humoral immunity.[19,21] In this regard, PNP inhibitors should be safer to use than adenosine deaminase inhibitors, which can evoke the symptoms of severe combined immunodeficiency. Since purines accumulate and are excreted chiefly as nucleosides in PNP deficiency, and purine nucleosides are much more water-soluble than urate, carefully controlled PNP inhibition might also find use in the treatment of acute primary or secondary gout.[19,21]

Considerable progress has been made in the identification of useful PNP inhibitors. Four analogs are currently available with K_i values ranging from 10^{-6} to 10^{-7} M and have been shown to inhibit PNP to varying degrees in different cell types. 8-Aminoguanine and its nucleoside, which are alternative PNP substrates but are not metabolized further, illustrate the enhancement of affinity for PNP that is afforded by an amino group at C(8). The C-nucleosides, 9-deaza-5′-iodoinosine and 5′-iodoformycin B exemplify the ability of a chloro or iodo substituent at C(5′) to improve the potency of PNP inhibitors. TCNR, a substituted triazole riboside, is a surprisingly good inhibitor which might be further improved by 8-amino or 5′-iodo substituents. It is probable that more potent inhibitors of PNP will be identified in the near future. An SAR exploration of the C(8) and C(5′) binding sites of PNP, similar to that carried out by Schaeffer[132] on adenosine deaminase, might prove especially fruitful and generate a wide range of new inhibitors with semi–tight, tight, or irreversible binding characteristics.

Selective immunosuppression has been induced in mice by administration of deoxyguanosine alone.[34] Although the i.p. injections may have favored lymphatic drainage, and mouse blood has significantly less PNP activity than human blood, it is possible that the currently available PNP inhibitors, particularly those such as 8-AGuo that have no secondary effects, might themselves cause immunosuppression or potentiate the activity of coadministered deoxyguanosine. However, more potent inhibitors are probably needed since patients with <1% of normal PNP activity exhibit much less severe symptoms of immunodeficiency.[16] In any case, the lesson learned from the clinical toxicity associated with the use of the tight-binding adenosine deaminase inhibitor, 2′-deoxycoformycin,[38] is that less potent inhibitors with K_i values ranging from 10^{-7} to 10^{-9} may be preferable, since they would allow better modulation of the duration of inhibition.

Since the lymphotoxicity caused by PNP deficiency appears to be chiefly related to the accumulation of 2′-deoxyguanosine, which may be directly phosphorylated and ultimately inhibit the synthesis of DNA precursors, it is reasonable to suppose that deoxyguanosine analogs might have unique cytotoxic effects provided that they are not cleaved by PNP. Of such analogs studied to date, only arabinosylguanine has been shown to possess HGPRT-independent cytotoxicity. This compound probably owes its effectiveness in the reported study and in antiviral testing[129] to its very poor affinity for PNP, which may make it resistant to cleavage at low concentrations. Although very limited tests have been conducted so far with deoxyguanosine analogs, several types of PNP-resistant deoxynucleosides have been identified. These include 2′-substituted guanosines, C-nucleosides, and the 8-aza-7-deaza purines (allopurinol and its guanosine-like analog). The last type of compound is especially interesting, because although these ribo– and 2′-deoxyribonucleosides are readily synthesized by PNP, once formed they undergo extremely slow phosphorolysis. This type of deoxynucleoside might prove active in tests for antiviral activity or with other tumor cell types. The enzymic synthesis of analog deoxynucleosides is easily accomplished with partially purified PNP and is favored by the equilibrium of the PNP reaction.[133] It may provide an alternative to difficult chemical syntheses provided some substrate activity is present with the base. PNP-synthesized analogs could be tested as antitumor agents in the presence of

PNP inhibitors. If deoxyguanosine analogs having good substrate activity with PNP are to be clinically useful, a potent PNP inhibitor may be required to prevent their cleavage in the bloodstream since rapid complete phosphorolysis of deoxyguanosine is seen in erythrocytes, even in the presence of 8-AG.[21] The high activity of PNP in human blood must be taken into consideration when tests are performed with laboratory animals that possess significantly lower activities.

The 5'-substituted inosines, which, like similarly modified methylthioadenosine, generate cytotoxic analogs of 5-methylthioribose 1-P, may be useful agents against tumors with high PNP, but low or absent MTA phosphorylase.[21,50-51] This type of compound has a very low V_{max} with isolated PNP and yet is fairly rapidly cleaved in intact cells.[21]

Studies of the protein structure of PNP are also in progress and have been aided by the use of chromatofocusing for large-scale enzyme purification. The combined use of X-ray and amino acid sequence analysis may provide information on the active site of human erythrocytic PNP within the near future. Hopefully, such information will be of value in the design of selective and potent inhibitors of this enzyme.

ACKNOWLEDGMENTS

The author is grateful to Dr. Robert E. Parks, Jr., who has for many years enthusiastically guided much of the work performed on human erythrocytic PNP and who proposed many of the concepts presented in this chapter. Thanks are also due to Dr. Shih-Fong Chen, Bonnie S. Robison, Dr. Diana J. Dowd, and Hye-Seon Choi for their valuable contributions to the PNP studies, to the medicinal chemists cited whose compounds made many of these studies possible, to Janice Ryden for technical assistance, and last but not least to Joyce Rose and Lorraine DeFusco for typing this manuscript.

This work was supported by USPHS grants CA 13943 and CA 20892 to the Roger Williams Cancer Center and American Cancer Society grant ACS CH-7W.

REFERENCES

1. **Choi, H.– S., Stoeckler, J. D., and Parks, R. E., Jr.,** unpublished observations.
2. **Kalckar, H. M.,** The enzymatic synthesis of purine ribosides, *J. Biol. Chem.,* 167, 477, 1947.
3. **Friedkin, M.,** Deoxyribose-1-phosphate. II. The isolation of crystalline deoxyribose-1-phosphate, *J. Biol. Chem.,* 184, 449, 1950.
4. **Yamada, E. W.,** The phosphorolysis of nucleosides by rabbit bone marrow, *J. Biol. Chem.,* 236, 3043, 1961.
5. **Parks, R. E., Jr. and Agarwal, R. P.,** Purine nucleoside phosphorylase, in *The Enzymes,* Vol. 7, 3rd ed., Boyer, P. D., Ed., Academic Press, New York, 1972, 483.
6. **Parks, R. E., Jr., Crabtree, G. W., Kong, C. M., Agarwal, R. P., Agarwal, K. C., and Scholar, E. M.,** Incorporation of analog purine nucleosides into the formed elements of human blood: erythrocytes, platelets, and lymphocytes, *Ann. N.Y. Acad. Sci.,* 255, 412, 1975.
7. **Moore, E. C. and Hurlbert, R. B.,** Regulation of mammalian deoxyribonucleotide biosynthesis by nucleotides as activators and inhibitors, *J. Biol. Chem.,* 241, 4802, 1966.
8. **Carson, D. A., Kaye, J., and Seegmiller, J. E.,** Lymphospecific toxicity in adenosine deaminase deficiency and purine nucleoside phosphorylase deficiency: possible role of nucleoside kinase(s), *Proc. Natl. Acad. Sci. U.S.A.,* 74, 5677, 1977.
9. **Van der Weyden, M. B. and Bailey, L.,** A micromethod for determining adenosine deaminase and purine nucleoside phosphorylase activity in cells from peripheral blood, *Clin. Chim. Acta,* 82, 179, 1982.
10. **Turner, B. M., Fisher, R. A., and Harris, H.,** The age related loss of activity of four enzymes in the human erythrocyte, *Clin. Chim. Acta,* 50, 85, 1974.
11. **Snyder, F. F., Mendelsohn, J., and Seegmiller, J. E.,** Adenosine metabolism in phytohemagglutinin-stimulated human lymphocytes, *J. Clin. Invest.,* 58, 654, 1976.

12. **Tax, W. J. M. and Veerkamp, J. H.,** Activity of adenosine deaminase and purine nucleoside phosphorylase in erythrocytes and lymphocytes of man, horse and cattle, *Comp. Biochem. Physiol.,* 61B, 439, 1978.

13. **Burgess, F. W., Stoeckler, J. D., and Parks, R. E., Jr.,** unpublished observation.

14. **Agarwal, K. C., Agarwal, R. P., Stoeckler, J. D., and Parks, R. E., Jr.,** Purine nucleoside phosphorylase. Microhetereogeneity and comparison of kinetic behavior of the enzyme from several tissues and species, *Biochemistry,* 14, 79, 1975.

15. **Giblett, E. R., Ammann, A. J., Wara, D. W., Sandman, R., and Diamond, L. K.,** Nucleoside-phosphorylase deficiency in a child with severely defective T-cell immunity and normal B-cell immunity, *Lancet,* i, 1010, 1975.

16. **Ammann, A. J.,** Immunological aberrations in purine nucleoside deficiencies, *Ciba Found. Symp.,* 68, 55, 1978.

17. **Gelfand, E. W., Dosch, H.-M., Biggar, W. D., and Fox, I. H.,** Partial purine nucleoside phosphorylase deficiency. Studies of lymphocyte function, *J. Clin. Invest.,* 61, 1071, 1978.

18. **Stoeckler, J. D. Cambor, C., Burgess, F. W., Erban, S. B., and Parks, R. E., Jr.,** Purine nucleoside phosphorylase inhibitors as potential chemotherapeutic and immunosuppressive agents, *Pharmacologist,* 22, 99, 1980.

19. **Parks, R. E., Jr., Stoeckler, J. D., Cambor, C., Savarese, T. M., Crabtree, G. W., and Chu, S.-H.,** Purine nucleoside phosphorylase and 5'-methylthioadenosine phosphorylase: Targets of chemotherapy, in *Molecular Actions and Targets for Cancer Chemotherapeutic Agents,* Sartorelli, A., Lazo, J. S., and Bertino, J. R., Eds., Academic Press, New York, 1981, 229.

20. **Kazmers, I. S., Mitchell, B. S., Dadonna, P. E., Wotring, L. L., Townsend, L. B., and Kelly, W. N.,** Inhibition of purine nucleoside phosphorylase by 8-aminoguanosine: selective toxicity for T lymphoblasts, *Science,* 214, 1137, 1981.

21. **Stoeckler, J. D., Cambor, C., Kuhns, V., Chu, S.-H., and Parks, R. E., Jr.,** Inhibitors of purine nucleoside phosphorylase, C(8) and C(5') substitutions, *Biochem. Pharmacol.,* 31, 163, 1982.

22. **Cohen, A., Doyle, D., Martin, D. W., Jr., and Ammann, A. J.,** Abnormal purine metabolism and purine overproduction in a patient deficient in purine nucleoside phosphorylase, *N. Engl. J. Med.,* 295, 1449, 1976.

23. **Siegenbeek van Heukelom, L. H., Akkerman, J. W. N., Staal, G. E. J., DeBruyn, C. H. M. M., Stoop, J. W., Zegers, B. J. M., DeBree, P. K., and Wadman, S. K.,** A patient with purine nucleoside phosphorylase deficiency: enzymological and metabolic aspects, *Clin. Chim. Acta,* 74, 271, 1977.

24. **Martin, D. W., Jr. and Gelfand, E. W.,** Biochemistry of diseases of immunodevelopment, *Ann. Rev. Biochem.,* 50, 845, 1981.

25. **Cohen, A., Gudas, L. J., Ammann, A. J., Staal, G. E. J., and Martin, D. W., Jr.,** Deoxyguanosine triphosphate as a possible toxic metabolite in the immunodeficiency associated with purine nucleoside phosphorylase deficiency, *J. Clin. Invest.,* 61, 1405, 1978.

26. **Rich, K. C., Mejias, E., and Fox, I. H.,** Purine nucleoside phosphorylase deficiency: improved metabolic and immunologic function with erythrocyte transfusions, *N. Engl. J. Med.,* 303, 973, 1980.

27. **Simmonds, H. A., Watson, A. R., Webster, D. R., Sahota, A., and Perrett, D.,** GTP depletion and other erythrocyte abnormalities in inherited PNP deficiency, *Biochem. Pharmacol.,* 31, 941, 1982.

28. **Chan, T.,** Deoxyguanosine toxicity on lymphoid cells as a cause for immunosuppression in purine nucleoside phosphorylase deficiency, *Cell,* 14, 523, 1978.

29. **Gudas, L. J., Ullman, B., Cohen, A., and Martin, D. W., Jr.,** Deoxyguanosine toxicity in a mouse T lymphoma: Relationship to purine nucleoside phosphorylase-associated immune dysfunction, *Cell,* 14, 531, 1978.

30. **Ullman, B., Gudas, L. J., Clift, S. M., and Martin, D. W., Jr.,** Isolation and characterization of purine-nucleoside phosphorylase-deficient T-lymphoma cells and secondary mutants with altered ribonucleotide reductase: genetic model for immunodeficiency, *Proc. Natl. Acad. Sci. U.S.A.,* 76, 1074, 1979.

31. **Morris, N. R., Reichard, P., and Fischer, G. A.,** Studies concerning the inhibition of cellular reproduction of deoxyribonucleosides. II. Inhibition of the synthesis of deoxycytidine by thymidine, deoxyadenosine and deoxyguanosine, *Biochim. Biophys. Acta,* 68, 93, 1963.

32. **Mitchell, B. S., Mejias, E., Daddona, P. E., and Kelley, W. N.,** Purinogenic immunodeficiency diseases: selective toxicity of deoxyribonucleosides for T cells, *Proc. Natl. Acad. Sci. U.S.A.,* 75, 5011, 1978.

33. **Gelfand, E. W., Lee, J. J., and Dosch, H.-M.,** Selective toxicity of purine deoxynucleosides for human lymphocyte growth and function, *Proc. Natl. Acad. Sci. U.S.A.,* 76, 1998, 1979.

34. **Dosch, H.-M., Mansour, A., Cohen, A., Shore, A., and Gelfand, E. W.,** Inhibition of suppressor T-cell development following deoxyguanosine administration, *Nature (London),* 285, 494, 1980.

35. **Carson, D. A., Kaye, J., Matsumoto, S., Seegmiller, J. E., and Thompson, L.,** Biochemical basis for the enhanced toxicity of deoxyribonucleosides toward malignant human T cell lines, *Proc. Natl. Acad. Sci. U.S.A.,* 76, 2430, 1979.

36. **Smith, C. M. and Henderson, J. F.,** Deoxyadenosine triphosphate accumulation in erythrocytes of deoxycoformycin-treated mice, *Biochem. Pharmacol.,* 31, 1545, 1982.

37. **Simmonds, H. A., Levinsky, R. J., Perrett, D., and Webster, D. R.,** Reciprocal relationship between erythrocyte ATP and deoxy-ATP levels in inherited ADA deficiency, *Biochem. Pharmacol.,* 31, 947, 1982.

38. **Siaw, M. F. E., Mitchell, B. S., Koller, C. A., Coleman, M. S., and Hutton, J. J.,** ATP depletion as a consequence of adenosine deaminase inhibition in man, *Proc. Natl. Acad. Sci. U.S.A.,* 77, 6157, 1980.

39. **Valentine, W. N., Fink, K., Paglia, D. E., Harris, S. R., and Adams, W. S.,** Hereditary hemolytic anemia with human erythrocytic pyrimidine 5'-nucleotidase deficiency, *J. Clin. Invest.,* 54, 866, 1974.

40. **Hershfield, M. S., Kredich, N. M., Ownby, D. R., and Buckley, R.,** In vivo inactivation of erythrocyte S-adenosylhomocysteine hydrolase by 2'-deoxyadenosine in adenosine deaminase-deficient patients, *J. Clin. Invest.,* 63, 807, 1979.

41. **Hershfield, M. S.,** Proposed explanation for S-adenosylhomocysteine hydrolase deficiency in purine nucleoside phosphorylase and hypoxanthine-guanine phosphoribosyltransferase-deficient patients, *J. Clin. Invest.,* 67, 696, 1981.

42. **Montgomery, J. A., Schabel, F. M., Jr., and Skipper, H. E.,** Experimental evaluation of potential anticancer agents. IX. The ribonucleosides and ribonucleotides of two purine antagonists, *Cancer Res.,* 22, 504, 1962.

43. **Paterson, A. R. P., Paran, J. H., Yang, S., and Lynch, T. P.,** Protection of mice against lethal dosages of nebularine by nitrobenzylthioinosine, an inhibitor of nucleoside transport, *Cancer Res.,* 39, 3607, 1979.

44. **Lynch, T. P., Jakobs, E. S., Paran, J. H., and Paterson, A. R. P.,** Treatment of mouse neoplasms with high doses of tubercidin, *Cancer Res.,* 41, 3200, 1981.

45. **LePage, G. A., Junga, I. G., and Bowman, B.,** Biochemical and carcinostatic effects of 2'-deoxythioguanosine, *Cancer Res.,* 24, 835, 1964.

46. **Krenitsky, T. A., Elion, G. B., Strelitz, R. A., and Hitchings, G. H.,** Ribonucleosides of allopurinol and oxoallopurinol. Isolation from human urine, enzymatic synthesis, and characterization, *J. Biol. Chem.,* 242, 2675, 1967.

47. **Nelson, D. J., Bugge, C. J. L., Krasny, H. C., and Elion, G. B.,** Formation of nucleotides of [6-14C]allopurinol and [6-14C]oxipurinol in rat tissues and effects on uridine nucleotide pools, *Biochem. Pharmacol.,* 22, 2003, 1973.

48. **Nishida, Y., Kamatani, N., Tanimoto, K., and Akaoka, I.,** Inhibition of purine nucleoside phosphorylase activity and of T-cell function with allopurinol-riboside, *Agents Actions,* 9, 549, 1979.

49. **Lee, S. H. and Sartorelli, A. C.,** Conversion of 6-thioguanine to the nucleoside level by purine nucleoside phosphorylase in Sarcoma 180 and Sarcoma 180/TG ascites cells, *Cancer Res.,* 41, 1086, 1981.

50. **Savarese, T. M., Chu, M. Y., Chu, S.-H., Crabtree, G. W., Dexter, D. L., Spremulli, E. N., Stoeckler, J. D., Calabresi, P., and Parks, R. E., Jr.,** 5'-Methylthioadenosine phosphorylase as a chemotherapeutic target enzyme, in *The Biochemistry of S-Adenosylmethionine and Related Compounds,* Usdin, E., Borchard, R. T., and Creveling C. R., Eds., Macmillan, New York, 1982, 709.

51. **Parks, R. E., Jr., Savarese, T. M., and Chu, S.-H.,** Analogs of 5'-methylthioadenosine as potential chemotherapeutic agents, in *New Approaches to the Design of Antineoplastic Agents,* Bardos, T. J. and Kalman, T. I., Eds., Elsevier, New York, 1982, 141.

52. **Kamatani, N. and Carson, D. A.,** Abnormal regulation of methylthioadenosine and polyamine metabolism in methylthioadenosine phosphorylase-deficient human leukemic cell lines, *Cancer Res.,* 40, 4178, 1980.

53. **Kim, B. Y., Cha, S., and Parks, R. E., Jr.,** Purine nucleoside phosphorylase. I. Purification and properties, *J. Biol. Chem.,* 243, 1763, 1968.

54. **Agarwal, R. P. and Parks, R. E., Jr.,** Purine nucleoside phosphorylase from human erythrocytes, IV. Crystallization and some properties, *J. Biol. Chem.,* 244, 644, 1969.

55. **Tsuboi, K. K. and Hudson, P. B.,** Enzymes of the human erythrocyte. I. Purine nucleoside phosphorylase; isolation procedure, *J. Biol. Chem.,* 224, 879, 1957.

56. **Abrams, R., Edmonds, M., and Libenson, L.,** Deoxyribosyl exchange activity associated with nucleoside phosphorylase, *Biochem. Biophys. Res. Commun.,* 20, 310, 1965.

57. **Lewis, A. S. and Glantz, M. D.,** Monomeric purine nucleoside phosphorylase from rabbit liver. Purification and characterization, *J. Biol. Chem.,* 251, 407, 1976.

58. **Lewis, A. S.,** Rabbit brain purine nucleoside phosphorylase. Physical and chemical properties. Inhibition studies with aminopterin, folic acid and structurally-related compounds, *Arch. Biochem. Biophys.,* 190, 662, 1978.

59. **Savage, B. and Spencer, N.,** Partial purification and properties of purine nucleoside phosphorylase from rabbit erythrocytes, *Biochem. J.,* 167, 703, 1977.

60. **Ikazawa, Z., Nishino, T., Murakami, K., and Tsushima, K.,** Purine nucleoside phosphorylase from bovine liver, *Comp. Biochem. Physiol.,* 60B, 111, 1978.

61. **Lewis, A. S. and Glantz, M. D.,** Bovine brain purine-nucleoside phosphorylase purification, characterization, and catalytic mechanism, *Biochemistry,* 15, 4451, 1976.

62. **Milman, G., Anton, D. L., and Weber, J. L.,** Chinese hamster purine-nucleoside phosphorylase: purification, structural, and catalytic properties, *Biochemistry,* 15, 4967, 1976.

63. **Murakami, K. and Tsushima, K.,** Crystallization and some properties of purine nucleoside phosphorylase from chicken liver, *Biochim. Biophys. Acta,* 384, 390, 1975.

64. **Carlson, J. D. and Fischer, A. G.,** Characterization of the active site of homogeneous thyroid purine nucleoside phosphorylase, *Biochim. Biophys. Acta,* 571, 21, 1979.

65. **Ghangas, G. and Rheem, G. H.,** Characterization of the subunit structure of human placental nucleoside phosphorylase by immunochemistry, *J. Biol. Chem.,* 254, 4233, 1979.

66a. **Cowen, M. E., Oegama, T. R., Sandberg, J. N., and Drach, J. C.,** Partial purification of purine nucleoside phosphorylase by affinity chromatography, *Fed. Proc.,* 35, 376, 1976.

66b. **Zannis, V., Doyle, D., and Martin, D. W., Jr.,** Purification and characterization of human erythrocyte purine nucleoside phosphorylase and its subunits, *J. Biol. Chem.,* 253, 504, 1978.

67. **McRoberts, J. A. and Martin, D. W., Jr.,** Submolecular characterization of a mutant human purine-nucleoside phosphorylase, *J. Biol. Chem.,* 255, 5605, 1980.

68. **Zannis, V. I., Gudas, L. J., and Martin, D. W., Jr.,** Characterization of the subunits of purine nucleoside phosphorylase from cultured normal human fibroblasts, *Biochem. Genet.,* 17, 621, 1979.

69. **Wiginton, D. A., Coleman, M. S., and Hutton, J. J.,** Characterization of purine nucleoside phosphorylase from human granulocytes and its metabolism of deoxyribonucleosides, *J. Biol. Chem.,* 255, 6663, 1980.

70. **Umemura, S., Nishino, T., Murakami, K., and Tsushima, K.,** Trimeric purine nucleoside phosphorylase from chicken liver having a proteolytic nick on each subunit and its kinetic properties, *J. Biol. Chem.,* 257, 13374, 1982.

71. **Osborne, W. R. A.,** Human red cell purine nucleoside phosphorylase. Purification by biospecific affinity chromatography and physical properties, *J. Biol. Chem.,* 255, 7089, 1980.

72. **Chen, S. F., Marcaccio, E., Stoeckler, J. D., and Parks, R. E., Jr.,** unpublished observation.

73. **Agarwal, R. P., Scholar, E. M., Agarwal, K. C., and Parks, R. E., Jr.,** Identification and isolation on a large scale of guanylate kinase from human erythrocytes, *Biochem. Pharmacol.,* 20, 1341, 1971.

74. **Agarwal, R. P., Agarwal, K. C., and Parks, R. E., Jr.,** A general method for the isolation of various enzymes from human erythrocytes, *Meth. Enzymol.,* 51, 581, 1978.

75. **Stoeckler, J. D., Agarwal, R. P., Agarwal, K. C., and Parks, R. E., Jr.,** Purine nucleoside phosphorylase from human erythrocytes, *Meth. Enzymol.,* 51, 530, 1978.

76. Pharmacia Fine Chemicals, Division of Pharmacia, Inc., Piscataway, N.J.

77. **Edwards, Y. H., Hopkinson, D. A., and Harris, H.,** Inherited variants of human nucleoside phosphorylase, *Ann. Hum. Genet. London.,* 34, 395, 1971.

78. **Ricciuti, F. and Ruddle, F. H.,** Assignment of nucleoside phosphorylase to D-14 and localization of X-linked loci in man by somatic cell genetics, *Nature New Biol.,* 241, 180, 1973.

79. **Hamerton, J. L., Douglas, G. R., Gee, P. A., and Richardson, B. J.,** The association of glucose phosphate isomerase expression with human chromosome 19 using somatic cell hybrids, *Cytogenet. Cell Genet.,* 12, 128, 1973.

80. **Klotz, I. M., Darnall, D. W., and Langerman, N. R.,** in *The Proteins,* Vol. 1, Neurath, H. and Hill, R. L., Eds., Academic Press, New York, 1975, 293.

81. **Agarwal, K. C., Agarwal, R. P., and Parks, R. E., Jr.,** Electrophoretic heterogeneity and physico-chemical properties of human erythrocytic purine nucleoside phosphorylase, *Fed. Proc.,* 32, 581, 1973.

82. **Stoeckler, J. D., Agarwal, R. P., Agarwal, K. C., Schmid, K., and Parks, R. E., Jr.,** Purine nucleoside phosphorylase from human erythrocytes: physicochemical properties of the crystalline enzyme, *Biochemistry,* 17, 278, 1978.

83. **Edwards, Y. H., Edwards, P. A., and Hopkinson, D. A.,** A trimeric structure for mammalian purine nucleoside phosphorylase, *FEBS Lett.,* 32, 235, 1973.

84. **Lewis, A. S. and Lowy, B. A.,** Human erythrocytic purine nucleoside phosphorylase: molecular weight and physical properties. A Theorell-Chance mechanism, *J. Biol. Chem.,* 254, 9927, 1979.

85. **Turner, B. M., Fisher, R. A., and Harris, H.,** An association between the kinetic and electrophoretic properties of human purine-nucleoside-phosphorylase isozymes, *Eur. J. Biochem.,* 24, 288, 1971.

86. **Radola, B. J.,** Isoelectric focusing in layers of granulated gels. I. Thin-layer isoelectric focusing of proteins, *Biochim Biophys. Acta,* 295, 412, 1973.

87. **Stoeckler, J. D. and Parks, R. E., Jr.,** unpublished observation.

88. **Cook, W. J., Ealick, S. E., Bugg, C. E., Stoeckler, J. D., and Parks, R. E., Jr.,** Crystallization and preliminary X-ray investigation of human erythrocytic purine nucleoside phosphorylase, *J. Biol. Chem.,* 256, 4079, 1981.

89. **Kim, B. K., Cha, S., and Parks, R. E., Jr.,** Purine nucleoside phosphorylase from human erythrocytes. II. Kinetic analysis and substrate-binding studies, *J. Biol. Chem.,* 243, 1771, 1968.

90. **Krenitsky, T. A.,** Purine nucleoside phosphorylase: Kinetics, mechanism and specificity, *Mol. Pharmacol.,* 3, 526, 1967.

91a. **Carlson, J. D. and Fischer, A. G.,** Thyroid purine nucleoside phosphorylase. II. Kinetic model by alternate substrate and inhibition studies, *Biochim. Biophys. Acta,* 566, 259, 1979.

91b. **Moyer, T. P. and Fischer, A. G.,** Purification and characterization of a purine-nucleoside phosphorylase from bovine thyroid, *Arch. Biochem. Biophys.,* 174, 622, 1976.

92. **Salamone, S. J., Jordan, F., and Jordan, R. R.,** ^{31}P NMR studies of purine nucleoside phosphorylase: determination of the scissile bond and the equilibrium constant, *Arch. Biochem. Biophys.,* 217, 139, 1982.

93. **Murakami, K. and Tsushima, K.,** Molecular properties and a nonidentical trimeric structure of purine nucleoside phosphorylase from chicken liver, *Biochem. Biophys. Acta,* 453, 205, 1976.

94. **Agarwal, R. P. and Parks, R. E., Jr.,** Purine nucleoside phosphorylase from human erythrocytes. V. Content and behavior of sulfhydryl groups, *J. Biol. Chem.,* 246, 3763, 1971.

95a. **Jordan, F. and Wu, A.,** Inactivation of purine nucleoside phosphorylase by modification of arginine residues, *Arch. Biochem. Biophys.,* 190, 699, 1978.

95b. **Salamone, S. J. and Jordan, F.,** Synthesis of 9-(3,4-dioxopentyl)hypoxanthine, the first arginine-directed purine derivative: an irreversible inhibitor for purine nucleoside phosphorylase, *Biochemistry,* 21, 6382, 1982.

96. **Agarwal, R. P., Spector, T., and Parks, R. E., Jr.,** Tight-binding inhibitors. IV. Inhibition of adenosine deaminases by various inhibitors, *Biochem. Pharmacol.,* 26, 359, 1977.

97. **Willis, R. C., Robins, R. K., and Seegmiller, J. E.,** An *in vivo* and *in vitro* evaluation of 1-β-D-ribofuranosyl-1,2,4-triazole-3-carboxamidine, *Molec. Pharmacol.,* 18, 287, 1980.

98. NCI, Drug Synthesis and Chemistry Branch, Div. of Cancer Treat., National Cancer Institute, Bethesda, Md.

99. **Cavalieri, L. F. and Bendich, A.,** The ultraviolet absorption spectra of pyrimidines and purines, *J. Am. Chem. Soc.,* 72, 2587, 1950.

100. **Parks, R. E., Jr., Stoeckler, J. D., Cambor, C., Savarese, T. M., Crabtree, G.W., and Chu, S.–H.,** Bristol-Meyers Cancer Symp., Yale University, New Haven, Conn., 1979.

101. **Holmes, R. E. and Robins, R. K.,** Purine nucleosides. IX. The synthesis of 9-β-D-ribofuranosyluric acid and other related 8-substituted purine ribonucleosides, *J. Am. Chem. Soc.,* 7, 1772, 1965.

102. **Stoeckler, J. D., Cambor, C., and Parks, R. E., Jr.,** Human erythrocytic purine nucleoside phosphorylase: Reaction with sugar-modified nucleoside substrates, *Biochemistry,* 19, 102, 1980.

103. **Jordan, F. and Wu, A.,** Stereoelectronic factors in the binding of substrate analogues and inhibitors to purine nucleoside phosphorylase isolated from human erythrocytes, *J. Med. Chem.,* 21, 877, 1978.

104. **Zimmerman, T. P., Gersten, N. B., Ross, A. F., and Miech, R. P.,** Adenine as substrate for purine nucleoside phosphorylase, *Can. J. Biochem.,* 49, 1050, 1971.

105. **Krenitsky, T. A., Elion, G. B., Henderson, A. M., and Hitchings, G. H.,** Inhibition of human purine nucleoside phosphorylase. Studies with intact erythrocytes and the purified enzyme, *J. Biol. Chem.,* 243, 2876, 1968.

106. **Stoeckler, J. D., Klein, R. S., and Parks, R. E., Jr.,** unpublished observation.

107. **Witkowski, J. T., Robins, R. K., Khare, G. P., and Sidwell, R. W.,** Synthesis and antiviral activity of 1,2,4-triazole-3-thiocarboxamide and 1,2,4-triazole-3-carboxamidine ribonucleosides, *J. Med. Chem.,* 16, 935, 1973.

108. **Srivastava, P. C., Pickering, M. V., Allen, L. B., Streeter, D. G., Campbell, M. T., Witkowski, J. T., Sidwell, R. W., and Robins, R. K.,** Synthesis and antiviral activity of certain thiazole C-nucleosides, *J. Med., Chem.,* 20, 256, 1977.

109. **Stoeckler, J. D., Robins, R. K., and Parks, R. E., Jr.,** unpublished observations.

110. **Koyama, G. and Umezawa, H.,** Formycin B and its relation to formycin, *J. Antibiot Tokyo,* 18A, 175, 1965.

111. **Sheen, M. R., Kim, B. K., and Parks, R. E., Jr.,** Purine nucleoside phosphorylase from human erythrocytes. III. Inhibition by the inosine analog formycin B of the isolated enzyme and of nucleoside metabolism in intact erythrocytes and Sarcoma 180 cells, *Mol. Pharmacol.,* 4, 293, 1968.

112. **Townsend, L. B., Cline, B. L., Panzica, R. P., Fagerness, P. E., Roti, L. W., Stoeckler, J. D., Crabtree, G. W., and Parks, R. E., Jr.,** Synthesis and studies on the structure-activity relationships of certain aza, deaza and aza/deaza guanine and guanosine analogs, in *Lectures in Heterocyclic Chemistry,* Vol. 4, Castle, R. N. and Lalezari, I., Eds., Hetero Corp., Orem, Utah, 1978, S79.

113. **Stoeckler, J. D., Townsend, L. B., and Parks, R. E., Jr.,** unpublished observation.

114. **Stoeckler, J. D., Schneller, S. W., and Parks, R. E., Jr.,** unpublished observation.

115. **Schneller, S. W., Luo, J.-K., Hosmane, R. S., Durrfeld, R. H., DeClercq, E., Stoeckler, J. D., Agarwal, K. C., Parks, R. E., Jr., and Saunders, P. P.,** Synthesis and bological evaluation of 6-amino-1H-pyrrolo[3,2-C]pyridin-4(5H)-one(3,7-dideazaguanine), *J. Med. Chem.,* submitted.

116. **Stoeckler, J. D., Chen, S. F., Panzica, R. P., and Parks, R. E., Jr.,** unpublished result.

117. **Chu, E., Stoeckler, J. D., and Parks, R. E., Jr.,** unpublished observation.

118. **Spremulli, E. N., Stoeckler, J. D., and Crabtree, G. W.,** unpublished data.

119. **Willemot, J., Martineau, R., DesRosiers, C., Kelly, S., Letourneau, J., and Lalanne, M.,** Inhibition of purine nucleoside phosphorylase and mitogen-stimulated transformation in immunocompetent murine spleen cells by formycin B, *Life Sci.,* 25, 1215, 1979.

120. **Osborne, W. R. A., Sullivan, J. L., and Scott, C. R.,** Formycin B, purine nucleoside phosphorylase and lymphocyte function, *Immunol. Commun.,* 9, 257, 1980.

121. **Cowan, M. J., Cashman, D., and Ammann, A. J.,** Effects of formycin B on human lymphocyte deoxyribonucleic acid synthesis, *Biochem. Pharmacol.,* 30, 2651, 1981.

122. **Stoeckler, J. D., Bell, C. A., Parks, R. E., Jr., Chu, C. K., Fox, J. J., and Ikehara, M.,** C(2′)-Substituted purine nucleoside analogs. Interactions with adenosine deaminase and purine nucleoside phosphorylase and formation of analog nucleotides, *Biochem. Pharmacol.,* 31, 1723, 1982.

123. **Dosanjh, A. K., Stoeckler, J. D., and Parks, R. E., Jr.,** unpublished observation.

124. **Stoeckler, J. D., Chen, S. F., Acton, E. M., and Parks, R. E., Jr.,** unpublished observations.

125. **Hakoshima, T., Omori, H., Tomita, K., Miki, H., and Ikehara, M.,** The crystal and molecular structure of 2′-deoxy-2′fluoroinosine monohydrate, *Nucl. Acids Res.,* 9, 711, 1981.

126. **Stoeckler, J. D., Ikehara, M., and Parks, R. E., Jr.,** unpublished results.

127. **Krenitsky, T. A., Tuttle, J. V., Koszalka, G. W., Chen, I. S., Beacham, L. M., III, Rideout, J. L., and Elion, G. B.,** Deoxycytidine kinase from calf thymus. Substrate and inhibitor specificity, *J. Biol. Chem.,* 251, 4055, 1976.

128. **Brink, J. J. and LePage, G. A.,** Metabolic effects of 9-D-arabinosylpurines in ascites tumor cells, *Cancer Res.,* 24, 312, 1964.

129. **Elion, G. B., Rideout, J. L., de Miranda, P., Collins, P., and Bauer, D. J.,** Biological activities of some purine arabinosides, *Ann. N.Y. Acad. Sci.,* 255, 468, 1975.

130. **Backlund, P. S., Jr. and Smith, R. A.,** Methionine synthesis from 5′-methylthioadenosine in liver, *J. Biol. Chem.,* 256, 1533, 1981.

131. **Kamatani, N., Willis, E. H., and Carson, D. A.,** Sequential metabolism of 5′-isobutylthioadenosine by methylthioadenosine phosphorylase and purine-nucleoside phosphorylase in viable human cells, *Biochem. Biophys. Commun.,* 104, 1335, 1982.

132. **Schaeffer, H. J. and Vogel, D.,** Enzyme inhibitors IX. Hydrophobic interactions of some 9-alkyladenines with adenosine deaminase, *J. Med. Chem.,* 8, 507, 1965.

133. **Stoeckler, J. D. and Parks, R. E., Jr.,** Synthesis of analog nucleosides with purine nucleoside phosphorylase immobilized on Sepharose, *Proc. Am. Assoc. Cancer Res.,* 18, 237, 1977.

134. **Dowd, D. J. and Chen, S.-F.,** unpublished data.

135. **Ealick, S. E., Cook, W. J., and Bugg, C. E., et al.,** Unpublished data.

136. **Goddard, J. M., Caput, D., Williams, S. R., and Martin, D. W., Jr.,** Cloning of human purine-nucleoside phospharylase cDNA sequences by complementation in *Escherichia coli, Proc. Natl. Acad. Sci. U.S.A.,* 80, 4281, 1983.

137. **Robison, B. S. and Parks, R. E., Jr.,** unpublished data.

Chapter 3

THE INTERACTION OF METHOTREXATE AND 5-FLUOROURACIL

Ed Cadman

TABLE OF CONTENTS

I. INTRODUCTION

Methotrexate (MTX), which is a tight-binding inhibitor of dihydrofolate reductase, will result in a reduction in the generation of thymidylate (dTMP) from deoxyuridylate (dUMP) and, therefore, indirectly inhibit the synthesis of DNA. This effect of MTX on dTMP synthesis demands that cells be actively synthesizing DNA. It is only during this active cell growth that dTMP synthesis occurs and, therefore, these are the only cells which would be affected by MTX. In many cells, this lethal effect of MTX can be prevented by the administration of thymidine, which is converted by thymidine kinase directly to dTMP, a reaction which does not require the folate cofactor 5-10 methylenetetrahydrofolate (CH_2FAH_4). Therefore, thymidine can circumvent the MTX block. Hryniuk[1] also documented that cells which had been exposed to MTX had a requirement for the purine base, hypoxanthine, in addition to thymidine, for total rescue from the cytotoxic effects of MTX. A thymidine-less state can persist and has been associated with the lethal effects of MTX for some cells when hypoxanthine was used alone following MTX exposure. Moran et al.[2] have documented that in the presence of hypoxanthine the amount of leucovorin (5-formyltetrahydrofolate) required for total amelioration of the lethal effects of MTX was reduced considerably. These observations clearly indicate that MTX has a much broader effect on intracellular metabolism than the simple inhibition of dTMP synthesis.

Besides biochemical reasons for investigating possible alterations in intracellular drug metabolism that follow MTX treatment, there are clinical reasons as well. MTX is a drug commonly used for the treatment of patients who have a malignancy. Most patients with cancer are given combinations of drugs, generally because, in most instances, the response rates are better when drug combinations are given compared to the use of single drugs.[3] The major reasoning used to support such combination therapy is that the drugs given must each have a different type of host toxicity and the mechanisms of action should be dissimilar. The intracellular biochemical interactions which can occur between drugs is generally not considered when the drug choice is conceived. Therefore, it would be quite useful to understand better these potential biochemical interactions among various drugs. There is no *a priori* reason to expect that all drug combinations will result in synergistic antitumor activity, certainly some combinations could be antagonistic. A further reason to investigate the biochemical interaction of drugs at the cellular level would be to determine the dose and timing of administration of drugs which would be most favorable for antineoplastic activity and least toxic for normal tissues. In addtion, from a better understanding of the biochemical and molecular pharmacology of drugs, the enzymatic differences between some normal and malignant cells could possibly be exploited.

II. BIOCHEMICAL CHANGES SUBSEQUENT TO MTX

The reduction of dTMP synthesis is an indirect effect of MTX treatment; the eventual result of the inhibition of dihydrofolate reductase by MTX. The inhibition of the methyl transfer to deoxyuridylate (dUMP) by dTMP synthetase to form dTMP occurs only when the methyl donor, CH_2FAH_4, has been reduced below levels which are necessary for this reaction to proceed. In the situation of limited dihydrofolate reductase activity, the result of MTX binding to this enzyme, the utilization of CH_2FAH_4 for methyl transfer to form dTMP will continue until the amount of CH_2FAH_4, which is being irreversibly consumed by this enzymatic process, can no longer sufficiently support this reaction. The folate byproduct produced from the synthesis of dTMP is dihydrofolate (FAH_2). This folate derivative, which was oxidized during the enzymatic conversion of dUMP to dTMP, is biologically inactive and must be chemically reduced (hydrogen added to the molecule) by dihydrofolate reductase, the enzyme which is inhibited by MTX. The ultimate consequence of this inhibition by

MTX of dihydrofolate reductase is a reduction of dTMP and the di- and triphosphate forms of this pyrimidine nucleotide, which is the immediate result of the depleted intracellular CH_2FAH_4 levels.[4-6]

The concentration of the substrate for dTMP synthetase, dUMP, is increased in response to this inhibition of dTMP synthesis and resultant decrease in dTTP.[7,8] The primary source of this dUMP accumulation is from the deamination of deoxycytidylate (dCMP) to dUMP.[9,10] Because dCTP has an inhibitory influence on the activity of deoxycytidine kinase[11,12] and is also a subtrate for DNA polymerase,[13,14] a reduction of dCTP potentially could influence metabolic pathways other than those directly altered by MTX treatment. This effect can be exploited in designing experiments which modulate cytosine arabinoside metabolism, a drug which resembles deoxycytidine.

A small component of the dUMP accumulation is likely to be from *de novo* pyrimidine synthesis of dUMP, however, other nucleosides and nucleotides within the *de novo* pyrimidine pathway do not appear to be increased in quantity following MTX exposure.[15] The dynamic flux of nucleotides along this synthetic pathway, however, may be slowed. This flow along the *de novo* pyrimidine pathway has been a difficult feature to quantitate with certainty. This reduction in flow along the *de novo* pyrimidine pathway could also be associated with a reduced need to salvage preformed pyrimidine nucleosides from the culture medium. This effect of MTX could explain the reduction of intracellular accumulation of uridine following MTX exposure, which otherwise is rapidly accumulated within unperturbed cells.[15] These MTX effects on the *de novo* pyrimidine flow may also account for the reduced accumulation of 5-fluorouridine (FUrd) within MTX-treated cells.[15] Under normal circumstances this fluoropyrimidine is converted to FUMP by uridine-cytidine kinase. If the *de novo* pyrimidine synthetic pathway is blocked at a point before UMP synthesis, for example with N-(phosphonacetyl)-L-aspartate[16] or pyrazofurin,[17] FUrd intracellular accumulation is enhanced. However, in MTX-treated cells FUrd accumulation is markedly reduced.

Intracellular folates are required for one carbon metabolism in the *de novo* synthesis of purines. The formation of formylglycinamide ribonucleotide from glycinamide requires 5,10-methenyltetrahydrofolate ($CHFAH_4$) and the synthesis of 5-formamidoimidazole-4-carboxamide ribonucleotide requires the transfer of the formyl group from 10-formyltetrahydrofolate ($CHOFAH_4$) to 5-aminoimidazole-4-carboxamide ribonucleotide. Neither one of these folate-requiring steps results in the oxidation of the tetrahydrofolate structure to a dihydrofolate derivative, which is in contrast to the oxidation which does occur during dTMP synthesis. Therefore, the tetrahydrofolate byproduct which remains after the one carbon transfer during *de novo* purine sythesis can undergo one carbon conversion without the requirements of the enzyme dihydrofolate reductase. The inhibitory effect of MTX on the *de novo* purines synthetic pathway is therefore indirect, and the consequence of the altered folate pools which result from continued dTMP synthesis in the presence of the reduced activity of dihydrofolate reductase which occurs from the binding of MTX to this enzyme. When dihydrofolate reductase is inhibited by MTX (K_i $10 - {}^{11}M$)[18] CH_2FAH_4 continues to be utilized and therefore consumed during the synthesis of dTMP from dUMP until this folate cofactor is reduced to such a level that this reaction is no longer sustained at a rate which allows DNA synthesis to continue. Presumably sufficient quantities of tetrahydrofolate (FAH_4), which would have undergone conversion to $CHFAH_4$ or $CHOFAH_4$, are now transformed to CH_2FAH_4 in an attempt to continue the synthesis of the dTMP (and ultimately dTTP) needed for DNA synthesis. Therefore, in response to the MTX inhibition of dihydrofolate reductase there is also a reduction in *de novo* purine synthesis because of this continud utilization without replenishment of tetrahydrofolates. The influence of MTX on the synthesis of purines had been appreciated by Sartorelli and LePage.[19] However, the cytotoxic effect of MTX has generally been considered to be the result of a thymidine-less state.[20,21] The subsequent interaction between MTX and 5-fluorouracil is dependent on this antipurine effect of MTX, which will be described in detail later.

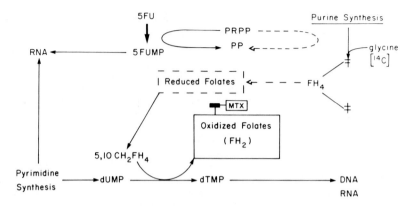

FIGURE 1.   Schematic representation of the effects of methotrexate (MTX) on folate metabolism, purine synthesis and deoxythymidylate formation. The MTX block of dihydrofolate
reductase is represented by the dark bar. The result of this block in folate conversions is a
depletion in the reduced folate pool (tetrahydrofolates, FH_4) and an expansion of the original
folate pool (dihydrofolate, FH_2).

Glycine is normally incorporated into the purine ring during formation of the purine
structure, glycinamide ribonucleotide, from phosphoribosylamine. In unperturbed cell growth
the $(1-{}^{14}C)$ label of radiolabeled glycine which had been added to the culture medium can
be found in the purine nucleotides which were synthesized and incorporated into DNA and
RNA. However, in the presence of MTX at concentrations which maximally inhibit dihydrofolate reductase for at least one cell-doubling time, this $(1-{}^{14}C)$ label is present in only
minimal amounts in these purine nucleotides. This observation is consistent with the concept
that MTX indeed has an indirect inhibitory effect on the synthesis of *de novo* purine[22] (Figure
1 and 2).

The various intracellular folates and their concentrations have been difficult to quantitate
with certainty and accuracy. We have recently documented, with the use of high performance
liquid chromatography, changes consistent with the presumed alterations of intracellular
folates following MTX which were described above. Although absolute elimination of
tetrahydrofolate derivatives was not observed,[23] the fraction of tetrahydrofolates was reduced
nearly 50%, while the dihydrofolate derivatives were essentially unchanged by the method
used for quantitation (Figure 3). There is no immediate explanation for the lack of dihydrofolate pool expansion in response to MTX. These effects of MTX on purine synthesis
are consistent with the previous observation that hypoxanthine, which is a purine base that
can be converted to inosine monophosphate (IMP) by hypoxanthine-guanine phosphoribosyltransferase, can enter the purine synthetic pathway beyond the need of folates and thus
sustain purine nucleotide formation in the presence of MTX.[1,17,24,25]

One consequence of the inhibition of the *de novo* purine synthetic pathway is an increase
in the availability of 5-phosphoribosyl-1-pyrophosphate (PRPP) (Figure 2). PRPP normally
contributes the phosphoribosyl portion of this molecule, with the amino group donated by
glutamine to form phosphoribosylamine. This enzymatic step is the first committed process
in the *de novo* purine pathway and susceptible to feedback inhibition by the final purine
products. PRPP can also þe utilized by orotate phosphoribosyltransferase, an enzyme used
in the *de novo* pyrimidine synthetic pathway and hypoxanthine-guanine phosphoribosyltransferase and adenine phosphoribosyltransferase, enzymes utilized in the salvage of the purines
hypoxanthine, guanine, and adenine, respectively. The intracellular activity of these enzymes
can be influenced by the availability this obligatory cosubstrate, PRPP.

The effects of MTX, therefore, depend on two primary factors. The first is that this agent
must inhibit the enzyme dihydrofolate reductase. The second is that the cell must be actively
synthesizing dTMP to result in the subsequent depletion of tetrahydrofolate pools. The

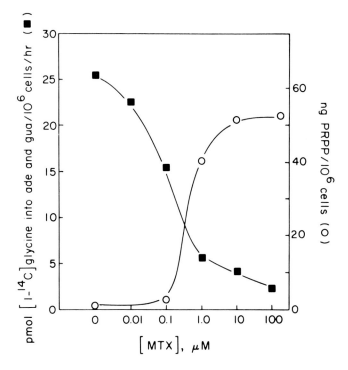

FIGURE 2.   The simultaneous changes in 5-phosphoribosyl-1-pyrophos-
phate (PRPP) levels and glycine incorporation into adenine and guanine
were determined in L1210 cells exposed to MTX for 3 hr.

antipurine MTX effect is the consequence of the alterations which subsequently occur in the folate pools. It is quite understandable, therefore, why MTX has little effect in populations of cells which are not actively dividing, in plateau growth, or have a small fraction of cells undergoing DNA synthesis (S-phase).[26] A corollary of this concept which has been recognized by Washtien,[27] is that cell populations with increased dTMP synthetase activity, as would be expected, are more likely to have perturbations of purine synthesis following MTX treatment because of the increased rate of CH_2FAH_4 utilization by this enhanced rate of dTMP synthesis. Likewise, if dTMP synthetase is inhibited directly by FdUMP and, therefore, not capable of utilizing CH_2FAH_4, the MTX-treated cells will require considerably less leucovorin (5-formyltetrahydrofolate) to reverse cytotoxicity.[2] Thymidine is necessary, under these circumstances, to maintain sufficient dTMP levels and, therefore, dTTP pools, so that DNA synthesis can continue. This observation also confirms that folate pool alterations in the presence of MTX can have significant antipurine effects.

Cells which are resistant to MTX either because of a reduced ability to transport MTX,[28] a reduced affinity of dihydrofolate reductase for MTX,[29-31] or contain excessive amounts of dihydrofolate reductase[32,33] would be protected from the intracellular modulatory effects just described. Obviously, these resistant cells would not respond as expected to other agents whose antitumor activity would otherwise have been enhanced by the biochemical alterations induced by MTX in non-MTX-resistant cells. Another major factor of which to remain cognizant when considering MTX as a modulating agent to be used with other drugs is that certain preformed nucleosides present in the culture medium or patient's blood can circumvent the biochemical effects of MTX and, therefore, ameliorate or prevent any anticipated modulating effects. For example, thymidine can replace the need for dTMP synthetase by being converted by thymidine kinase to dTMP. Hypoxanthine, as mentioned above, can be converted to IMP and thus circumvent the inhibition of purine synthesis induced by the

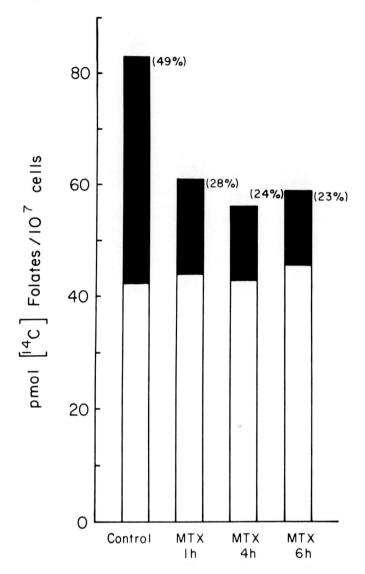

FIGURE 3.   The intracellular folates were evaluated in L1210 cells following
10 μ*M* MTX. Cell cultures were grown in media which contained ^{14}C-folate,
after 48 hr of cell growth when the cells were in logarithmic growth, the folate
pools were determined by an HPLC method recently described.[23] The folates
were categorized as dihydrofolates (open bars) or tetrahydrofolates (dark bars).
The percent at the top of each bar represents what percent of the total folates
were tetrahydrofolates.

altered folate pools subsequent to MTX treatment. The degree to which either of these
compounds can prevent MTX cytotoxicity is dependent upon the salvage pathway enzyme
activity of thymidine kinase and hypoxanthine-guanine phosphoribosyl transferase, respectively, and the concentration of the preformed compound. The complexity of the multiple
enzymatic steps needed for reversal of MTX effect, does, in fact, provide a potential basis
for selective toxicity among normal and malignant cells when differences in the utilization
of these salvage compounds can be identified.[23,34] For example, if a malignant cell had
reduced activity of, or absent thymidine kinase, while the normal cell had the capacity to
utilize thymidine, then MTX would have an advantage for causing damage to the malignant
cell.

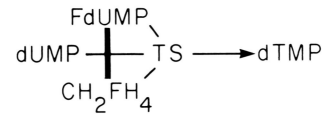

FIGURE 4. Schematic representation of the covalent bonding of 5-fluoro-2'-deoxyuridylate (FdUMP) and 5,10-methylenetetrahydrofolate (CH₂FH₄) with thymidylate synthetase (TS).

These effects of MTX on the folate pools and the subsequent indirect effects on pyrimidine and purine synthesis provide a basis for combination therapy with purine and pyrimidine analogs and is the foundation from which the following studies and observations were made.

III. EFFECT OF MTX ON FLUOROPYRIMIDINE METABOLISM

The major metabolite which has been considered to be responsible for the cytotoxicity of the fluoropyrimidines is 5-fluoro-2'-deoxyuridylate (FdUMP). For FdUMP to maximally inhibit the synthesis of dTMP it must form a covalent bond with dTMP synthetase in the presence of CH_2FAH_4 (Figure 4).[35-37] It was suggested, therefore, by Ullman et al.,[38] that this inhibition of dTMP synthetase would be suboptimal following MTX exposure because the CH_2FAH_4 pools would have been depleted by the continued activity of dTMP synthetase which would have consumed CH_2FAH_4 in the continued conversion of dUMP to dTMP. Under such conditions, when FdUMP was formed after MTX exposure there could be no covalent bonding to dTMP synthetase because of the reduction or absent CH_2FAH_4 pools. Therefore, the sequence of MTX before a fluoropyrimidine theoretically should have been antagonistic. The converse sequence of a fluoropyrimidine before MTX was also considered antagonistic by Bowen et al.[39] because the FdUMP would have directly inhibited the only enzymatic reaction which would have utilized and consumed CH_2FAH_4. In this circumstance, the subsequent administration of MTX would presumably have little effect on the folate pools because the mechanism by which the alteration of these pools would have occurred (continued synthesis of dTMP) was now blocked by FdUMP.

These biochemical interactions between FdUMP and MTX on dTMP synthetase were accurate assessments of what would happen to folate pools and dTMP synthesis. However, 5-fluorouracil (FUra), the most commonly used fluoropyrimidine for the treatment of patients with cancer, is metabolized to many other nucleotide derivatives in addition to FdUMP. For example, 5-fluorouridine triphosphate (FUTP) can be incorporated into RNA[40] although the extent to which this incorporation is cytotoxic has not been clearly delineated.

A. 5-Fluorouracil

FUra is converted to the nucleotide, 5-fluorouridylate (FUMP), by orotate phosphoribosyltransferase (OPRTase) (step 1, Figure 5). This initial ribosylphosphorylation is generally considered to be the rate-limiting step in the total intracellular accumulation of FUra ribonucleotide derivatives. This enzymatic process is, therefore, an important step which could influence the overall effects of FUra. OPRTase requires PRPP, from which the phosphoribosyl moiety is transferred to FUra to form FUMP. The subsequent formation of other FUra ribonucleotides and deoxyribonucleotides occurs, including the formation of FdUMP and FUTP.[41] FUra can also be acted upon by uridine phosphorylase in the presence of ribose-1-phosphate[42] to form FUrd (step 3, Figure 5), and by deoxyribose (thymidine) phosphorylase in the presence of a deoxyribose donor to form 5-fluoro-2'-deoxyuridine (FdUrd) (step 2,

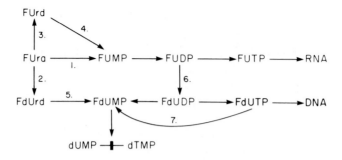

FIGURE 5.   Schematic representation of the metabolic conversions of the
fluoropyrimidines. The enzymes are (1) orotate phosphoribosyltransferase,
(2) thymidine phosphorylase, (3) uridine phosphorylase, (4) uridine-cytidine kinase, (5) thymidine kinase, (6) ribonucleotide reductase, (7) deoxyuridine triphosphate nucleotide hydrolase.

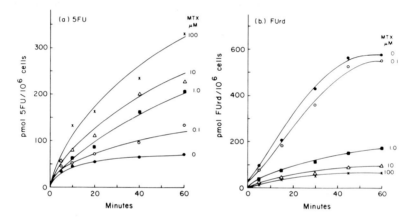

FIGURE 6.   The intracellular accumulation of 5-fluorouracil (5FU) and 5-fluorouracil (FUrd)
into L1210 cells following methotrexate (MTX) treatment. After 3 hr of exposure to the
indicated concentration of MTX, [³H]-FUra or [³H]-FUrd was added to the cultures to a
concentration of 1 μ*M* and the intracellular accumulation of drug determined by a rapid
microfuge method.[17]

Figure 5).[43] Both of these nucleoside analogs can then be converted to their monophosphate
derivative by uridine-cytidine kinase[44] and thymidine kinase,[45] respectively (Figure 5). These
later two phosphorylase mechanisms, however, are not considered to be the predominate
method of metabolic conversion of FUra in most cells.

In cells exposed to MTX, the subsequent elevation of PRPP levels can be used to convert
FUra in greater quantities to FUMP by OPRTase. When MTX was given in sufficient amounts
to L1210 cells, which resulted in intracellular concentrations that saturated dihydrofolate
reductase, thymidine triphosphate pools (dTTP) were reduced, purine synthesis was halted
and PRPP levels eventually increased five- to ten-fold (Figure 3). The rate and total intracellular accumulation of FUra metabolites increased nearly fivefold including FUTP and
free (soluble) FdUMP in MTX-treated cells.[15,17] Figure 6 demonstrates that FUra (5FU)
accumulation was enhanced in MTX-treated cells while the fluoropyrimidine nucleoside,
FUrd, accumulation was reduced under identical conditions. Figure 7 demonstrates that the
majority of the FUra accumulation was in nucleotide forms, indicating that a metabolic
process was enhanced which favored FUra conversion to nucleotides.

The following experiments were performed with L1210 cells (which were the cells used
in the above studies) and support the notion that it is the increased PRPP levels following

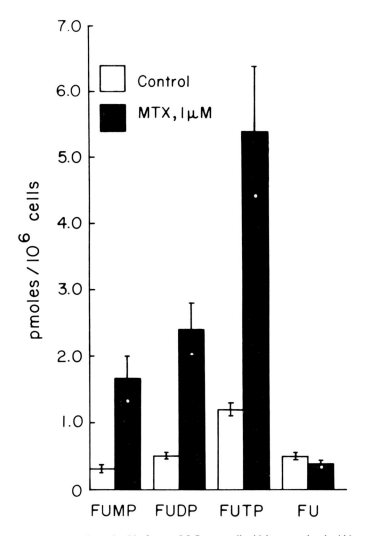

FIGURE 7. Ribonucleotide forms of 5-fluorouracil which accumulated within L1210 cells exposed for 3 hr to 1 μ*M* methotrexate (MTX). Conditions were identical to those described in Figure 6. (From Cadman, E. C., Heimer, R., and Davis, L., *Science,* 205, 1135, 1979. With permission. Copyright 1979 by the American Association for the Advancement of Science.

MTX treatment which accounts for the enhanced intracellular FUra accumulation and metabolism. The first evidence that supports this contention is that when orotate is allowed to increase within the cells, intracellular FUra accumulation is dramatically reduced. This can be achieved by using pyrazofurin which, as the monophosphate derivative, is a tight-binding inhibitor of orotate decarboxylase (K_i $10^{-9} M$).[46,47] The consequence of pyrazofurin exposure is an elevation of intracellular orotate which then competes with FUra for PRPP at the enzyme, OPRTase. Because orotate is a better substrate than FUra for OPRTase, PRPP levels were reduced following pyrazofurin treatment, even in cells exposed to MTX. The enhanced FUra accumulation, which normally occurs with MTX treatment, was also prevented when pyrazofurin was given. Pyrazofurin, which is phosphorylated by adenosine kinase, does not utilize PRPP and therefore will not affect PRPP alone. The K_m of orotate conversion to OMP by OPRTase is 12 to 14 n*M* while the K_m of FUra conversion to FUMP is 520 u*M*.[17] Therefore, the increase in orotate levels will be preferentially utilized by OPRTase and thus consume the cosubstrate, PRPP. In Table 1, the effects of various drugs

Table 1
THE EFFECT OF VARIOUS DRUGS ON 5-PHOSPHORIBOSYL-1-PYROPHOSPHATE (PRPP) LEVELS AND INTRACELLULAR 5-FLUOROURACIL (FUra) ACCUMULATION IN LOGARITHMICALLY GROWING L1210 CELLS

		Concentration (μM)		Exposure (hr)		PRPP ($ng/10^6cells$)	FUra ($pmol/min/10^6cells$)
Drug 1	Drug	Drug 1	Drug 2	Drug 1	Drug 2		
Single drug							
Control	—	—	—	—	—	7 ± 1.2	0.025
MTX	—	10	—	3	—	52.2	0.108
Hyp	—	10	—	1	—	3.8	0.020
PF	—	5	—	3	—	12.2	UD
Tbc	—	10	—	1	—	<0.7	UD
MMPR	—	1	—	3	—	110.2	0.108
Combinations							
MTX	Hyp	10	10	3 →	1	6.3	0.022
MTX	PF	10	5	3 +	3	40.0	UD
Tbc	MTX	10	10	2 →	1	2.0	UD

Note: After the indicated exposure time, PRPP levels were determined as we have described using the conversion of [³H]-adenine to [³H]-AMP.[17] [³H]-FUra (2 Ci/mmol) was added to achieve a concentration of $3\mu M$ and the rate of intracellular [³H]-FUra measured by the microfuge methods we recently described.[17] The FUra rates were linear for the hour during which the studies were performed. All experiments were done in duplicate twice; the mean values are shown; the greatest range was ± 8%. The arrow (→) indicates drug 1 was given for the indicated time before adding the second drug. The plus (+) indicates both drugs were added simultaneously to the L1210 cell culture. MTX — methotrexate; Hyp — hypoxanthine; PF — pyrazofurin; Tbc — tubercidin; MMPR — 6-methylmercaptopurine riboside; UD — undetectable.

on both PRPP levels and the rate of intracellular FUra accumulation are presented. Three important concepts are supported by the data contained in this table. Hypoxanthine (Hyp), which can also utilize PRPP, will compete for PRPP with FUra and, therefore, negate the effect of MTX on enhanced FUra accumulation. 7-Deazaadenosine (tubercidin, Tbc) directly inhibits PRPP synthetase[48] and does not allow an increase in PRPP levels to occur following MTX treatment. This drug, therefore, also prevents the MTX enhancement of FUra accumulation. Finally, the direct inhibitor of early *de novo* purine synthesis, methylmercaptopurine riboside (MMPR), can mimic the effects of MTX.

The use of *N*-(phosphonacetyl)-L-aspartate (PALA), which inhibits aspartate transcarbamylase and therefore reduces orotate synthesis, will also enhance FUra metabolism for any given availability of PRPP providing the PRPP levels do not already greatly exceed the K_m of the enzymatic reaction for conversion of FUra to FUMP.[17] However, the rate of FUra accumulation was only enhanced 20% in the presence of PALA, indicating that when PRPP levels are below the K_m of FUra conversion to FUMP, a reduction in orotate concentrations will not result in the optimum enhancement of FUra phosphorylation.

If elevation of the PRPP concentrations is the important aspect of this initial FUra metabolic step, then other drugs which inhibit *de novo* purine synthesis and elevate PRPP levels should also be associated with an enhanced FUra metabolism in a similar fashion as that observed following MTX. This would indicate (1) that it was the antipurine effect of MTX which was responsible for the elevated PRPP levels, and (2) that it was the increased PRPP levels that resulted in the enhanced FUra accumulation and metabolism and not some other MTX effect. Methylmercaptopurine ribonucleoside (MMPR) is a purine analog which is phosphorylated by adenosine kinase. In the nucleotide form this drug inhibits amidophosphoribosyltransferase,[49] the initial committed step in *de novo* purine synthesis which combines

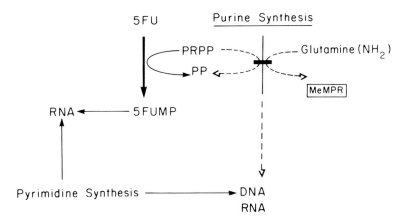

FIGURE 8.   Schematic representation of the direct inhibition of amidophosphoribosyltransferase by methylmercaptopurine riboside (McMPR). The result is a reduced utilization of 5-
phosphoribosyl-1-pyrophosphate (PRPP) and the subsequent enhanced conversion of 5-fluo-
rouracil (5FU) to 5-fluorouridylate (5FUMP) by orotate phosphoribosyltransferase.

Table 2

THE EFFECT OF INHIBITORS OF *DE NOVO* PURINE SYNTHESIS ON [1-¹⁴C]-GLYCINE INCORPORATION INTO ADENINE AND GUANINE, PRPP LEVELS, AND THE INTRACELLULAR ACCUMULATION OF FUra

Drug	(μM)	(Hr)	[1-^{14}C]-glycine into adenine and guanine (%control ± 10%)	PRPP (ng/10⁶ cells)	FUra (pmol/min/10⁶ cells)
Control	—	—	100	7 ± 1.2	0.025
MTX	10	3	16	52.2	0.108
MMPR	10	3	7	110.2	0.108
DON	10	3	4	ND	0.086
AZA	10	3	14	15	0.075
L-ALA	10	3	60	25	0.048
Tbc	10	1.5	17	0.1	UD

Note: See Table 1 for methods; MTX — methotrexate, MMPR — 6-methylmercaptopurine riboside, DON — 6-diazo-5-oxo-L-norleucine, AZA — azaserine, L-ALA — L-alanosine,
Tbc — tubercidin.

the phosphoribosyl moiety of PRPP with the amino group from glutamine to form phosphoribosylamine (Figure 8). As expected PRPP levels were increased in cells exposed to
MMPR (Table 1).[22] In addition, intracellular FUra accumulation and metabolism was enhanced to the same extent as that which followed MTX exposure providing both drug
concentrations were sufficient to elevate the PRPP similar concentrations (Table 1). The
addition of MMPR to MTX-treated cells did not increase further the PRPP levels or result
in a greater accumulation of FUra than that observed when either drug was used alone at
the maximum concentration required for these alterations. Similar findings have been noted
following the use of several other agents which inhibit purine synthesis: 6-diazo-5-oxo-L-
norleucine (DON), azaserine, and L-alanosine (Table 2).[22]

Hypoxanthine is a base which is converted to IMP by HGPRTase. This reaction also
requires PRPP as a cosubstrate. When hypoxanthine was added after MTX but before FUra,
the PRPP levels were reduced and the enhanced FUra accumulation and metabolism was

Table 3
**THE EFFECT OF MTX EXPOSURE ON PRPP LEVELS
AND INTRACELLULAR FUra ACCUMULATION INTO
THE HUMAN TUMOR CELL LINES, HUMAN COLON
TUMOR HCT-8 AND THE BREAST CANCER CELL
47-DN**

Human cell line MTX Time	(μM)	(Hr)	PRPP (ng/10^6 cells)	FURA (pmol/min/10^6 cells)
HCT-8	0	—	20	1.11
	10	24	72	2.76
47-DN	0	—	20	4.1
	10	24	3500	11.1

eliminated.[17,22] Similarly, tubercidin, which is also phosphorylated by adenosine kinase, results in lowered PRPP levels by inhibiting PRPP synthetase.[50] This drug will prevent the MTX effect on PRPP levels and FUra metabolism.[17,22] These observations are consistent with the concept that PRPP is quite necessary for the enhancement of FUra accumulation following MTX treatment.   Leucovorin, when given after MTX, will also ameliorate the enhancement of FUra accumulation and metabolism, which indicates that the effect of MTX in producing these alterations in FUra metabolism was the result of the altered folate metabolism as indicated previously in the above section.

The sequential administration of MTX before FUra was initially studied in L1210 cells.[15,17,22] Similar modulation of FUra metabolism and enhanced cytotoxicity has also been observed in the human colon carcinoma, HCT-8, and the human breast cancer cell line, 47-DN (Table 3).[51,52] Major et al.[53] have made recent observations in the human breast carcinoma cell line MCF-7 which also are similar to those just outlined between FUra and MTX. Donehower et al.[54] noted enhanced cytotoxicity in the human breast cancer cell line, ZR-75-1, with sequential MTX and FUra. The maximum effect on FUra metabolism, PRPP elevation, and cytotoxicity of sequential MTX and FUra was between 3 and 6 hr for the L1210 cells. The optimal interval for the human cancer cell lines was following an 18- to 24-hr continuous exposure to MTX. The most obvious reason for this difference is that the L1210 cells have a 12-hr doubling time, whereas the human cells studied had a doubling time of 24 to 36 hr. As previously noted, MTX is maximally effective in cells which are actively synthesizing DNA (making dTMP). Therefore, the longer the exposure to MTX in a slowly dividing cell population, the greater the proportion of the total cell population that will begin to synthesize DNA and, therefore, be affected by MTX.[51] Other factors, such as changes in MTX transport and polyglutamate formation and retention, may be related to growth patterns and be quite important as well.[55-57] Mechanisms by which cells can be synchronized or encouraged to undergo division (enter S-phase) could possibly enhance the sequential use of MTX and FUra. Estrogen stimulation of the breast cancer cell line, 47-DN, does in fact enhance the cytotoxicity of this drug sequence; although the doubling time is decreased by this estrogen treatment other factors could also be occurring which could result in further enhancement of the sequential MTX-FUra cytotoxicity.[136]

The precise mechanism by which this sequence of MTX prior to FUra results in synergistic cytotoxicity is unknown. As will be discussed below, it is unlikely that this enhanced antitumor activity is the result of an altered and more tightly bound and inhibited ternary complex with dTMP synthetase. FUTP is incorporated into RNA at increased rates and quantity in cells exposed to MTX,[15,17,58] and FUra does interfere with RNA processing.[59-65] The specific nature of the synergistic cytotoxicity, however, remains to be elucidated.

B. 5-Fluorouridine

FUrd is generally phosphorylated by uridine-cytidine kinase to FUMP, from which all other nucleotide derivatives are synthesized. MTX treatment reduces the intracellular accumulation of this analog of uridine, presumably from a reduction in the *de novo* pyrimidine synthetic pathway induced by the indirect block at the conversion of dUMP to dTMP.[15] These results are opposite to those observed for FUra and indicate that the enhanced intracellular accumulation of FUra following MTX treatment is not mediated by an intermediate accumulation of FUra following MTX treatment is not mediated by an intermediate conversion by pyrimidine phosphorylase of FUra to FUrd (Figure 6).

C. 5-Fluoro-2′-Deoxyuridine

FdUrd intracellular accumulation within MTX-treated cells occurs much more quickly than either FUra or FUrd; however, the total amount of FdUrd and its major metabolite, FdUMP, is not increased following MTX exposure.[137] In addition, the sequence of MTX before FdUrd does not result in synergistic cytotoxicity.[5,17] Because FUra is markedly synergistic with MTX in this sequence, the effect of the MTX-FUra sequence must be mediated by a mechanism other than inhibition of dTMP synthesis. Since FdUMP can directly inhibit dTMP synthetase, and prevent utilization of tetrahydrofolate, FdUrd, which is nearly completely converted to FdUMP, can influence the effect of MTX on the tetrahydrofolate pools. This will be discussed in the subsequent section.

IV. EFFECT OF MTX ON THYMIDYLATE SYNTHETASE

Thymidylate synthetase, which transfers the methyl group from CH_2FAH_4 to dUMP to form dTMP is absolutely necessary for cell proliferation in the absence of exogenous thymidine. This enzymatic process, therefore, has been a site of exceptional interest by molecular biologists. MTX inhibits dihydrofolate reductase, the enzyme which converts dihydrofolate (FAH_2) to tetrahydrofolate (FAH_4). The former folate is a product of dTMP synthesis, which results when the methyl group and hydrogen transfer (oxidation) of CH_2FAH_4 occurs. MTX, therefore, indirectly inhibits this reaction by preventing the regeneration of the utilized FAH_4 (Figure 1). All the fluoropyrimidines can inhibit dTMP synthetase directly after conversion to FdUMP, the analogue of dUMP. The inhibition of this enzyme activity requires the formation of a ternary complex among FdUMP, dTMP synthetase, and the folate cofactor, CH_2FAH_4 (Figure 4).[35,37] This information provided the basis by which the enzyme, dTMP synthetase, could be easily isolated and quantified in the presence of radiolabeled FdUMP. This knowledge was capable of being used to determine what in vivo influences the fluctuation of folates might have on this enzymatic process. Another consequence of this inhibition is an elevation of dUMP levels in a similar fashion to that observed following MTX.[8,39,66-68] It is important to remain aware of the interactions required for the optimal inhibition of dTMP synthetase since dUMP, CH_2FAH_4, and FdUMP can all vary considerably, depending on factors such as type of drug used, exposure time, and cell growth rates. In spite of concentrations of FdUMP and CH_2FAH_4 in excess of that needed to form the ternary complex with dTMP synthetase, elevations in dUMP levels can result in a resumption of dTMP synthesis and have been associated with resumption of cellular recovery from the toxicity of the inhibition of this enzyme.[8]

The L1210 cells studied had amounts of dTMP synthetase which ranged from 80 to 120 ng/10^6 cells and varied in a consistent fashion with the doubling time or percentage of cells in S-phase.[5] The more rapidly dividing and the greater the percent of cells in S, the higher was the value for dTMP synthetase. When MTX was added to cell cultures at 5 μM for 3 hr before adding 100 μM[^{14}C]-FdUrd, which was rapidly converted to [^{14}C]-FdUMP, the amount of binding of FdUMP to the enzyme was less than 20% of that observed in non-

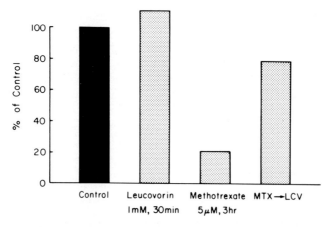

FIGURE 9.   The changes in the amount of the thymidylate synthetase —
FdUMP — CH_2FAH_4 ternary complex in L1210 cells were evaluated
following exposure to methotrexate. The amount of complex formed was
determined as indicated in the text and is reported as percent of control.

Table 4
THE EFFECT OF FdUrd ON PURINE SYNTHESIS, PRPP LEVELS, AND THE INTRACELLULAR ACCUMULATION OF FUra

	Concentration time		[1-^{14}C]-glycine into adenine and guanine (% control ± 10%)	PRPP ng/10^6 cells	FUra pmol/min/10^6 cells
Drug	**(μM)**	**(Hr)**			
Control	—	—	100	7 ± 1.2	0.025
MTX	10	3	16	52.2	0.108
FdUrd	100	3	100	10	0.023
FdUrd + MTX	10 + 100	3	130	10	0.023

Note: see Tables 1 and 2 for methods and definitions.

MTX-treated cells (Figure 9). If leucovorin at 100 μ*M* was added after the MTX exposure period, but before the addition of [^{14}C]-FdUrd, the binding was normal, indicating that the same amount on dTMP synthetase was present in the MTX-exposed cells but it was not properly binding FdUMP. The logical explanation for this observation is that the required cofactor, CH_2FAH_4, was reduced in MTX-treated cells to levels which would not promote covalent binding of FdUMP to TMP synthetase. This interaction had been previously hypothesized by Bowen et al. (Figure 9).[39]

The effect of inhibiting dTMP synthetase with FdUMP prior to MTX had the predicted results. By inhibiting this enzyme, CH_2FAH_4 could not be utilized and converted to the oxidized, biologically inactive FAH_2. Therefore, MTX treatment after this inhibition of dTMP synthetase by FdUMP would have little effect on the folate pools and distribution. Under such circumstances, purine synthesis continued as indicated by normal accumulation of [1-^{14}C]-glycine incorporation to purine bases; there also was no elevation of PRPP levels.[17,22] The data of these experiments are contained in Table 4. The schematic representation of the proposed interaction between these drugs is represented in Figure 10. The ability of MTX to enhance FUra accumulation and metabolism was also abrogated by FdUrd treatment before MTX administration. The cytotoxicity when FdUrd was given before MTX was no greater than that observed with FdUrd alone,[17] indicating that the antipurine effect of MTX is indeed quite important for maximal MTX cytotoxicity.

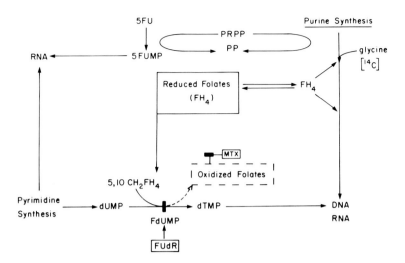

FIGURE 10. Schematic representation of the inhibition of thymidylate synthetase by 5-fluoro-2-'-deoxyuridylate (FdUMP) in folate pools. The inhibition of thymidylate synthetase before methotrexate (MTX) administration prevents the utilization of the reduced folates (FH$_4$). Therefore, the antipurine effect of MTX is prevented because of these preserved FH$_4$ pools.

MTX, which is a folate analog, has been considered by some investigators to be able to substitute for CH$_2$FAH$_4$ in forming the ternary complex with FdUMP and dTMP synthetase. Santi et al.[69] have shown, with in vitro biochemical studies, that MTX could substitute for CH$_2$FAH$_4$ in the complex, but at a considerably reduced efficiency. Heimer and Cadman[70] and Heimer et al.[5] subsequently exposed L1210 cells to [³H]-MTX and [¹⁴C]-FdUrd and then isolated from the treated cells the ternary complex. In the region of dTMP synthetase, only [¹⁴C] radioactivity was observed. The specific activity of [³H]-MTX was such that if only 1% of the complex contained [³H]-MTX it should have been quantitated. Experiments were also done with unlabeled FdUrd and [³H])-MTX to reduce the possible interference in counting radioactivity from both [¹⁴C] and [³H] in the same sample. [³H]-MTX was present only in the regions which corresponded to dihydrofolate reductase and free MTX. The radioactivity in the dihydrofolate reductase region disappeared following the addition of dihydrofolate reductase specific antibody, indicating that this was indeed MTX which was bound to the reductase enzyme (Figure 11). In vitro studies by Fernandes and Bertino[71] indicate that dihydrofolate polyglutamates can promote binding of FdUMP to thymidylate synthetase. Whether this has a significant contribution to the interaction of MTX and FUra in vivo remains to be determined. The fact that less FdUMP was found associated with thymidylate synthetase following MTX treatment would suggest that the dihydrofolate effect on the stability of ternary complex is minimal in the whole cell.

It appears, therefore, that the interaction of MTX and the fluoropyrimidines are antagonistic with respect to the inhibition of dTMP synthetase. Therefore, using the same L1210 cells, we also evaluated the cytotoxicity of MTX given before FUra or FdUrd. The doses of both fluoropyrimidines were chosen such that identical intracellular concentrations of FdUMP would result. Our assumption was that if the entire reason for the synergistic cytotoxicity of sequentially administered MTX and FUra were mediated from the inhibition of thymidylate synthetase, then the identical cytotoxicity should result when FdUrd was substituted for FUra. The results of these cloning studies are presented in Figure 12. The sequence of MTX before FdUrd was not synergistic. Therefore, the enhanced cytotoxicity observed when MTX precedes FUra is probably mediated primarily by another mechanism other than inhibition of dTMP synthesis.

Attempts at prolonging the inhibition of FdUMP at dTMP synthetase have been made by

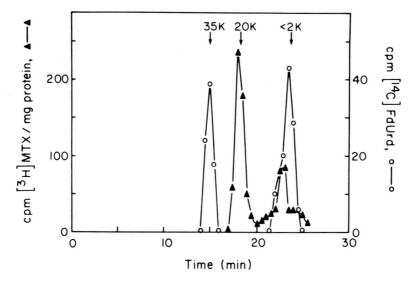

FIGURE 11.   G2000SW steric exclusion column chromatography from extracts of L1210 cells treated with 10 μ*M* [³H]-methotrexate (MTX) for 6 hr before adding 100 μ*M* [¹⁴C]-FuUrd. Thymidylate synthetase — CH₂FAH₄ — FdUMP complex normally resides at the area corresponding to 35k. The peak at 20k represents dihydrofolate reductase and the radioactivity at less than 2k represent nucleosides and nucleotides. For details of methods see Reference 69.

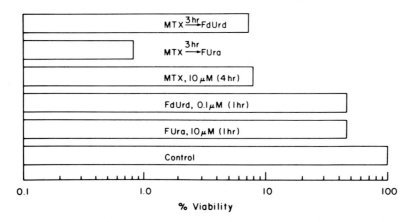

FIGURE 12.   The viability of L1210 cells following the indicated drug treatments revealed that only methotrexate (MTX) before 5-fluorouracil (FUra) resulted in synergistic cytotoxicity. If 5-fluoro-2′-deoxyuridine was substituted for FUra at a dose which resulted in identical intracellular 5-fluoro-2′-deoxyuridylate (FdUMP) levels, there was no enhanced cytotoxicity.

using high doses of exogenous leucovorin (5-formyltetrahydrofolate). Under these conditions CH₂FAH₄ levels would be expected to be increased, which presumably would lead to the stabilization and prolongation of the ternary complex. The results have been conflicting in that some studies indicate a slightly increased cytotoxicity; others do not. Ullman et al.[38] demonstrated that the CH₂FAH₄ levels were important for maximizing the cytotoxicity of FdUrd in L1210 cells. They also documented that the reduction of these folates by MTX treatment antagonized the cytotoxicity of FdUrd. Waxman et al.[72] had also reported an increase in FUra cytotoxicity with leucovorin. Heppner and Calabresi[73] had previously shown that the administration of leucovorin resulted in increased antitumor activity of FUra against mammary tumor growth in mice. Recently, Evans et al.[74] confirmed once again, this time in S180 and human carcinoma cells (Hep-2), that FUra cytotoxicity could be enhanced with leucovorin. Houghton and Houghton[75] also have documented the importance of excessive CH$_2$FAH$_4$ levels in promoting maximum ternary complex formation in human tumor xenographs. These basic observations have resulted in phase I clinical trials in which patients with cancer were given leucovorin with FUra. There appeared to be increased toxicity to the patients compared to what would have been expected from FUra alone.[76] In our own biochemical evaluation, the addition of leucovorin to cells given FUra did prolong the time at which maximum binding of dTMP synthetase occurred, however, this was not associated with enhanced cytotoxicity in the L1210 cells studies.[77] Klubes et al.[78] also have been unable to show an increased tumorcidal effect of FUra in mice bearing L1210 when leucovorin was administered with this fluoropyrimidine. The lack of consistent results among these reports could be a reflection of the fact that the inhibition of dTMP synthetase is only one of several possible cytotoxic effects of FUra. If this DNA-directed effect of FUra were primarily responsible for FUra cytotoxicity in a given cell line, then prolonging the inhibition of this enzyme would be expected to result in greater antitumor activity. If this is not the primary cytotoxic site of action for some cell lines, however, then prolonging this inhibition in these cells may not be associated with an enhanced tumorcidal effect. Obviously, if differences for maximum cytotoxicity were found to be significant between normal and malignant cells, it would provide a rational basis for a selective antitumor effect with this drug combination.

Therefore, there are two methods by which the binding of FdUMP to the dTMP synthetase can be influenced. Ideally, if the CH$_2$FAH$_4$ levels are maintained in excess of the molar concentration of the enzyme dTMP synthetase (the optimal amount is unknown) and dUMP levels are kept at a minimum, the maximum amount of enzyme-inhibition complex would be maintained for the longest possible time. These alterations in CH$_2$FAH$_4$ and dUMP concentrations could prolong the inhibition of dTMP formation and therefore the DNA-directed effects of the fluoropyrimidines. The CH$_2$FAH$_4$ levels can easily be maintained by administering leucovorin. The reduction of dUMP levels theoretically could also be achieved easily. As recently discussed, dUMP accumulates to high levels before the resumption of dTMP synthesis indicating that this deoxynucleotide is crucial for the resumption of DNA synthesis in fluoropyrimidine-treated cells.[8,79] Inhibiting *de novo* pyrimidine metabolism by agents such as PALA would be expected to help achieve this goal by reducing the *de novo* synthesis of dUMP.[80] Since the majority of dUMP is derived from deoxycytidylate (dCMP) by the action of dCMP deaminase,[9,10,81,82] inhibitors of this enzyme would be expected to prevent even further the accumulation of dUMP that normally occurs in response to dTMP synthesis inhibition. Studies have not been reported utilizing these modulating techniques to maximize the inhibition of dTMP synthesis; therefore, the biological consequences of these biochemical alterations are only speculative.

V. EFFECT OF MTX ON FLUOROPYRIMIDINES AND RNA FUNCTION

Many investigators have documented that fluoropyrimidines residues can be incorporated into RNA, presumably as FUTP.[40,64,65] It is still uncertain, however, if this is the cause of cytotoxicity. The major alteration is the interference in RNA processing.[59-63] But this may not be a cause of cytotoxicity, either. However, the observation that many cells require both thymidine and uridine to be protected or rescued from the lethal effects of FUra suggest that some RNA effect is occurring which is important. What influence pretreating cells with MTX has on this presumed RNA effect of FUra is currently unknown. Such MTX-treated cells do accumulate more FUra into RNA, which may be one of several factors occurring in MTX-pretreated cells that result in synergistic cytotoxicity. The use of newer molecular biological techniques, including gene isolation and cloning, may help determine with more specificity the effects of incorporating fluorinated uracil residues into RNA. We have recently observed that FUrd treatment results in a marked reduction in the 1.6 kb mRNA specific for dihydrofolate reductase. These studies were done with the C_3L518Y cell line which has amplified gene copies for this enzyme and contains a 200-fold increase in the corresponding mRNA.[83]

VI. EFFECT OF MTX ON FLUOROPYRIMIDINE INCORPORATION INTO DNA

The incorporation of FdUTP into DNA and the effects this may have on DNA structure and function are potentially quite fascinating. This interaction could possibly be of therapeutic importance when considering biochemical modulation as a means for designing combination drug trials. The documentation of the existence of FdUDP and FdUTP or FUra residues in DNA had eluded detection until recently.[84,85] The enzymes are present in mammalian cells for dUTP and FdUTP synthesis; however, deoxyuridine triphosphate nucleotide hydrolase (dUTPase) efficiently converts dUTP to dUMP. The K_m for this reaction varies from 0.27 to 8 μM for dUTP[84,86] and from 1.2 to 5.5 μM for FdUTP.[84,85] This enzyme does not act on any of the standard four deoxy-ribo, mono, di, or triphosphates[33,87] and explains why the dUTP pools have not been easily detectable and why FdUTP has been thought not to exist. Such a highly specific and active enzyme, which has been estimated capable of hydrolyzing 3500 dUTP molecules per minute at 37°,[88] will markedly reduce the chance of incorporating uracil (or 5-fluorouracil) residues into DNA.

The K_m for dTTP and dUTP of DNA polymerase is 10 μM[86,89] Therefore, there is no discrimination by the polymerases, for either deoxynucleotide and the ratio of dUTP to dTTP will determine the amount of uracil incorporated into DNA.[90,91] The dTTP pools in most cells range between 40 and 60 pmol/10^6 cell and at steady-state conditions there is approximately 1 dUTP/300 dTTP.[88] Therefore, the amount of dUTP (or FdUTP) incorporated into DNA can be regulated by changes in these pool sizes. Cells pretreated with 10 μM MTX for 6 hr had a reduction of dTTP to 1 pmol/10^6 cells and an increase in dUTP to 0.2 pmol/10^6 cells,[92] thus favoring dUTP entry into newly sythesized DNA.

The incorporated uracil into DNA is very dynamic and is rapidly removed by uracil-DNA glycosylase,[93] which results in an apyrimidinic site that is then cleaved by an endonuclease. Subsequent exonuclease activity removes the damaged segment of the DNA, which it then repaired by polymerase and ligase.[94-96] This efficient repair process undoubtedly has made the detection of the presence of FdUTP in DNA rather difficult. Although recently Goulian et al.,[92] Caradonna and Cheng,[84] and Major et al.[97,98] have found FdUTP in DNA of cells treated with high doses of radiolabeled FdUrd. We have examined three cell lines (L1210, L5178Y, and S-180) for the incorporation of FUra residues into DNA and in each instance small amounts were detected.

The consequence of uracil or 5-fluorouracil residues in the DNA structure are unknown. In *Escherichia coli* deficient in both dUTPase and uracil-DNA glycosylase, uracil could readily be detected in DNA.[91,99] In cells deficient of dUTPase, there was an interruption of DNA synthesis and an increase of small pieces of DNA in the 4 to 5S region, often referred to as Okazaki fragments.[65,90,100-103] The actual disturbance and, possibly, function of DNA synthesis is therefore apparently the result of the repair mechanism initiated by the uracil removal by uracil-DNA glycosylase. Nakayama and Cheng[104] have recently presented preliminary studies demonstrating that these effects do occur following FdUrd treatment. They noted disruption of DNA synthesis and an increase in small DNA fragments.

The significance of the incorporation of fluorouracil into DNA is unknown. However, with high doses or prolonged exposure to the fluoropyrimidines, especially FdUrd, this effect could be important for cytotoxicity. Since the nucleotide pools can be altered by MTX, the use of this agent could enhance these effects by lowering the competing dTTP levels prior to the administration of the fluoropyrimidine.

VII. EFFECT OF MTX ON FLUOROPYRIMIDINES AND MEMBRANES

There have been no investigations evaluating the effect of MTX and FUra, when given together, on cell membrane structure and function. It is an area that needs study based on at least the following observations, however. Kessel[105] has recently noted structural changes in membranes of cells treated with FUra. This is not entirely unexpected, since uridine diphosphate sugars may be a component used in membrane formation. The fluorinated uridine can indeed become a diphosphate sugar, and has been detected by Rustum.[106] Pretreatment with MTX in our studies also increased this fraudulent nucleotide severalfold within L1210 cells[107] and could be a component leading to enhanced antitumor activity with this drug sequence. Since some uridine phosphate sugars are also involved in energy transfer and glycogen synthesis, other effects of these drugs could also be occurring which heretofore have not been considered important sites of cytotoxicity for FUra.

VIII. REVIEW OF CYTOTOXICITY STUDIES USING MTX-FURA

Table 5 outlines the available information on studies performed in cancer cells to determine the cytotoxicity between MTX and FUra. The first indication that these two drugs might result in greater than additive cytotoxicity was noted by Kline et al.[108] Most studies have found that when MTX precedes FUra the result is enhanced cytotoxicity, and when the sequence is reversed antagonism occurs. Based on the biochemical studies which were previously presented, it is quite apparent that the dose of MTX must be such that all the dihydrofolate reductase is inhibited and that the MTX exposure be of such a duration that a substantial portion of the cancer cell population will require the synthesis of dTMP, i.e., enter S-phase of the cell cycle. If these two criteria are not met then the effect of MTX will be suboptimal and the modulatory effect on FUra metabolism minimized. These considerations could account for the differences noted in Table 5. What also remains to be determined is if this drug sequence has any selectivity for cancer cells. If identical biochemical alterations are occurring simultaneously and at the same magnitude in normal tissues, then most toxicity obviously will also be enhanced. There are some preliminary studies in humans which indicate that a 24-hr interval between MTX and the administration of FUra is quite safe.[109]

IX. SEQUENTIAL METHOTREXATE 5-FLUOROURACIL IN HUMANS

The extension of the biochemical experiments attempting to understand the interaction between MTX and FUra has led to several clinical studies. Many of these investigations are preliminary and inconclusive; however, some things can be learned from these results. The data are presented in Table 6. The two major groups of patients treated have been those with colon tumors (154) and breast tumors (99). This is a reflection of the observations that these two drugs are commonly used for breast cancer and that FUra is the drug of choice for the treatment of colon cancer. The initial animal studies which were published indicated that a 1-hr interval between MTX and FUra was optimal. This information influenced some of the first protocol designs for the use of these drugs in patients. Later, biochemical studies and cytotoxic evaluation of human tumor cells emphasized that a longer interval between drugs was actually better for both optimizing the biochemical modulatory effects of MTX and enhancing tumor cell killing. This observation has now begun to impact on the newer clinical cancer treatment protocols, which have increased the interval from 4 to 24 hr.

Most of the patients with colon cancer were not treated with other agents before being given MTX and FUra. The overall response rate was 35%. Of these patients, 93 were treated with a 4-hr interval or longer, which was associated with a 43% response rate. The remaining 31 patients received the drugs at an interval of 1 hr or less and only 10% had a response.

Table 5

ANTITUMOR STUDIES EVALUATING COMBINATIONS OF MTX AND FUra

Cell line	Drug doses	Timing	Antagonistic	Additive	Synergistic	Ref.
L1210 (culture)	M—6 × 10⁻⁸ M	M 6 hr F	+		+	68
	F-2 × 10⁻⁷ M	Simultaneous	+			
		F 6 hr M	+			
L1210 (in mice)	M-1 mg/kg	Daily together			+	108
	F-60 mg/kg					
Immunocompetence (in mice)	M-1 mg/kg	M 1 hr F			+	116
	F-60 mg/kg					
Immunocompetence (in mice)	M-1 mg/kg	M 1/4 hr F			+	117
	F-60 mg/kg	F 2—6 hr M	+			
C3H/HeJ mammary tumors (in mice)	M-1 mg/kg	M 1/4 hr L3/4 hr F			+	73
	L-1 mg/kg					
	F-50 mg/kg					
13762 Mammary tumor (in rats)	M-0.4 mg/kg	M 6 hr F			+	118
	F-30 mg/kg	F 6 hr M	+			
L1210 (culture)	M->10 × 10⁻⁶ M × 4 hr	M 3 hr F			+	15
	F-10 × 10⁻⁶ M × 1 hr	F 3 hr M	+			17
S180 (in mice)	M-42 mg/kg	M 2 hr F			+	4
	F-60 mg/kg	F 2 hr M	+			
L1210 (in mice)	M-40 mg/kg	M 24 F			+	119
	F-100 mg/kg	F 24 M	+			
C221R osteosarcoma (in mice)	M-7.5 mg/kg × 3 over 24 hr	M 24 F		+	+	117
	F-100 mg/kg	F 24 M	+			
ZR-75-1 human breast cancer (culture)	50% Response isobolograms	M 2 hr F			+	54
		F 2 hr M	+			
47-DN human breast cancer (culture)	M-1 × 10⁻⁷ M × 24 hr	M 18 F			+	52
	F-10 × 10⁻⁶ M × 6 hr	M + F	+			109
MCF-7 human breast cancer (culture)	M-1 × 10⁻⁶ M × 6 hr	M 6 hr F			+	53
	F-10 × 10⁻⁶ M × 3 hr					
HCT-8 human colon cancer (culture)	M-1 × 10⁻⁷ M × 24 hr	M 18 F			+	51
	F-10 × 10⁻⁶ M × 6 hr					

The accepted response rate in colon cancer patients from FUra treatment is 20%. Therefore, these preliminary clinical results are of major interest. Obviously, further clinical studies are needed to better define the dose and timing required to achieve maximum therapeutic benefit from this drug sequence.

A total of 99 patients with breast cancer were treated with this drug sequence; 45% had a response. Since nearly all of these patients had been previously treated, it is difficult to know if this drug sequence would result in a higher response rate if used before other drug therapy (Table 7).

X. THE EFFECT OF MTX ON THE PURINE ANALOGS, 6-THIOGUANINE AND 6-MERCAPTOPURINE

Because the primary MTX modulating effect on FUra metabolism is the consequence of the *de novo* purine synthesis inhibition by MTX, purine analogs which utilize PRPP for phosphorylation should also have an enhanced intracellular metablism. We evaluated both 6-mercaptopurine (6-MP) and 6-thioguanine (6-TG). The schematic interaction is represented in Figure 13. 6-MP is a synthetic purine base which is converted to 6-MP monophosphate by hypoxanthine-guanine phosphoribosyltransferase in the presence of PRPP.[11,90] Therefore, since MTX results in elevated intracellular PRPP levels it was not unexpected to find that there was a marked enhanced intracellular accumulation of 6-MP into cells pretreated with MTX. MTX at 10 μM for 3 hr resulted in a sixfold increase in intracellular 6-MP.[138]

The MTX pretreatment-increased intracellular quantity of PRPP is associated with this increased intracellular accumulation of 6-MP. Since the rate-limiting step in the accumulation of 6-MP is apparently the formation of nucleoside monophosphate, the increased availability of this cosubstrate, PRPP, which is necessary for this initial phosphorylation process, is most likely the explanation of this MTX effect of 6-MP accumulation. Although the optimum dose and time of this drug sequence have not been explored, it is likely that they may vary considerably depending on the cell-doubling time and enzymatic characteristics for 6-MP conversion to 6-MP-monophosphate. The triphosphate derivative of methylmercaptopurine riboside, a nucleoside purine analog which is phosphorylated by adenosine kinase and inhibits amidophosphoribosyltransferase is the first committed step in *de novo* purine synthesis.[110] Like the indirect inhibition of purine synthesis induced by MTX, it increases PRPP levels.[17] Scholar et al.[111] have shown that methylmercaptopurine riboside could also result in an enhancement of intracellular accumulation of 6-MP, and most likely explains earlier experiments which indicated that these drugs could act synergistically in killing cells.[112,113] As has been previously described in this review, methylmercaptopurine riboside will also allow for an enhanced intracellular accumulation of 5-fluorouracil.[17] These former results all support our contention that the enhancing effect of MTX on 6-MP intracellular accumulation is mediated from the indirect inhibition of purine synthesis.

Because MTX and 6-MP are widely used antimetabolites for the treatment of cancer, particularly acute lymphocytic leukemia in children, the potential interaction between these two agents may provide useful information to aid in the design of future clinical research protocols.

Similar results were obtained when MTX-treated cells were exposed to 6-thioguanine (6-TG). This drug is also dependent upon the action of hypoxanthine-guanine phosphoribosyltransferase and the availability of PRPP, which converts 6-TG to 6-TG monophosphate. This nucleotide has been shown to have inhibitory effects on several enzymes involved in *de novo* purine synthesis.[114] 6-TG, however, can be incorporated into DNA and RNA, although the mechanism of cytotoxicity has not been established.

6-TG accumulated within MTX-treated cells slightly more than threefold greater than in control cells. The sequence of MTX before 6-TG also resulted in synergistic cytotoxicity.[115]

Table 6
EFFECT OF SEQUENTIAL METHOTREXATE AND 5-FLUOROURACIL IN CANCER PATIENTS

Author	MTX (mg/m²)	FUra (mg/m²)	Interval (hr)	Freq.	LV at 24 hr (mg/m²)	Evaluable patients			Response%						Total pts.	Ref.
						Colon	Breast	Head and neck	Colon CR	Colon PR	Breast CR	Breast PR	Head and neck CR	Head and neck PR		
Plotkin	100	600	0	?	25 × 1	—	7(?)[a]	—	—	—	0	15[b]	—	—	7	120
Plotkin	200	600	0	?	10 q 6 × ?	—	11(?)	—	—	—	0	36	—	—	11	120
Gewirtz	200	600	1	day 1 & 8	10 q 6 × 6	—	17(13)	—	—	—	0	53	—	—	17	121
Panasci	200	600	1	2 wk	10 q 6 × 6	5(4)	5(3)	—	0	0	0	0	—	—	10	122
Panasci	200	1000	1	2 wk	10 q 6 × 6	7(0)	3(2)	—	0	28	0	0	—	—	10	122
Cantrell	250	600	1	3 wk	10 q 6 × 12	16(10)	—	—	0	6	—	—	—	—	16	123
Tisman	1500	1500	1	3—4 wk	10 q 6 × 8	—	13(13)	—	—	—	0	23	—	—	13	124
Blumerreich	200	600	1	day 1 & 8	10 q 6 × 6	7(0)	—	—	—	0	—	—	—	—	7	125
Allegra[c]	200	600	1	q 18 day	10 q 6 × 6	—	25(7)	—	—	—	56	16	—	—	25	126
Pitman	125—250	600	1	2 wk	10 q 6 × 5	—	—	10(0)	—	—	—	—	(40)	(60)	10	127
Solan[d]	200	600	4	wk × 4	10 q 6 × 6	11(5)	—	—	—	(30)18[b]	—	—	—	—	11	128
Solan[d]	40	600	4	then 2 wk	—	14(16)	—	—	—	(37)21	—	—	—	—	14	128
Herrmann	200—300[e]	900	7	2 wk	14 q 6 × 8	10(2)	—	—	—	(62)50	—	—	—	—	10	129
Drapkin	200—600[e]	300—600	7	2 wk	12 q 6 × 6	19(13)	—	—	—	(60)33	—	—	—	—	19	130
Herrmann	150[f]	900	7	2—3 wk	12—15 q 6 × 8	—	18(18)	—	—	—	—	50	—	—	18	131
Mehrotra	100	600	18	1 wk	10 q 6 × 11	3(0)	—	—	—	0	—	—	—	—	3	132
Mehrotra	100	600	4	1 wk	10 q 6 × 1	10(0)	—	—	—	80	—	—	—	—	10	132
Weinerman[g]	20 mg/kg[h]	600	3	3—4 wk	10 q 6 × 4	29(?)	—	—	7	28	—	—	—	—	29	133
Kemeny	40	600	24	day 1 & 8	0	23(0)	—	—	—	34	—	—	—	—	23	134
Benz[i]	50 q 6 × 5 p.o.	600	24	wk	10 q 6 × 6	—	—	—	—	—	—	—	—	—	7	135

[a]   Number in ( ) represents number of patients previously treated with chemotherapy.

[b]   Percent in ( ) represents the percent response seen in previously untreated patients. The response without brackets is the overall total percent response.

[c]   Patients also received tamoxifen 10 mg p.o. bid for 10 days followed by premarin 0.625 mg p.o. bid for 4 days and then MTX and FUra given as indicated; 11 of 14 patients with estrogen-positive tumors responded and 3 of 7 patients with estrogen-negative tumors responded; all 4 patients with unknown estrogen status responded.

d   Several hematological toxicity noted in 8 of 13 patients receiving the higher dose MTX.

e   MTX infused over 4 hr.

f   150 mg/m^2 i.v. push then 150 mg/m^2 infused over 4 hr.

g   Two patients had severe hematologic toxicity.

h   20 mg/kg Infused over 4 hr.

i   Toxicity study only, no response data given; mild toxicity in seven patients treated.

Table 7
SUMMARY OF SEQUENTIAL
MTX-FUra CLINICAL STUDIES

Colon Cancer

Patients		% Response
Total	154	29
Utreated	124	35

Interval between MTX and FUra

	≥4 hr	≤1 hr
Untreated patients	93	31
% Response	43	10

Breast Cancer

Patients		% Response
Total	99	45

Interval between MTX and FUra

	≥4 hr	≤1 hr
Total patients	18	81
% Response	50	44

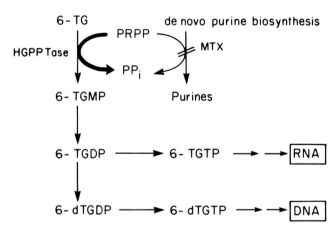

FIGURE 13.   The schematic representation of 6-thioguanine (6-TG) metabolism. Methotrexate (MTX), by indirectly inhibiting *de novo* purine synthesis, leads to increased levels of 5-phosphoribosyl-1-pyrophosphate (PRPP) which results in enhanced conversion of 6-TG to the monophosphate derivative (6-TGMP) by hypoxanthine-guanine phosphoribosyltransferase (HGPTase). 6-Methylmercaptopurine is metabolized in a similar fashion and would be affected as 6-TG following MTX exposure.

Therefore, as with FUra, MTX can have a modulation effect on the metabolism and subsequent cytotoxic activity of 6-MP and 6-TG. Since all of these drugs (MTX, FUra, 6-MP, and 6-TG) are currently available and used for the treatment of patients with cancer, these biochemical interactions can provide the rationale for the design of combination therapy with this agent.

XI. SUMMARY

When methotrexate (MTX) precedes 5-fluorouracil (FUra) the result is an enhanced intracellular accumulation of FUra nucleotide derivatives and synergistic cytotoxicity. The biochemical rationale for this altered FUra metabolism is based on the antipurine effect of MTX which results in increased availability of phosphoribosylpyrophosphate (PRPP), which is used to convert FUra to FUMP. Because this is the rate-limiting step in the metabolic conversion of FUra, increased intracellular quantities of all FUra nucleotides results. Although the precise mechanism by which the enhanced cytotoxicity occurs has not been delineated, it appears that the greater antitumor activity is not the consequence of a greater or more prolonged inhibition of thymidylate synthetase. Similar modulating effects on the metabolism of nucleoside and base analogs can result following MTX treatment. This information provides a basis and framework that may be very important when considering drug combination therapy.

ACKNOWLEDGMENTS

This review was supported in part from grants CA-27130 and CA-08341 from the National Cancer Institute and grant CH-145 from the American Cancer Society. Dr. Cadman is also a recipient of a Faculty Cancer Research Award from the American Cancer Society. Thanks to Hillary Raeffer for editorial assistance.

REFERENCES

1. **Hryniuk, W. M.,** Purineless death as a link between growth rate and cytotoxicity by methotrexate, *Cancer Res.*, 32, 1506, 1972.
2. **Moran, R. G., Mulkins, M., and Heidelberger, C.,** Role of thymidylate synthetase activity in development of methotrexate cytotoxicity, *Proc. Natl. Acad. Sci. U.S.A.*, 11, 5924, 1979.
3. **Canellos, G. P., DeVita, V. T., Gold, G. L., Chabner, B. A., Schein, P. S., and Young, R.C.,** Combination chemotherapy for advanced breast cancer: response and effect on survival, *Ann. Intern. Med.*, 84, 389, 1976.
4. **Bertino, J. R.,** Methotrexate: molecular pharmacology, *Cancer Chemother.*, III, 311, 1981.
5. **Heimer, R., Burger, D., and Cadman, E.,** Levels of thymidylate synthetase during unperturbed growth of L1210 cells, *Proc. Am. Assoc. Cancer Res.*, 23, (Abstr.), 88, 1982.
6. **Kinahan, J. J., Otten, M., and Grindey, G. B.,** Evaluation of ribonucleotides and deoxyribonucleoside triphosphate pools in cultured leukemia cells during exposure to methotrexate or methotrexate plus thymidine, *Cancer Res.*, 39, 3531, 1979.
7. **Jackson, R. C.,** Modulation of methotrexate toxicity by thymidine: sequence dependent biochemical effects, *Mol. Pharmacol.*, 18, 281, 1980.
8. **Myers, C. E., Young, R. C., and Chabner, B. A.,** Biochemical determinants of 5-fluorouracil response in vivo, *J. Clin. Invest.*, 56, 1231, 1975.
9. **Fridland, A.,** Effect of methotrexate on deoxyribonucleotide pools and DNA synthesis in human lymphocytic cells, *Cancer Res.*, 34, 1883, 1974.
10. **Maley, F. and Maley, G.F.,** On the nature of a sparing effect by thymidine on the utilization of deoxycytidine, *Biochemistry*, 1, 847, 1962.
11. **Furth, J. J. and Cohen, S. S.,** Inhibition of mammalian DNA polymerase by the 5'-triphosphate of 1- -D-arabinofuranosylcytosine and the 5'-triphosphate of 9- -arabinofuranosyladenine, *Cancer Res.*, 28, 2061, 1968.

12. **Graham, F. L. and Whitmore, G. F.,** Studies in mouse L-cells on the incorporation of 1- -D-arabino-furanosylcytosine 5'-triphosphate, *Cancer Res.,* 38, 2636, 1970.

13. **Ives, D. H. and Durham, I. P.,** Deoxycytidine kinase. III. Kinetic and allosteric regulation of the calf thymus enzyme, *J. Biol. Chem.,* 245, 2285, 1970.

14. **Plagemann, P. G.W., Marz, R., and Wohlheuter, R. M.,** Transport and metabolism of 1- -D-arabino-furanosylcytosine into cultured Novikoff rat hepatoma cells. Relationship to phosphorylation, and regulation of triphosphate synthesis, *Cancer Res.,* 38, 978, 1978.

15. **Cadman, E. C., Heimer, R., and Davis, L.,** Enhanced 5-fluorouracil nucleotide formation after methotrexate administration: Explanation for drug synergism, *Science,* 250, 1135, 1979.

16. **Anukarahanonta, T., Holstege, A., and Keppler, D. O. R.,** Selective enhancement of 5-fluororidine uptake and action in rat hepatomas in vivo following pretreatment with D-galactosamine and 6-azauridine or *N*- (phosphonacetyl)-L-aspartate, *Eur. J. Cancer,* 16, 1171, 1980.

17. **Cadman, E., Heimer, R., and Benz, C.,** The influence of methotrexate pretreatment on 5-fluorouracil metabolism in L1210 cells, *J. Biol. Chem.,* 256(4), 1695, 1981.

18. **Cha, S., Kim, S. Y. R., Kornstein, S. G., Kantoff, P. W., Kim, K. H., and Nagub, F. N. M.,** Kinetic parameters of dihydrofolate reductase inhibited by methotrexate, an example of equilibrium study, *Biochem. Pharmacol.,* 30(12), 1507, 1981.

19. **Sartorelli, A. C. and LePage, G. A.,** A methopterin on the purine biosynthesis of susceptible and resistant TA3 ascites cells, *Cancer Res.,* 18, 1336, 1958.

20. **Borsa, J. and Whitmore, G. F.,** Studies relating to the mode of action of methotrexate. II. Studies in sites of action on L-cells in vitro, *Mol. Pharmacol.,* 5, 303, 1969.

21. **Cohen, S. S.,** On the nature of thymineless death, *Ann. N. Y. Acad. Sci.,* 186, 292, 1971.

22. **Cadman, E., Benz, C., Heimer, R., and O'Shaughnessy, J.,** Effect of de novo purine synthesis inhibitors on 5-fluorouracil metabolism and cytotoxicity, *Biochem. Pharmacol.,* 30(17), 2469, 1981.

23. **Heimer, R., Benz, C., and Cadman, E.,** 5-Fluoro-2'-deoxyuridine antagonizes the antifolate activity of methotrexate by preserving reduced folate pools, *Mol. Pharmacol.,* submitted, 1982.

24. **Harrap, K. R., Taylor, G. A., and Browman, G. P.,** Enhancement of the therapeutic effectiveness of methotrexate and protection of normal proliferating tissues with purines and pyrimidines, *Chem. Biol. Interact.,* 18, 119, 1977.

25. **Pinedo, H. M., Zaharko, D. S., Bull, J. M., and Chabner, B. A.,** The reversal of methotrexate cytotoxicity to mouse bone marrow cells by leucovorin and nucleosides, *Cancer Res.,* 36, 4418, 1976.

26. **Hryniuk, M. W., Fischer, G. A., and Bertino, J. R.,** S-phase cells of rapidly growing and resting populations: differences in response to methotrexate, *Mol. Pharmacol.,* 5, 557, 1969.

27. **Washtien, W. L.,** Thymidylate synthetase levels as a factor in 5-fluorodeoxyuridine and methotrexate cytotoxicity in gastrointestinal tumor cells, *Mol. Pharmacol.,* 21, 723, 1981.

28. **Sirotnak, F. M., Kurita, S., and Hutchison, D. J.,** On the nature of a transport alteration determining resistance to amethopterin in the L1210 leukemia, *Cancer Res.,* 28, 75, 1968.

29. **Flintoff, W. F., Davidson, S. V., and Siminovitch, L.,** Isolation and partial characterization of three methotrexate-resistant phenotypes from Chinese hamster ovary cells, *Somatic Cell Genet.,* 2(3), 245, 1976.

30. **Gupta, R. S., Flintoff, W. F., and Siminovitch, L.,** Purification and properties of dihydrofolate reductase from methotrexate-sensitive and methotrexate-resistant Chinese hamster ovary cells, *Can. J. Biochem.,* 55, 445, 1977.

31. **Jackson, R. C. and Harrup,K. R.,** Studies with a mathematical model of folate metabolism, *Arch. Biochem. Biophys.,* 158, 827, 1973.

32. **Schimke, R. T., Alt, F. W., Kellems, R. E., Kaufman, R. J., and Bertino, J. R.,** Amplification of dihydrofolate reductase genes in methotrexate-resistant cultured mouse cells, *Cold Spring Harbor Symp. Quant. Biol.,* 42, 649, 1977.

33. **Schrecker, A. W., Mead, J. A. R., Greensberg, N. H., and Goldin, A.,** Dihydrofolate reductase activity of leukemia L1210 during development of methotrexate resistance, *Biochem. Pharmacol.,* 20, 716, 1971.

34. **Grindey, G. B., Semon, J. H., and Pavelic, Z. P.,** Modulation versus rescue of antimetabolite toxicity by salvage metabolites administered by continuous infusion, *Antibiot. Chemother.,* 23, 295, 1978.

35. **Danenberg, P. V. and Lockshin, A.,** Fluorinated pyrimidines as tight-binding inhibitors of thymidylate synthetase, *Pharmacol. Ther.,* 13, 69, 181.

36. **Lockshin, A. and Danenberg, P. V.,** Biochemical factors affecting the tightness of 5-fluorodeoxyuridylate binding to human thymidylate synthetase, *Biochem. Pharmacol.,* 30, 247, 1981.

37. **Santi, D. V.,** Perspectives on the design and biochemical pharmacology of inhibitors of thymidylate synthetase, *J. Med. Chem.,* 23, 103, 1980.

38. **Ullman, B., Lee, M., Martin, D. W., Jr., and Santi, D. V.,** Increased L1210 sensitive FdUrd with LCV in vitro, *Proc. Natl. Acad. Sci. U.S.A.,* 75, 980, 1978.

39. **Bowen, D., White, J. C., and Goldman, I. D.,** A basis for fluoropyrimidine-induced antagonism to methotrexate in Ehrlich ascites tumor cells in vitro, *Cancer Res.,* 38, 219, 1978.

40. **Mandel, H. G.,** The incorporation of 5-fluorouracil into RNA and its molecular consequences, in *Progress in Molecular and Subcellular Biology,* Hahn, F. E., Ed., Springer-Verlag, New York, 1969.

41. **Myers, C. E.,** The pharmacology of the fluoropyrimidines, *Pharmacol. Rev.* 33(1), 1, 1981.

42. **Ullman, B. and Kirsch, J.,** Metabolism of 5-fluorouracil in cultured cells. Protection from 5-fluorouracil cytotoxicity by purines, *Mol. Pharmacol.,* 15, 357, 1979.

43. **Skold, O.,** Enzymic ribosidation and ribotidation of 5-fluorouracil by extracts of the Ehrlich-ascites tumors, *Biochim. Biophys. Acta,* 29, 651, 1958.

44. **Chaudhuri, N. K., Montag, B. J., and Heidelberger, C.,** Studies on fluorinated pyrimidines. III. The metabolism of 5-fluorouracil-2-C^{14} and 5-fluoro-orotic-2-C^{14} acid in vitro, *Cancer Res.,* 18, 318, 1958.

45. **Harbers, E., Chaudhuri, N. K., and Heidelberger, C.,** Studies on fluorinated pyrimidines. VIII. Further biochemical and metabolic investigations, *J. Biol. Chem.,* 234, 1255, 1959.

46. **Cadman, E. C., Dix, D. E., and Handschumacher, R. E.,** Clinical, biological and biochemical effects of pyrazofurin, *Cancer Res.,* 38, 682, 1978.

47. **Dix, D. E., Lehman, C. P., Jakubowski, A., Moyer, J. D., and Handschumacher, R. E.,** Pyrazofurin metabolism, enzyme inhibition, and resistance in L5178Y cells, *Cancer Res.,* 39, 4485, 1979.

48. **Henderson, J. F. and Khoo, M. K. Y.,** On the mechanisms of feedback inhibition of purine biosynthesis de novo in Ehrlich ascites tumor cells in vitro, *J. Biol. Chem.,* 240, 3104, 1965.

49. **Nelson, J. A. and Parks, R. E., Jr.,** Biochemical mechanisms for the synergism between 6-thioguanine and 6-(methylmercapto) purine ribonucleoside in sarcoma 180 cells, *Cancer Res.,* 32, 2034, 1972.

50. **Henderson, J. F. and Khoo, M.,** On the mechanism of feedback inhibition of purine biosynthesis de novo in Ehrlich ascites tumor cells in vitro, *J. Biol. Chem.,* 240, 3104, 1965.

51. **Benz, C. and Cadman, E.,** Modulation of 5-fluorouracil metabolism and cytotoxicity by antimetabolite pretreatment in human colorectal adenocarcinoma HCT-8, *Cancer Res.,* 41, 994, 1981.

52. **Benz, C., Schoenberg, M., Choti, M., and Cadman, E.,** Schedule dependent cytotoxicty of hotrexate and 5-fluorouracil in human colon and breast tumor cell lines, *J. Cell Invest.,* 66, 1162, 1980.

53. **Major, P. P., Egan, E. M., Sargent, L., and Kufe, D. W.,** Modulation of 5-fluorouracil metabolism in human MCF-7 breast carcinoma cells, *Cancer Chemother. Pharmacol.,* 8, 87, 1982.

54. **Donehower, R. C., Allegra, J. C., Lippman, M. E., and Chabner, B. A.,** Combined effects of methotrexate and 5-fluoropyrimidine on human breast cancer cells in serum-free culture, *Eur. J. Cancer,* 16, 655, 1980.

55. **Chello, P. L., Sirotnak, F. M., and Dorick, D. M.,** Alterations in the kinetics of methotrexate transport during growth of L1210 murine leukemia cells in culture, *Mol. Pharmacol.,* 18, 274, 1980.

56. **Fry, D. W., Yalowich, J. C., and Goldman, I. D.,** Rapid formation of polyglutamyl derivatives of methotrexate and their association dihydrofolate reductase as assessed by high pressure liquid chromatography in the Ehrlich ascites tumor cell in vitro, *J. Biol. Chem.,* 257(4), 1890, 1982.

57. **Jolivet, J., Schilsky, R. L., Bailey, B. D., and Chabner, B. A.,** The synthesis and retention of methotrexate polyglutamates in cultured human breast cancer cells, *Ann. N.Y. Acad. Sci.,* 397, 184, 1982.

58. **Kufe, D. W. and Major, P. P.,** 5-Fluorouacil incorporation into human breast carcinoma RNA correlates with cytotoxicity, *J. Biol. Chem.,* 256(19), 9802, 1981.

59. **Carrico, C. K. and Glazer, R. I.,** Effect of 5-fluorouracil on the synthesis and translation of polyadenylic acid-containing RNA from regenerating rat liver, *Cancer Res.,* 39, 3694, 1979.

60. **Cory, J. G., Breland, J. C., and Carter, G. L.,** Effect of 5-fluorouracil on RNA metabolism in Novikoff hepatoma cells, *Cancer Res.,* 39, 4905, 1979.

61. **Glazer, R. I. and Hartman, K. D.,** The effect of 5-fluorouracil on the synthesis and methylation of low molecular weight nuclear RNA in L1210 cells, *Mol. Pharmacol.,* 17, 245, 1980.

62. **Glazer, R. I. and Legraverend, M.,** The effect of 5-flourouride 5'-triphosphate on RNA transcribed in isolated nuclei in vitro, *Mol. Pharmacol.,* 17, 279, 1980.

63. **Glazer, R. I. and Peale, A. L.,** The effect of 5-flourouracil on the synthesis on nuclear RNA in L1210 cells in vitro, *Mol. Pharmacol.,* 16, 270, 1979.

64. **Wilkinson, D. S. and Crumley, J.,** The mechanism of 5-fluorouridine toxicity in Novikoff hepatoma cells, *Cancer Res.,* 36, 4032, 1976.

65. **Wilkinson, D. S., Cihak, A., and Pitot, H. C.,** Inhibition of ribosomal ribonucleic acid maturation in rat liver by 5-fluoroorotic acid resulting in the selective labeling of cytoplasmic messenger ribonucleic acid, *J. Biol. Chem.,* 246(21), 6418, 1971.

66. **Jackson, R. C.,** The regulation of thymidylate biosynthesis in Novikoff hepatoma cells and the effects of amethopterin, 5'-fluorodeoxyuridine and 3-deazauridine, *J. Biol. Chem.,* 253, 7440, 1978.

67. **Klubes, P., Connelly, K., Cerna, I., and Mandel, H. G.,** Effects of 5-fluorouracil on 5-fluorodeoxyuridine 5'-monophosphate and 2-deoxyuridine 5'-monophosphate pools, and DNA synthesis in solid mouse L1210 and rat Walker 256 tumors, *Cancer Res.,* 36, 2325, 1978.

68. **Tattersall, M. H. N., Jackson, R. G., Connors, T. A., and Harrup, K. R.,** Combination chemotherapy: the interaction of methotrexate and 5-fluorouracil, *Eur. J. Cancer,* 9, j733, 1973.

69. **Santi, D. V., McHenry, C. S., and Sommer, H.,** Mechanism of interaction of thymidylate synthetase with 5-fluorodeoxyuridylate, *Biochemistry,* 13, 471, 1974.

70. **Heimer, R. and Cadman, E.,** Analysis of the thymidylate synthetase ternary complex by high-performance liquid steric exclusion chromatography, *Anal. Biochem.,* 118, 322, 1981.

71. **Fernandes, D. J. and Bertino, J. R.,** 5-Fluorouracil-methotrexate synergy: enhancement of 5-fluoro-deoxyuridylate binding to thymidylate synthetase by dihydropteroylpolyglutamates, *Proc. Natl. Acad. Sci. U.S.A.,* 77(10), 5663, 1980.

72. **Waxman, S., Bruckner, H., Wagles, A., and Schreiber, C.,** Increased FUra cytotoxicity with LCV in vitro, *Proc. Am. Assoc. Cancer Res.,* 19, 149, 1978.

73. **Heppner, G. H. and Calabresi, P.,** Increased antitumor activity with methotrexate prior to LCV 1 hr prior to FUra in vivo — mammary tumor in C3H mice, *Cancer Res.,* 37, 4580, 1977.

74. **Evans, R. M., Laskin, J. D., and Hakala, M. T.,** Increased growth inhibited by FUra with LCV in vitro, *Cancer Res.,* 41, 3288, 1981.

75. **Houghton, J. A. and Houghton, P. J.,** Availability of N^5, N^{10}Methylenetetrahydrofolate (CH_2:FH_4) as a determinant of 5-fluoropyrimidine sensitivity in xenografts of human colorectal adenocarcinomas, *Proc. Am. Assoc. Cancer Res.,* 22(Abstr.), 974, 1981.

76. **Bruckner, H. W., Ohnuma, T., Hart, R., Jaffrey, I., Spiegelman, M., Ambinder, E., Stoch, J. A., Wilfinger, C., Goldberg, J., Biller, H., and Holland, J. F.,** LCV increases toxicity of FUra in patients on Phase I trial, *Proc. Am. Assoc. Cancer Res.,* 23(Abstr.), 434, 1982.

77. **Danhauser, L., Heimer, R., Bobrow, S., and Cadman, E.,** Effect of leucovorin on the activity of 5-fluorouracil in cultured in L1210 cells pretreated with methotrexate, *Proc. Am. Assoc. Cancer Res.,* 23(Abstr.), 741, 1982.

78. **Klubes, P., Cerna, L., and Meldon, M. A.,** Effect of concurrent calcium leucovorin infusion on 5-fluorouracil cytotoxicity against murine L1210 leukemia, *Cancer Chemother. Pharmacol.,* 6, 121, 1981.

79. **Berger, S. H. and Hakala, M. T.,** Role of cellular dUMP and FdUMP pools and of excess folinic acid (CF) in recovery of thymidylate synthetase (dTMP-S) activity after 5-fluorouracil (FUra) treatment, *Proc. Am. Assoc. Cancer Res.,* 23(Abstr.), 857, 1982.

80. **Moyer, J. D. and Handschumacher, R. F.,** Selective inhibition of pyrimidine synthesis and depletion of nucleotide pools by *N*-(phosphonacetyl)-L-aspartate, *Cancer Res.,* 39, 3089, 1979.

81. **Maley, G. F. and Maley, F.,** Nucleotide interconversions in embryonic and neoplastic tissues. I. The conversion of deoxycytidylate acid to deoxyuridylic acid and thymidylic acid, *J. Biol. Chem.,* 234,(11), 2975, 1959.

82. **Maley, G. F. and Maley, F.,** The purification and properties of deoxycytidylate deaminase from chick embryo extracts, *J. Biol. Chem.,* 239, 1168, 1964.

83. **Armstrong, R. D. and Cadman, E.,** Effect of fluoropyrimidine incorporation into ribosomal (r), small molecular weight (4 to 10S) and messenger (m) RNA, *Proc. Am. Assoc. Cancer Res.,* Abstract, submitted 1982.

84. **Caradonna, S. J. and Cheng, Y.,** The role of deoxyuridine triphosphate nucleotidylhydrolase, uracil-DNA glycosylase, and DNA polymerase in the metabolism of FUdR in human tumor cells, *Mol. Pharmacol.,* 18, 513, 1980.

85. **Ingraham, H. A., Tseng, B. Y., and Goulian, M.,** Mechanism for exclusion of 5-fluorouracil from DNA, *Cancer Res.,* 40, 998, 1980.

86. **Grindey, G. B. and Nichol, C. A.,** Mammalian deoxyuridine 5′-triphosphate pyrophosphate, *Biochim. Biophys. Acta,* 240, 180, 1971.

87. **Williams, M. V. and Cheng, Y.,** Human deoxyuridine triphosphate nucleotidohydrolase, *J. Biol. Chem.,* 254, 2897, 1979.

88. **Shlomai, J. and Kornberg, A.,** Deoxyuridine triphosphatase of *Escherichia coli,* *J. Biol. Chem.,* 253, 3305, 1978.

89. **Arima, T., Aklyoshi, H., and Fujii, S.,** A new deoxyuridine-5′-triphosphatase in Yoshida sarcoma cells involved in deoxyuridine 5%-triphosphate metabolism, *Cancer Res.,* 37, 1598, 1977.

90. **Olivera, B. M.,** DNA intermediates at the *Escherichia coli* replication fork: effect of dUTP, *Proc. Natl. Acad. Sci. U.S.A.,* 75(1), 238, 1978.

91. **Tye, B. K., Chien, J., Lehman, I. R., Duncan, B. K., and Warner, H. R.,** Uracil incorporation: a course of pulse-labeled DNA fragments in the replication of the *Escherichia coli* chromosome, *Proc. Natl. Acad. Sci. U.S.A.,* 75, 233, 1978.

92. **Goulian, M., Bleile, B., and Tseng, B. Y.,** The effect of methotrexate on levels of dUTP in animal cells, *J. Biol. Chem.,* 255(22), 10630, 1980.

93. **Lindahl, T.,** DNA glycosylases, endonucleases for apurinic/apyrimidinic sites, and base excision-repair, *Prog. Nucl. Acid Res. Mol. Biol.,* 22, 135, 1979.

94. **Hanawalt, P. C., Cooper, P. K., Ganesan, A. K., and Smith, C. A.,** DNA repair in bacteria and mammalian cells, *Ann. Rev. Biochem.,* 48, 783, 1979.

95. **Kuhnlein, U., Lee, B., and Linn, S.,** Human uracil DNA N-glycosidase: studies in normal and repair defective cultured fibroblasts, *Nucl. Acids Res.,* 5(1), 117, 1978.
96. **Linsley, W. S., Penhoet, E. E., and Linn, S.,** Human endonuclease specific for apurinic/apyrimidinic sites in DNA, *J. Biol. Chem.,* 252(2), 1235, 1977.
97. **Major, P. P., Egan, E. M., Beardsley, G. P., Minden, M. D., and Kufe, D. W.,** Lethality of human myeloblasts correlates with the incorporation of arabinofuranosylcytosine into DNA, *Proc. Natl. Acad. Sci. U.S.A.,* 78, 3235, 1981.
98. **Major, P. P., Egan, E., Herrick, D., and Kufe, D. W.,** 5-Fluorouracil incorporation in DNA of human breast carcinoma cells, *Cancer Res.,* 42, 3005, 1982.
99. **Olivera, B. M., Ramos, P. M., Warner, H. R., and Duncan, B. K.,** DNA intermediates at the *Escherichia coli* replication fork. II. Studies using dut and ung mutants in vitro, *J. Mol. Biol.,* 128, 265, 1979.
100. **Tye, B. K., Nyman, P. O., Lehman, I. R., Hochhauser, S., and Weiss, B.,** Transient accumulation of Okazaki fragments as a result of uracil incorporation into nascent DNA, *Proc. Natl. Acad. Sci. U.S.A.,* 74(1), 154, 1977.
101. **Brynolf, K., Eliasson, R., and Reichard, P.,** Formation of Lkazaki fragments in polyoma DNA synthesis caused by misincorporation of uracil, *Cell,* 13, 573, 1978.
102. **Tamanoi, F. and Okazaki, T.,** Uracil incorporation into nascent DNA of thymine-requiring mutant of *Bacillus subtilis* 168, *Proc. Natl. Acad. Sci. U.S.A.,* 75, 2195, 1978.
103. **Tye, B. K. and Lehman, I. R.,** Excision repair of uracil incorporated in DNA as a result of a defect in dUTPase, *J. Mol. Biol.,* 117, 293, 1977.
104. **Nakayama, K. and Cheng, Y.-C.,** Mechanism of action of 5-fluorodeoxyuridine in HeLa cells-''self potentiation'', *Proc. Am. Assoc. Cancer Res.,* 23(Abstr.), 844, 1982.
105. **Kessel, D.,** Cell surface alterations associated with exposure of leukemia L1210 cells to fluorouracil, *Cancer Res.,* 40, 322, 1980.
106. **Rustum, Y. M.,** High-pressure liquid chromatography. I. Quantitative separation of purine and pyrimidine nucleosides and base, *Anal. Biochem.,* 90, 289, 1978.
107. **Dreyer, R. and Cadman, E.,** Use of periodate and methylamine for the quantitation of intracellular 5-fluoro-2'-deoxyuridine-5'-monophosphate by high-performance liquid chromatography, *J. Chromatogr.,* 219, 273, 1981.
108. **Kline, I., Venditti, J. M., Mead, J. A. R., Tyrer, D. D., and Goldin, A.,** The antileukemic effectiveness of 5-fluorouracil and methotrexate in the combination chemotherapy of advanced leukemia L1210 in mice, *Cancer Res.,* 26, 848, 1966.
109. **Benz, C., Tillis, T., Tattelman, E., and Cadman, E.,** Optimal scheduling of methotrexate and 5-fluorouracil in human breast cancer, *Cancer Res.,* 42, 2081, 1982.
110. **Paterson, A. R. P. and Tidd, D. M.,** in *Antineoplastic and Immunosuppressive Agents, Part II,* Sartorelli, A. C. and Johns, D. G., Eds., Springer-Verlag New York, 1975, 385.
111. **Scholar, E. M., Brown, P. R., and Parks, R. E., Jr.,** Synergistic effects of 6-mercaptopurine and 6-methylmercaptopurine ribonucleoside on the levels of adenine nucleotides of sarcoma 180 cells, *Cancer Res.,* 32, 259, 1972.
112. **Paterson, A. R. P. and Wang, M. C.,** Mechanism of the growth inhibition potentiation arising from combination of 6-mercaptopurine with 6-(methylmercapto) purine ribonucleoside, *Cancer Res.,* 30, 2379, 1970.
113. **Paterson, A. R. and Moriwaki, A.,** Combination chemotherapy — synergistic inhibition of lymphoma L5178Y cells in culture and in vivo with 6-mercaptopurine and 6-(methylcapto) purine ribonucleoside, *Cancer Res.,* 29, 681, 1969.
114. **Pratt, W. B. and Reddon, R. W.,** *The Anticancer Drugs,* Oxford University Press, London, 1979, 98.
115. **Armstrong, R. D., Vera, R., Snyder, P., and Cadman, E.,** Enhancement of 6-thioguanine cytotoxic activity with methotrexate, *Biochem. Biophys. Res. Commun.,* 109(2), 595, 1982.
116. **DiLorenzo, J. A., Griswold, D. E., Bareham, C. R., and Calabaresi, P.,** Selective alteration of immunocompetence with methotrexate and 5-fluorouracil, *Cancer Res.,* 34, 124, 1974.
117. **Bareham, C. R., Griswold, D. E., and Calabresi, P.,** Synergism of methotrexate with imuran and with 5-fluorouracil and their effects on hemolysin plaque-forming cell production in the mouse, *Cancer Res.,* 34, 571, 1974.
118. **Lee, Y.-T.N. and Khwaja, T.A.,** Adjuvant postoperative chemotherapy with 5-fluorouracil and methotrexate: effect of schedule of administration on metastasis of 13762 mammary adenocarcinoma, *J. Surg. Oncol.,* 9, 469, 1977.
119. **Mulder, J. H., Smink, T., and Van Putten, L. M.,** 5-Fluorouracil and methotrexate combination chemotherapy: the effect of drug scheduling, *Eur. J. Cancer Clin. Oncol.,* 17(7), 831, 1981.
120. **Plotkin, D., and Waugh, W. J.,** Sequential methotrexate-5 fluorouracil (M F) in advanced breast carcinoma, *Proc. Am. Soc. Clin. Oncol.,* 23(Abstr.), C-309, 1982.
121. **Gewirtz, A. M. and Cadman, E.,** Preliminary report on the efficacy of sequential methotrexate and 5-fluorouracil in advanced breast cancer, *Cancer,* 47, 2552, 1981.

122. **Panasci, L. and Margolese, R.,** Sequential methotrexate (MTX) and 5-fluorouracil as (FU) in breast and colorectal cancer. Results of increasing the dose of FU, *Proc. Am. Soc. Clin. Oncol.,* 23(Abstr.), C-393, 1982.

123. **Cantrell, J. E., Jr., Brunet, R., Lagarde, C., Schein, P. S., and Smith, F. P.,** Phase II study of sequential methotrexate-5-FU therapy in advanced measurable colorectal cancer, *Cancer Treat. Rep.,* 66(7), 1563, 1982.

124. **Tisman, G. and Wu, S. J. G.,** Effectiveness of intermediate-dose methotrexate and high-dose 5-fluorouracil as sequential combination chemotherapy in refractory breast cancer and as primary therapy in metastatic adenocarcinoma of the colon, *Cancer Treat. Rep.,* 64(8,9), 829, 1980.

125. **Woodcock, T. M., Allegra, M., Richman, S. P., Kubota, T. T., and Allegra, J. C.,** Sequential therapy with methotrexate (MTX) and 5-flourouracil (5FU) for adenocinoma of the colon, *Proc. Am. Soc. Clin. Oncol.,* 23 (Abstr.), C-398, 1982.

126. **Allegra, J. C., Woodrock, T. M., Richman, S. P., Bland, K. I., and Wittlff, J. L.,** A phase II trial of tamoxifen, premarin, methotrexate and 5-fluorouracil in metastatic breast cancer, *Breast Cancer Res., Treat.,* 2, 93, 1982.

127. **Pitman, S. W., Kowal, C., Papac, R. J., and Bertino, J. R.,** Sequential methotrexate-5-fluorouracil: a highly active drug combination in advanced squamous cell carcinoma of the head and neck, *Proc. Am. Soc. Clin. Oncol.,* 21(Abstr.), C-607, 1980.

128. **Solan, A., Vogl, S. E., Kaplan, B. H., Berenzweig, M., Richard, J., and Lanham, R.,** Sequential chemotherapy of advanced colorectal cancer with standard of high-dose methotrexate followed by 5-fluorouacil, *Med. Pediatr. Oncol.,* 10, 145, 1982.

129. **Herrmann, R., Manegold, C., Rittinghausen, R., Fritze, D., and Schettler, G.,** Sequential methotrexate (MTX) and 5-fluorouracil (FU) in colo-rectal adenocarcinoma. Results of a pilot study, *Proc. Am. Soc. Clin. Oncol.,* 22(Abstr.), C-487, 1981.

130. **Drapkin, R., Griffiths, E., McAloon, E., Paladine, W., Sokol, G., and Lyman, G.,** Sequential methotrexate (MTX) and 5-fluorouracil (5FU) in adenocarcinoma of the colon and rectum, *Proc. Am. Soc. Clin. Ocol.,* 22(Abstr.), C-471, 1981.

131. **Herrmann, R., Westerhausen, M., Bruntsch, U., Jungi, F., Manegold, C., and Fr1tze, D.,** Sequential methotrexate (MTX) and 5-fluorouracil (FU) is effective in extensively pretreated breast cancer, *Proc. Am. Soc. Clin. Oncol.,* 23(Abstr.), C-334, 1982.

132. **Mehrotra, S., Rosenthal, C. J., and Gardner, B.,** Biochemical modulation of antineoplastic response in colorectal carcinoma: 5 fluorouracil (F), high dose methotrexate (M) with calcium leucovorin (L) rescue (FML) in two sequences of administration, *Proc. Am. Soc. Clin. Oncol.,* 23(Abstr.), C-387, 1982.

133. **Weinerman, B., Schacter, B., Schipper, H., Bowman, D., and Levitt, M.,** Sequential methotrexate and 5-FU in the treatment of colorectal cancer, *Cancer Treat. Rep.,* 66(7), 1553, 1982.

134. **Kemeny, N. and Michaelson, R.,** Phase II trial of low dose methotrexate and sequential 5-fluorouracil in the treatment of metastatic colorectal carcinoma, *Proc. Am. Soc. Clin. Oncol.,* 23(Abstr.), C-370, 1982.

135. **Benz, C., Tattelman, E., and Cadman, E.,** Phase I pilot study using 24-hour sequenced methotrexate and 5-fluorouracil, *Proc. Am. Soc. Clin. Oncol.,* 23(Abstr.), C-49, 1982.

136. **Benz, C. and Cadman, E.,** unpublished observation.

137. **Heimer, R. and Cadman, E.,** unpublished observations.

138. **Cadman, E.,** unpublished data.

Chapter 4

INHIBITION OF CYTIDINE DEAMINASE: MECHANISM AND EFFECTS ON THE METABOLISM OF ANTITUMOR AGENTS

Victor E. Marquez

TABLE OF CONTENTS

I. INTRODUCTION

Cytidine deaminase (CDA) or cytidine aminohydrolase EC 3.5.4.5 is a widely distributed enzyme that catalyzes the hydrolytic deamination of cytosine nucleosides to the corresponding uracil nucleosides. The enzyme was first described in 1950 after its isolation from yeast extracts.[1] In addition to its presence in microorganisms and yeast,[1,2] it is found in mammalian tissues as well.[3] High CDA activity has been detected in human tissues (liver, kidney, spleen, heart, and muscle) and in animal tissues from many species including monkey, rabbit, mouse, dog, cat, etc.[3] It is also present in normal and neoplastic tissues of both man and mouse. Specifically, high levels of CDA have been detected in chronic myelogenous leukemic (CML) cells and human peripheral white cells and marrow.[4] It can also be selectively induced in cells after a viral infection, possibly through a virus-specified enzyme.[5] CDA is not found in some common experimental tumor systems such as L1210, but it is detectable in S180, HeLa cells, and several other tumor lines.[6-9] The position of CDA in catabolic and salvage pathways combined with its wide substrate specificity allows this enzyme to exercise a unique control on the availability of nucleic acid precursors and their antimetabolites. Inhibition of CDA, therefore, will have an indirect effect on the cytotoxicity of several pyrimidine antimetabolites which otherwise would be rapidly deaminated. It is the purpose of this article to review the consequences of CDA inhibition in antitumor therapy and to describe the activity and possible advantages of a new generation of very powerful CDA inhibitors.

II. SUBSTRATE SPECIFICITY — STRUCTURE-ACTIVITY RELATIONSHIP

Despite some differences in the specificity of this enzyme for its natural substrates cytidine and deoxycytidine, which vary according to the enzyme source,[10,11] the behavior of the enzyme and its preference for different substrates is fairly constant and predictable.

A. Changes in the Sugar Moiety

The presence and integrity of a pentofuranose configuration at pyrimidine position 1 is required for substrate activity (Figure 1). Therefore, compounds such as cytosine (C), 1-methyl-C, 1-β-D-glucopyranosyl-C, and the acyclic nucleoside analog 1-[(2-hydroxyethyoxy)methyl]-C were not deaminated by CDA.[12,13] Similarly, the resulting cytidine dialdehyde derived from the periodate scission of the 2′,3′-diol and the correspondingly reduced acyclic triol, were devoid of either substrate or inhibitory properties for CDA.[14,15] Within the required pentofuranose structure, the stereochemistry is very important. For example, neither α-cytidine (1-α-D-ribofuranosyl-C) nor the L-enantiomer of 1-β-D-arabinofuranosyl-C (ara-C,**2**)* are substrates for the enzyme.[15,16] Replacement of the furan ring by the cyclopentane ring in cytidine, however, does not destroy substrate properties since the carbocyclic analog, carbodine, is deaminated by the enzyme.[17] In the pentofuranose series, the relative substrate preference decreases from the ribo- to the arabinofuranosyl analog (ara-C) and drops to zero for the xylo- and lyxofuranosyl derivatives.[18] These findings have led to the still valid postulate that the 3′-OH group in the "down" configuration is essential for substrate activity.

1. Position 2′ of the Pentofuranose

The 2′-OH is not absolutely essential for substrate activity. The relative preference follows the order of 2′-H ~ 2′-OH$_{trans}$ > 2′-OH $_{cis}$ where *trans* (ribo) and *cis* (ara) refer to the configuration relative to the 4′-CH$_2$OH. If a halogen replaces the 2′-OH, the same trend of

---

*   All chemical compounds for which a structure is given are identified by boldface Arabic numerals. The structures are found either in the text or in the accompanying figures.

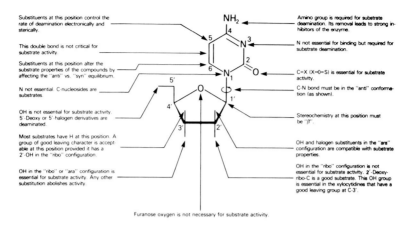

FIGURE 1. Structure-activity relationships for CDA.

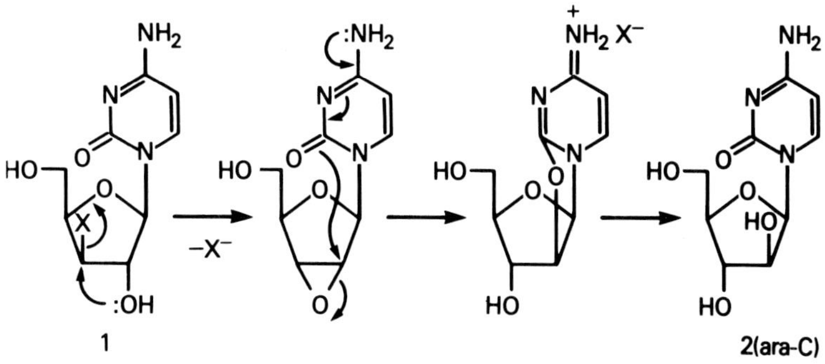

FIGURE 2. Chemical conversion of xylofuranosyl analogs to ara-C.

ribo > ara is maintained.[18] As the size of the 2'-substituent increases, the ara analogs rapidly become inert towards deamination, probably due to a conformational change from "anti" to "syn".[18] The general order of substrate activity for the 2'-position in the ara series is HO>F>Cl>Br ~ mesyloxy ~ methoxy ~ N_3. The last four compounds are not deaminated by CDA.[18-20]

2. Position 3' of the Pentofuranose

The 3'-OH position in the "down" (ribo or ara) configuration appears to be essential for enzyme activity. 3'-Deoxy-ara-C, β-D-xylo-C, and β-lyxo-C are not substrates for CDA. Substitution of the 3'OH in either the ribo or ara series by F, Cl, NH_2, or methoxy groups produces compounds resistant to enzymatic deamination.[18,19] Interestingly, xylofuranosyl analogs (1) bearing a good leaving group at the 3'-position (i.e., Br, mesyloxy, tosyloxy) are deaminated. These compounds appear to undergo a prior chemical reaction which transforms them into the corresponding arabinofuranosyl derivatives (2) with the required 3'-OH in the "down" configuration (Figure 2).[18] This reaction, however, requires the integrity of the 2'-OH in the "down" configuration to form the necessary epoxide. Since F is not a good leaving group, 3'-deoxy-3'-F-xylo-C is not a substrate for CDA.[18]

3. Position 5' of the Pentofuranose

Substitution or removal of the 5'-OH does not destroy the substrate properties of the compounds. For example, 5'-deoxy-ara-C is deaminated as well as ara-C by the mouse kidney enzyme and the 5'-O-methyl-ribo-C derivative is a reasonable substrate for the enzyme

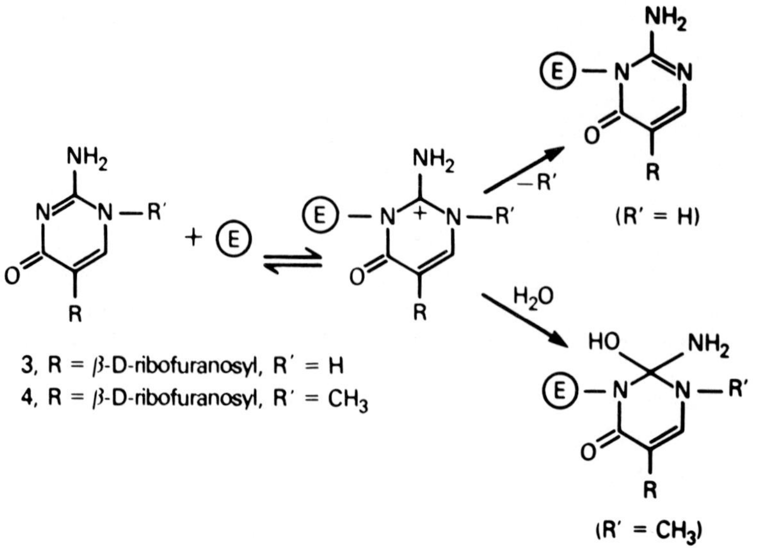

FIGURE 3.   Resistance and susceptibility towards deamination by isocytidine C-nucleosides.

from *Salmonella thyphimurium* and human granulocytes.[19] Data obtained from the corresponding cytosine nucleotides (CMP, dCMP, etc.) suggest that these compounds must be dephosphorylated prior to deamination by CDA.[12]

B. Changes in the Pyrimidine Aglycon

1. Pyrimidine Position 1 (N-1)

A C–N glycosidic linkage does not appear to be critical for substrate deamination despite the fact that C-nucleosides such as ψ-isocytidine (3), 2′-deoxy-ψ-isocytidine, and ara-ψ-isocytosine are not deaminated by CDA.[21] The stability of these compounds contrasts with the susceptibility of another C-nucleoside, N^1-methyl-ψ-isocytidne (4) to undergo enzymatic deamination. The reason for this difference is inherent to the mechanism of reaction of CDA. The N-1 hydrogen in the resistant C-nucleosides, a position equivalent to the 5-position of cytidine (Figure 3), can dissociate after binding at the active site, thereby preventing charge localization and subsequent hydration at the adjacent carbon atom bearing the amino function.[21] In the case of the nondissociable N^1-methyl compound (4), charge localization is rapidly followed by enzymatic hydration and deamination. The mechanism of CDA deamination will be discussed in Section III.

2. Pyrimidine Position 2

Presence of a carbonyl function at this position appears critical. Neither 2-amino-ribouridine (isocytidine) nor its corresponding arabinoside behaved as substrates or inhibitors of CDA.[12] 2-Thiopyrimidine-β-D-ara-C (thio-Ara-C) has been synthesized and studied.[22,23] The fact that thio-ara-C is very similar to ara-C in its mechanism of action and cytotoxicity would indicate that it is also a good substrate for CDA.[23]

3. Pyrimidine Position 3 (N-3)

Early observations about the substrate specificity for CDA indicated the necessity of an unsubstituted nitrogen at this position.[12] Chemically, substitution at N-3 in a cytosine nucleoside would induce formation of a 4-iminocytidine analog which is inherently resistant to deamination. In addition to this effect, the mere presence of the N-3 nitrogen appears to be essential for the "electronic" fit of the substrate. For example, 3-deazacytidine does not undergo deamination by mouse kidney CDA.[21] This nitrogen atom, however, appears more critical for the deamination reaction than for binding, since both 3-deazauridine and 1-β-D-ribofuranosyl 2-pyridone behaved as moderate competitive inhibitors of the enzyme.[24,25]

4. Pyrimidine Position 4

For obvious reasons a 4-amino group at this position is essential for substrate activity. Complete removal of the 4-amino group gave rise to compounds that behaved as strong competitive inhibitors,[25] while the 4-keto(uridine) and 4-thio (thiouridine) derivatives displayed moderate inhibitory properties.[12] About the only change tolerated by the enzyme at this position is the substitution of one hydrogen by a methyl group. However, N^4-methyl cytidine is a very poor substrate for CDA.[26] Interestingly, the enzyme catalyzes its formation in appreciable amounts from uridine and methylamine at an alkaline pH.[26] Other substitutions at C-4, such as in 4-hydrazino and 4-hydroxylamino cytidines, destroyed substrate activity.[12] 4-Hydroxylaminocytidine behaved as a competitive inhibitor of CDA.[6]

5. Pyrimidine Position 5

Substituents at this position affect the rate of deamination of cytosine nucleosides sterically and electronically. For the halogen series Cl, Br, and I, the rate of deamination is not markedly different. For example, 5-Cl-ara-C was deaminated approximately 1.5-fold faster than ara-C, while the bromo derivative was deaminated at a rate comparable to that of ara-C.[12] The iodo derivative was deaminated at an even lower rate than that of ara-C, but similar to that of the 5-methyl derivative.[12] Clearly, the effect of iodine was largely steric and comparable to the effect of the methyl group. The introduction of a fluorine atom, however, brings about a dramatic increase in the rate of deamination in every cytosine nucleoside tested.[18] In this case, the effect is exclusively electronic. The order of deamination for 5-substituted cytosine nucleosides is F>>>Cl>H>Br> I~CH$_3$. The fluorine atom not only increases the rate of deamination for the substrates but it also enhances the affinity towards CDA for some of the inhibitors.[25] Other substituents, such as OH, reduced the rate of deamination[27] and replacement of the aromatic C-5 carbon by a nitrogen, as in 5-aza-cytidine, did not destroy the substrate properties of the compound.[28]

6. Pyrimidine Position 6

The effects of substitution at this position are mainly steric and the substituent at C-6 directly influences the relative equilibrium between the natural "anti" form and the unnatural "syn" conformation. Therefore, 6-methyl-ribo-C is a poor substrate for CDA, probably because it is more stable in the "syn" conformation.[18,29] On the contrary, replacement of C-6 by a nitrogen, as in 6-aza-cytidine, significantly reduces the barrier to rotation around the glycosidic bond and the conformation of the nucleoside appears to be in the "high anti" form rather than in the conventional "anti" conformation of cytidine.[30] This compound was an effective substrate for CDA which bound weakly to the enzyme, but was deaminated at a higher rate than cytidine.[31]

7. Pyrimidine 5,6 Double Bond

Presence of this double bond is not critical for either substrate binding or deamination. Both 5,6-dihydrocytidine and 5,6-dihydro-5-aza-cytidine are good substrates for CDA.[32,33] Powerful inhibitors of CDA, such as tetrahydrouridine (THU), also lack the 5,6-double bond.[31,34]

III. MECHANISM OF REACTION OF CDA

The deamination reaction of cytidine and cytosine nucleoside analogs is an equilibrium reaction heavily favoring the direction of hydrolysis:[10,11]

$$\text{Cytidine} + \text{H}_2\text{O} \rightleftharpoons \text{uridine} + \text{NH}_3$$

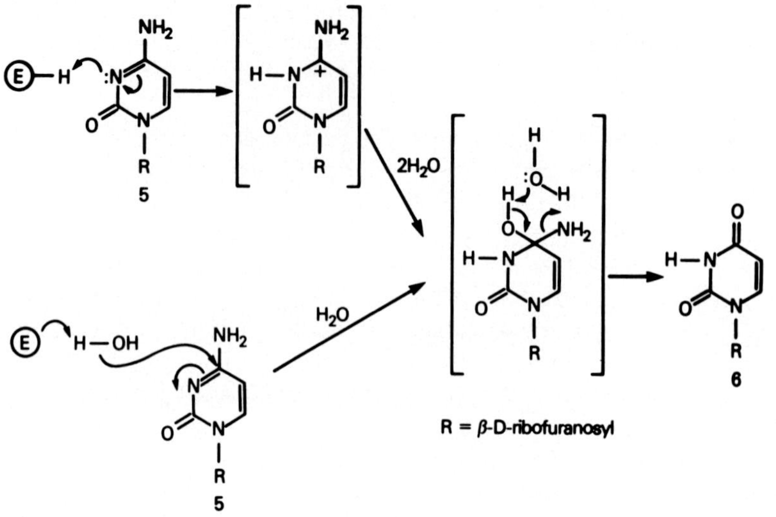

FIGURE 4. Mechanisms of the deamination reaction by CDA.

The enzyme operates well within a wide range of pH (6.5 to 10) with little change in activity.[10,11,34] It is not deactivated by EDTA addition or borohydride reduction.[10,11] Presence of SH groups are essential for activity and consequently divalent cations inhibit the enzyme.[35]

The half-life for the spontaneous rate of hydrolysis of cytidine in neutral solution at room temperature is calculated to be in the order of years,[36] whereas that of 5,6-dihydrocytidine was approximately 105 min.[32] This increased reactivity of the reduced analog, coupled with the known role of inorganic anions[36-38] to induce rapid deamination of cytidine after addition to the 5,6-double bond, suggested that enzymic nucleophilic attack at C-6 was a possible first step in CDA deamination. However, this does not appear to be the case since 5,6-dihydrocytidine and 6-azacytidine, which preclude the formation of such an adduct, served as substrates for CDA.[32] In addition, whereas the citrate-catalyzed deamination of cytidine was accompanied by incorporation of solvent deuterium at position C-5,[37] such was not the case for the reaction catalyzed by CDA.[34] It appears, therefore, that the reaction proceeds via an addition-elimination mechanism commencing with water attack at the C-4 position of cytidine to give a high-energy tetrahedral intermediate.[40] This transition-state intermediate rapidly eliminates ammonia in a fashion similar to that postulated for adenosine deaminase.[40,41] Water addition at C-4 can also occur via hydration following the electrophilic attack of the enzyme at the N-3 of cytidine.[21] Recent work with cytidine C-nucleosides supports this mechanism, which also proceeds through the intermediacy of a tetrahedral hemiaminal.[21] Elimination of ammonia from the transition-state intermediate could be spontaneous or assisted by a second molecule of water (Figure 4). This possibility exists in the chemical deamination of 1-methyl-5,6-dihydrocytosine where a large negative entropy was consistent with a proposed highly ordered intermediate.[42] Interestingly, a significant negative entropy was also calculated for the binding of CDA to the transition-state inhibitor, tetrahydrouridine(THU).[43]

IV. INHIBITORS OF CDA

The structural requirements for CDA inhibitors are varied and related to their mechanism of inhibition. In general, the enzyme is very sensitive to inhibition by SH reagents of different structures such as *p*-hydroxymercuribenzoate, *N*-ethyl-maleimide, as well as by Hg^{+2} and Cu^{+2} salts.[35,44] A rhodium complex has shown a mixed type of inhibition consistent with its binding in the proximity of the catalytic site[45] and an acridine derivative inhibited the enzymatic reaction by forming a complex with the substrate, which, in turn, competed for the active site.[46] The first reported competitive inhibitor of CDA was N^4-hydroxy-5-methyl-2′-deoxycytidine (**7**).[12] The problem with this and other N^4-hydroxy inhibitors was that although they were not directly deaminated, they underwent reduction in vivo to the parent cytidine substrates.[6] The synthesis of 3,4,5,6-tetrahydrouridine (THU, **8**) prepared by the overreduction of cytidine,[47] afforded the first potent inhibitor of CDA which was believed to behave as a transition-state analog.[32,34]

A. Tetrahydrouridine (THU) as an Inhibitor of CDA

The significant and specific inhibitory properties of THU against CDA quickly made it the inhibitor of choice and provided further support to the existence of a tetrahedral intermediate in the enzymatic mechanism of deamination.[31,32,34,40] In view of its structural resemblance to the hypothetical transition-state intermediate, THU binds very strongly to the enzyme with a 2- to 3-log higher affinity than cytidine. The kinetic behavior of THU appears to vary according to the enzyme source. It is instantaneous, purely competitive, and reversible for the bacterial enzyme,[34] and subject to a short incubation period with a slow onset of inhibition in the case of the human liver enzyme.[31] THU ($K_i = 2.4 \times 10^{-7} M$) is bound to the bacterial enzyme 875 times more tightly than the substrate cytidine ($K_m = 2.1 \times 10^{-4} M$).[10] For the human enzymes, however, THU appears less effective in view of the higher affinity of these enzymes for cytidine. The K_m values for cytidine with CDA from human liver and normal or leukemic granulocytes are $9.6 \times 10^{-6} M$ and $1.1 \times 10^{-5} M$, respectively.[11,48] On the other hand, the K_i value for THU against these enzymes is $2.9 \sim 5.4 \times 10^{-8} M$, which is equivalent to an increase in binding of only 200 to 230 times with respect to cytidine.[11,47] Other investigators have reported even higher values for the K_i of THU ($2.0 \times 10^{-7} M$) with enzymes isolated from mouse kidney and monkey serum.[25,49]

One of two recently synthesized analogs of THU, bearing heteroatoms to mimic a tetrahedral configuration, showed good inhibitory activity against CDA.[50,51] The phosphorus-containing pyrimidine nucleoside (**10**), as opposed to the sulfur analog (**9**), competed for the active site and appeared to bind covalently to CDA.[51]

THU inhibition of CDA has been sought as a way of overcoming the rapid deamination of cytidine analogs, particularly ara-C, used in anticancer therapy. As discussed in the next section, this and other combinations with different antimetabolites have yet to prove their practical advantages in the clinic and in the laboratory. In relation to THU, the problems associated with the lack of success in combination chemotherapy could be several. For example, THU is cleared very fast from plasma and tissues of animals and humans, and has a relatively short half-life.[8,52-54] These properties make it necessary to use very high doses of the inhibitor (~1 g/kg) to achieve a significant but transient inhibition of CDA.[8,54] In addition, CDA from the human liver has a tremendous deaminating capacity and THU may be incapable of saturating all of the body deaminases.[3] A residual deaminase activity has been measured in mouse kidney CDA even after the addition of THU.[33] THU has also been found to be relatively unstable under acidic conditions.[55] Presence of acid catalyzes the conversion of the sugar moiety from the active 1-β-D-ribofuranoside form to the totally inactive 1-β-D-ribopyranoside form.[55] This reaction reaches a rapid equilibrium heavily in favor of the more stable pyranoside-THU. Prolonged storage and moisture are also responsible for the formation of the pyranoside form.[55] This reaction, and the formation of a suspected THU dimer, may be responsible in part for the different half-life values reported for THU in the literature.[54,56] Particular importance should be given to this acid-catalyzed reaction in cases of orally administered THU.[56,57] The discrepancy found between blood level values determined by radioactive and enzymatic assays, following the oral administration of ^{14}C-2-THU in humans,[56] could be explained by this reaction, which would be most likely to occur in the stomach. Blood levels from the radioactive assay showed that only 23% of the drug possessed inhibitory properties against CDA.[56] This is particularly interesting in view of the fact that perhaps the only successful association of THU with ara-C in which an increase in therapeutic index was evident resulted from a combination study using the oral route for both agents.[57] The scope of this rearrangement has been studied using a series of pyrimidinone and diazepinone nucleosides (Figure 5).[55] The nature of the pyranoside forms have been confirmed by proton NMR which showed a shift to higher field ($\delta_{1'}$) and an increase value for the coupling constant ($J_{1',2'}$) of the corresponding anomeric protons. The stability of extra conjugation provided by the 4-keto group of dihydrouridine and the aromatic uracil, cytosine, and 2-pyrimidinone nucleosides permitted these compounds to remain as ribofuranosides under acidic conditions. As shown in Figure 5, the opening of the five-member furanose ring is quickly followed by the attack of the primary 5'-OH at C-1' to form the ribopyranoside structure.

B. Pyrimidin-2-One Nucleosides as Inhibitors of CDA

Evidence for the covalent hydration of simple pyrimidines indicated that the hydrated species were present in appreciable quantities (approximately 0.05%).[58-60] This fact led to the investigation of pyrimidin-2-one ribosides (**11**) as potential inhibitors of CDA since hydration was expected to generate a tetrahedral analog similar to THU.[25,31] Indeed, the parent compound behaved as a good inhibitor of the mouse kidney and yeast enzymes ($K_i = 2.0 \times 10^{-6}$ M) but still less potent than THU ($K_i = 2.2 \times 10^{-7}$ M).[25] Substitution for chlorine or bromide at C-5 produced little change, but fluorine substitution, which probably facilitated hydration, gave a compound that was as active as THU against both enzymes.[25] Both the parent compound (**11a**) and the 5-fluoro analog (**11b**) were cytotoxic to L1210 cells in culture;[25] however, in vivo studies showed the fluoro analog to be extremely toxic.[61] Further studies with the parent pyrimidin-2-one riboside (NSC-309132) indicated moderate antitumor activity against P388 (T/C 152), L1210 (T/C 175), and B16 melanoma (T/C 180) at 400 mg/kg.[61] Obviously, this activity was not related to its inhibitory properties of CDA, since THU is rather innocuous and nontoxic both in vitro and in vivo.[62,63] This pyrimidin-2-one nucleoside could be phosphorylated, and as such it may inhibit cytidylate deaminase in a similar fashion as 3-deazauridine monophosphate.[24] The acid stability of this compound, coupled with its inherent cytotoxicity, makes it a suitable candidate for drug combination studies with readily deaminated antimetabolites.

11a, X = H
b, X = F

12a, R = OH
b, R = H

16

C. Diazepin-2-One Nucleosides as Inhibitors of CDA

For the analogous aminohydrolase, adenosine deaminase, the fermentation products co-formycin (**12a**) and 2'-deoxycoformycin (**12b**) behaved as extremely powerful inhibitors. These compounds were 10^5 to 10^6 times more tightly bound to the enzyme than the substrate adenosine or the deamination product inosine.[61] These structures suggested that the compounds behaved as transition-state inhibitors of adenosine deaminase.[41,64] The puckered and enlarged 7-member ring of the coformycins may have provided a better fit as a "stretched" substrate during the transition state.[64,65] Similarly, the ring-expanded counterparts in the pyrimidine series were also reported to be potent inhibitors of CDA.[66-68] This improvement, however, was not as dramatic as in the coformycin series against adenosine deaminase since the inhibitory potency of these compounds increased only by tenfold with respect to THU (Table 1).[63,65] A structure-activity study in this series revealed that the optimal ring size was seven and that a specific stereochemistry of the hydroxyl at C-5 was associated with a 1-log difference in inhibitory activity.[66,68] In addition, two unsaturated diazepinone nucleosides, **15** and **18** showed comparable or slightly superior activity in comparison with the most active C-5 hydroxy diastereoisomer, **16**.[68,69] It is possible that these compounds are hydrated stereoselectively at the active site, generating the transition-state analogs *in situ*. From structural considerations, compound **15** corresponds to a ring-enlarged version of the "anhydro" form of THU.[31] As with THU, these compounds were also inactivated by the acid-catalyzed ribofuranose to ribopyranose interconversion (Figure 5).[55]

V. CONSEQUENCES OF CDA INHIBITION

A. Ara-C Therapy

1. Metabolism and Properties of Ara-C

1-β-D-Arabinofuranosyl cytosine (ara-C,**2**) is a cytidine analog in which the configuration of the 2'-hydroxy group is inverted. It is one of the most successful antimetabolites yet prepared and possesses a wide spectrum of activity against experimental murine tumors as well as good clinical activity against acute myelocytic leukemia (AML).[70,71] It also shows antiviral and immunosuppressive activities.[72,73] It is predominantly an S-phase cell-cycle-specific agent, which accounts for the schedule dependency in relation to its antitumor activity.[74,75] Effects on cellular proliferation in normal host tissue also occur, especially in the bone marrow.[75,76] The metabolic fate of ara-C has been investigated extensively, particularly in relation to the formation of the key phosphorylated metabolite, ara-CTP. A rapid cellular uptake and intracellular phosphorylation by deoxycytidine kinase (dCK) are considered essential steps for good antiproliferative activity (Figure 6).[77] However, an even more rapid catabolic deamination by CDA quickly depletes plasma levels of ara-C, transforming it into the metabolically inert ara-U.[3,77] Following i.v. administration, drug levels fall rapidly in a biphasic mode ($t_{1/2}$ 12 and 111 min, respectively), and after 20 min the drug is practically undetectable.[78] This effect of CDA is of great magnitude in view of its wide distribution in mammalian tissues.[3] In addition, even after surviving systemic and hepatic deamination, ara-C can likewise be deaminated by intracellular CDA present in leukemic myeloblasts.[4,48] Despite this tremendous catabolic activity, ara-C is still phosphorylated intracellularly and its biological response is commensurate with the ability of cells to take up and retain ara-C as its phosphoryated metabolites.[79] Once ara-C enters the cell, it is converted to its active metabolite ara-CTP by the sequential action of dCK and two other kinases (Figure 6). It is this metabolite that is responsible for the inhibition of cellular DNA polymerase ($K_i = 1.0 \times 10^{-6}$ M) by competing with the natural substrate dCTP.[80] Other mechanisms of cytotoxicity of ara-C include inhibition of ribonucleotide reductase and incorporation into low-molecular-weight RNA.[77,81] Whatever the mechanism of cytotoxicity, the steps leading toward ara-CTP are crucial. These steps have been investigated with isolated

Table 1
INHIBITION CONSTANTS (K$_i$) AGAINST CDA FOR A
SERIES OF DIAZEPINONE NUCLEOSIDES

Compound	Ref. #	K$_i$, M	
		Mouse Kidney	Human Liver
8(THU)	66	2.2×10^{-7}	1×10^{-7}
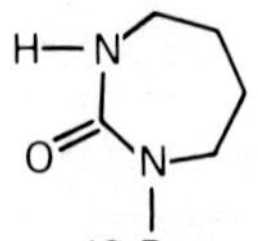 13,R	68	3×10^{-7}	4×10^{-7}
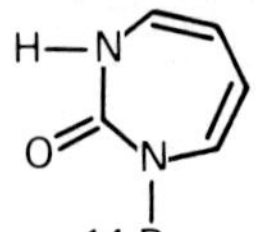 14,R	69	4×10^{-7}	2×10^{-7}
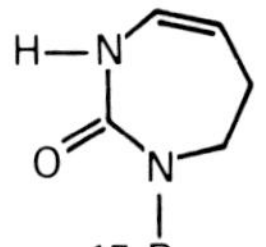 15,R	69	8×10^{-8}	3×10^{-7}
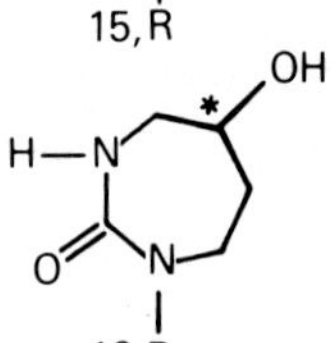 16,R	66	2×10^{-8}	4×10^{-8}
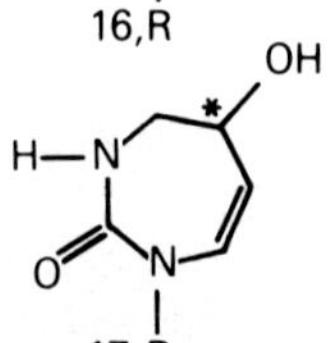 17,R	67,69	5.5×10^{-8}	—
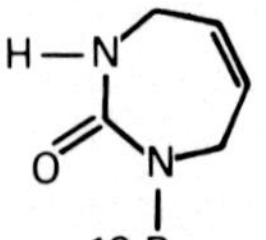 18,R	68	7×10^{-8}	2.5×10^{-8}

R = β-D-ribofuranosyl

*Most active diastereoisomer

enzymes and whole cells and are summarized in Figure 6. The first phosphorylating enzyme, dCK, is a very complex enzyme which appears to be rate limiting and subject to many regulatory mechanisms.[82-84] The other two phosphorylating enzymes are present in much higher concentration and their K$_m$ values are at least 1 log greater.[84,85] Ara-C affinity for dCK is poorer (K$_m$ = 2.56 × 10^{-5} M) than that of deoxycytidine (K$_m$ = 7.8 × 10^{-6} M), but its maximum velocity is only 10% less.[82] The phosphorylation of ara-C is strongly

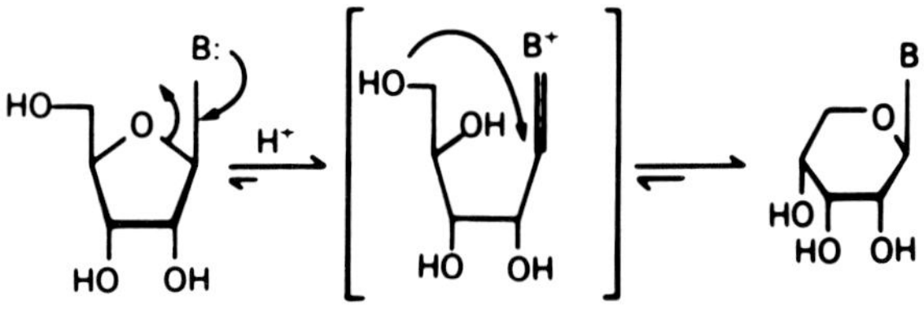

B	$\delta_{1'}$	$J_{1'2'}$(Hz)	$\delta_{1'}$	$J_{1'2'}$(Hz)
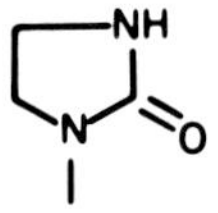	5.40	6	5.00	10
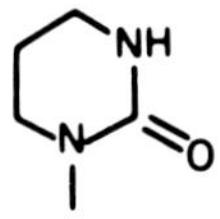	5.80	6	5.40	10
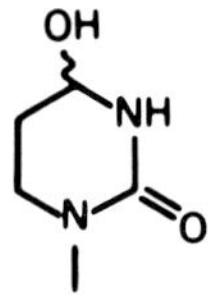	5.80	6	5.40	10
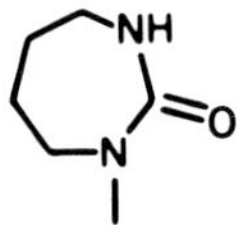	5.40	7	5.10	10.5
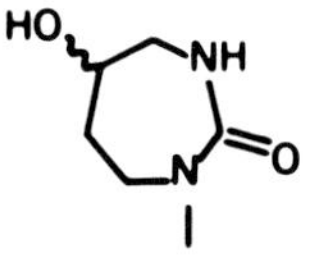	5.40	7	5.10	10

FIGURE 5. Acid-catalyzed conversion of ribofuranoside nucleosides to the corresponding ribopyranoside forms.

inhibited by dCTP ($K_i = 7.3 \times 10^{-6}$ M) and deoxycytidine ($K_i = 1.7 \times 10^{-7}$ M).[82] In addition, high ara-CTP levels also exert a negative feedback, and too-high levels of ara-C seem to decrease the rate of ara-CTP production.[83,86] One of the reasons for the clinical selectivity of ara-C against AML leukemias is that dCK levels in leukemic granulocytes from AML patients are greater than those found in normal granulocytes.[4,82] This suggests that dCK levels are a direct function of cell proliferation, a fact that agrees well with the cell-cycle specificity of ara-C. The concentration levels of the catabolic enzyme, CDA, vary in the opposite direction, being higher in normal granulocytes than in AML cells.[82] This enzyme, likewise, has a greater affinity for cytidine ($K_m = 1.1 \times 10^{-5}$ M) than for ara-C ($K_m = 8.8 \times 10^{-5}$ M).[48] Within each category of cells, normal or AML, CDA levels are greater than dCK levels.[48,82] In addition, the situation is further complicated by the fact that both CDA and dCK levels change during cell maturation.[82] The kinase deaminase ratio has been correlated with drug sensitivity in many instances, and it could explain why, for

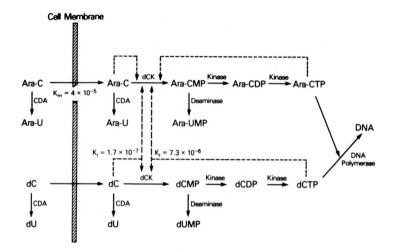

FIGURE 6. Biological mechanisms of activation and deactivation of ara-C.

example, AML cells produce more ara-CTP than CML, ALL, CLL, and normal granulocytes.[86] Unfortunately, the situation appears to be more complex since this ratio itself, or the properties of the enzyme, appear to be different after prolonged incubation or cell lysis.[82,83,86-88] In intact cells, the initial phosphorylation of ara-C is very rapid and only after prolonged incubation, which depletes the levels of high-energy triphosphate donors, does deamination become predominant.[86] There are thus many problems associated with the interpretation of results in these closed systems.

2. Ara-C Resistance

Resistance to ara-C therapy is frequently encontered in the clinic and a number of biochemical mechanisms have been postulated on the basis of studies with experimental animal tumors and human leukemic cells. Initial results suggested that a deficiency in dCK levels, or an increase in intracellular CDA activity, were responsible for lowering the intracellular levels of the active metabolite ara-CTP.[89,90] However, in the case of AML cells, the concentration of these enzymes varies considerably from patient to patient and no clear conclusions can be drawn with certainty.[82,91,92] There is no doubt that these two enzymes play a role in cells resistant to ara-C, but they do not appear to be directly responsible as the cause of resistance.[92] Despite the fact that some experimental studies have established a relationship between successful therapy and the ability of the leukemic cell to form and retain ara-CTP,[93,94] some AML cells from relapsed patients, previously sensitive to ara-C, became resistant to the drug in spite of their continued ability to synthesize high levels of ara-CTP.[86,95] These cells with such high ara-CTP concentrations may also have high dCTP pools, in which case a greater ara-CTP production does not necessarily correlate with greater inhibition of DNA synthesis.[83,92] This situation may be further complicated by the fact that an increase in dCTP pools may arise via an increase in cytidine triphosphate (CTP) synthetase and ribonucleotide reductase activities, as opposed to simply higher dCK levels.[96] As seen in Figure 6, dCTP is, in turn, a powerful feedback inhibitor of dCK and could later induce a lower ara-CTP production.[97] Other enzymes could very well be involved in the mechanism of resistance. For example, the second kinase (dCMP kinase), although present in high concentrations, has a poor affinity for ara-CMP ($k_m = 7.4 \times 10^{-4}$ M); therefore, at low ara-CMP concentrations, this step could become rate-limiting.[98] Low ara-CMP levels could be accounted for by high dCMP deaminase activity which is significantly increased in leukemic myeloblasts and has a higher affinity for ara-CMP than dCMP kinase.[99]

In light of more recent studies, the role of CDA appears to be less important as a mechanism of resistance to ara-C.[88,92] The lack of consensus in this regard probably results from the experimental models used to study the problem.[87,88,100,101] In in vitro studies the importance of the intracellular degradative pathway catalyzed by CDA may have been overestimated by the nature of the test system itself where the essential steady supply of high energy triphosphates and ara-C are absent.[86-87]

It can be concluded that there are several critical steps in the metabolic pathway of ara-C that can be related to drug resistance. As a result, some drug-combination studies have taken advantage of this knowledge to enhance ara-C activation. Tetrahydrouridine produced consistent increases in intracellular ara-CTP levels by competing with CDA;[103] hydroxyurea[104,105] and thymidine[106] decreased the synthesis of dCTP by interfering with ribonucleotide reductase activity, and 3-deazauridine interfered either with CTP synthetase or deoxycytidylate deaminase.[24,107,108] Recent evidence suggests that some of these pharmacological combinations, which in addition take into account the kinetic features of AML cells, may show great promise in dealing with relapsing acute leukemia.[109] Perhaps the main factor for the development of resistance is the selection of a cell population with a low mitotic rate.[92] Secondary factors, singly or in combination, could be low dCK levels, high CDA activity, and increased dCTP pools. Despite these very interesting observations, the mechanism of ara-C resistance remains to be defined with certainty.

3. Ara-C and CDA Inhibitors

Strong inhibition of CDA has been experimentally and clinically achieved with THU. In vitro combination studies with ara-C using AML cells reported consistent increases in intracellular ara-CTP.[86,87,103] Other studies, however, found only a moderate increase in ara-CTP production despite the complete inhibition of ara-U formation.[88] In synchronized cultures of normal rat kidney cells and S-180 cells, which like AML cells contain high levels of CDA, THU enhanced the cytotoxicity of sublethal doses of ara-C.[108,110] Similar combination studies, however, have not met with the expected success in the treatment of animal and human leukemias, due perhaps to the complexity of the metabolic activation of ara-C. In four experimental mouse tumors with high deaminase/kinase ratios, the combination of ara-C plus THU produced significant increases in survival only in the S180J ascites-bearing animals.[8]

Other studies suggest that perhaps inhibition of the host's deaminase is more critical in maintaining an adequate supply of ara-C. After systemic administration, THU has been shown to increase the plasma half-life of ara-C in both animal species and humans.[8,54,111,112] Ideally, sustained higher blood levels of ara-C would have increased the activity of the drug towards the tumor cells; but, unfortunately, there was also a parallel increase in toxicity, especially in dogs and monkeys.[112] In other species the effect of the inhibition was rapid and transient, possibly because of the fast clearance of THU itself.[8] A combination of ara-C and a new diazepinone nucleoside **18** shown previously to be ten times more potent than THU as a CDA inhibitor,[68] produced a comparable increase in life-span to that obtained with THU, but at a dose ten times lower (Table 2).[113] Since L1210 cells are completely devoid of CDA,[6] this effect is strictly related to inhibition of the host's deaminase. It would be of interest to know if this and other more powerful inhibitors of CDA are capable of maintaining lower and sustained levels of ara-C. The successful results with the oral administration of THU and ara-C seem to indicate that after inhibition of bacterial or intestinal CDA, a gradual absorption of ara-C produced lower but more effective levels of the drug.[57] When THU is given systemically, or i.p., blood levels of ara-C tend to be higher, but of short duration. The latter situation is not only inefficient but it may enhance toxicity as well. Another reported pharmacokinetic association of ara-C and THU that may have therapeutic applicability in humans because of its lack of toxicity was represented by the intrathecal administration of both drugs in monkeys.[114] In clinical phase I studies, 25 to 50 mg/kg of

Table 2
INCREASED THERAPEUTIC
ACTIVITY OF ARA-C IN
COMBINATION WITH CDA
INHIBITORS

Ara-C (dose)	Inhibitor (dose)	T/C
3 mg/kg	—	136
10 mg/kg	—	160
3 mg/kg	THU (1 g/kg)	166
3 mg/kg	**18** (100 mg/kg)	161

THU in combination with 0.1 to 0.2 mg/kg of ara-C produced appreciable but tolerable myelosuppression expected for a higher dose of ara-C alone.[115] The combination of 25 mg/kg of THU and 0.1 mg/kg of ara-C was equivalent to a 5-day course of 3 mg/kg of ara-C alone.[115] In view of the lack of real therapeutic advantages with the use of THU, the trend appears to have shifted towards the development and study of CDA-resistant ara-C prodrugs.[116,117]

B. 5-Azacytidine (5-AC) Therapy

1. Metabolism and Properties of 5-AC

5-Azacytidine (5-AC) is a cytidine analog which possesses a nitrogen atom at the 5-position of the heterocyclic aglycon.[118] It is converted to the monophosphate derivative (5-ACMP) by uridine-cytidine kinase (UCK) and subsequently transformed into its presumed active metabolite, 5-azacytidine triphosphate (5-ACTP), through the action of two nucleotide kinases.[119] 5-AC has been shown to be an effective cytostatic agent for the treatment of AML leukemia and some human solid tumors.[120,121] There is no single mechanism responsible for its cytotoxicity, which possibly occurs as a result of a combination of actions at different sites. Incorporation of 5-AC into RNA has been correlated with inhibition of protein synthesis.[122,123] Such inhibition could result directly from destabilization of ribosomal RNA or as a consequence to the inhibition of cytosine-5-methyl transferase.[124,125] More recently, other mechanisms of cytotoxicity such as incorporation of the drug in nuclear RNA and its interference with the processes of methylation and transcription have been investigated.[126] Additionally, 5-AC is capable of inhibiting DNA synthesis.[123]

As in the case of ara-C, the first step leading to the phosphorylated metabolite 5-ACMP is considered crucial; and deletion of the UCK enzyme system is responsible for the appearance of resistance to the drug.[127] This kinase is a complex salvage enzyme of the pyrimidine pathway which is subject to feedback regulation by UTP and CTP.[123,128] As expected, uridine and cytidine are capable of reversing the cytotoxicity of 5-AC.[129] The phosphorylating step, as opposed to transport, is considered to be rate limiting.[130] Several UCKs from different sources such as calf thymus, L1210 extracts, HeLa cells, and human AML cells, are capable of phosphorylating 5-AC.[33,123,128,131,132] However, the drug behaved as a much poorer substrate (K_m = 0.2 to 11 × 10^{-3} M) than the natural nucleosides (K_m = 5 × 10^{-5} M).[131,132]

2. 5-AC and THU

As expected from its chemical structure, 5-AC is also a substrate for CDA. It is a poorer substrate for the mouse kidney enzyme (K_m = 2.1 × 10^{-3} M)[33] than for the deaminase from human leukemic cells (K_m = 4.3 × 10^{-4} M);[28] however, at saturating substrate concentrations it is deaminated more rapidly than cytidine.[28] Results from combination studies of 5-AC with THU in L1210 mice were not significantly better when compared with the use of 5-AC alone and only toxicity was enhanced.[133] Consistent with the inhibition of kidney CDA, the urinary excretion of unchanged drug was increased significantly.[133] With the oral coadministration of 5-AC and THU, the results showed that the combination was as effective as 5-AC used singly by the i.p. route. No difference in therapeutic index was evidenced.[134] In the case of 5-AC, the results of combination studies with THU may be even more complex than those with ara-C due to the rapid nonenzymatic degradation of 5-AC and its deamination product.[135] In HeLa cells, despite the presence of measurable amounts of CDA, THU was unable to enhance the cytostatic activity of slightly inhibitory concentrations of 5-AC.[131] Other drug combination studies with inhibitors of *de novo* pyrimidine synthesis, as well as with inhibitors of CTP synthetase, both of which activate the UCK system towards 5-AC, appear to hold more promise in 5-AC antitumor therapy.[130,136,137]

C. Dihydro-5-Azacytidine (DH5-AC) Therapy
1. Metabolism and Properties of DH5-AC

In an effort to overcome the instability of 5-AC, the hydrolytically unstable 5,6-imino double bond was chemically reduced to give 5,6-dihydro-5-azacytidine (DH5-AC).[138] This new compound was no longer susceptible to hydrolytic attack and concomitant ring opening and was much more stable in aqueous solutions.[138] In comparative studies against L1210 leukemia in mice, the reduced analog showed the same level of activity as that of 5-AC in terms of extension of life-span, but at a dose level approximately 30 times higher.[138] The therapeutic index, however, appeared to be more favorable for DH5-AC.[138] Additionally, the compound was superior to 5-AC in the intracerebrally implanted L1210 system, indicating some ability to cross the blood-brain barrier.[138] In tissue culture studies with L1210 cells, both 5-AC and DH5-AC were phosphorylated by UCK, but only at 5% the rate of the natural substrates.[33] Although the drug was originally conceived as a prodrug of 5-AC, most studies indicate that the phosphorylated metabolites of DH5-AC are, in themselves, responsible for the cytotoxicity of the drug.[139-141] To date, no 5-AC has been detected as a metabolite of DH5-AC.[139] Both 5-AC and DH5-AC appear to have the same mechanism of action in relation to their incorporation, inhibition of synthesis, and methylation of nuclear RNA.[126,140] Their relative differences in relation to their incorporation and inhibition of synthesis of ribosomal RNA correlated well with their antitumor potencies.[141] Cytotoxic effects of both drugs were overcome by cytidine or uridine, and addition of thymidine potentiated their effect in L1210 cells in culture.[33] As substrates for UCK from HeLa cells, however, 5-AC appeared to be a better substrate than DH5-AC and, in L1210 cells, deoxycytidine was capable of enhancing the activity of 5-AC, but had no effect with DH5-AC.[33] 5-AC was also capable of inhibiting DNA methylation in mouse embryo cells, whereas DH5-AC was virtually devoid of activity.[142]

2. DH5-AC and THU

The reduced analog is definitely a substrate for CDA. However, the nature of its substrate properties appears to be more complex than those of cytidine and 5-AC. With the mouse kidney enzyme, DH5-AC binds to CDA with an affinity comparable to that of cytidine (K_ms 2.9×10^{-5} M and 4.2×10^{-5} M, respectively), which is significantly greater than the affinity for 5-AC ($K_m = 1.81 \times 10^{-3}$ M).[33] At saturating substrate concentrations, however, the V_{max} values showed that 5-AC was deaminated at about the same rate as cytidine and approximately ten times faster than DH5-AC.[33] A similar trend was observed for CDA from HeLa cells, where DH5-AC binding to the enzyme was superior to that of cytidine and tenfold better than 5-AC.[131] Nevertheless, at saturating substrate concentrations the relative rates of deamination were very similar and followed the order of cytidine >5-AC>DH5AC.[131] The results with the mouse kidney enzyme are in agreement with a mechanistic interpretation that predicts that DH5-AC should be a poorer substrate than either cytidine or 5-AC.[21]

Similarly, another laboratory has reported that, with the mouse kidney enzyme, DH5-AC is also a poor substrate for CDA and that it is capable of effectively inhibiting the deamination of cytidine.[143] Not surprisingly, the results of DH5-AC in combination with THU are widely different. With the mouse kidney enzyme, even at saturating THU concentrations that reduced 5-AC deamination to almost nil, significant deamination of DH5-AC still occurred.[33] On the contrary, in the HeLa cells the effect of THU appeared to be more pronounced in inhibiting DH5-AC deamination than 5-AC deamination. In this system, doses of 100 and 200 μM of DH5-AC, which were not inhibitory, completely arrested cell growth in the presence of 100 μM of THU.[131] A similar effect was not evidenced with 5-AC.[131] It is possible that since DH5-AC has a better affinity for CDA than either cytidine or 5-AC, it undergoes deamination faster at the lower concentrations typical of physiological conditions.[9,33] Recently it has been found that CDA from human liver does not deaminate DH5-AC to an appreciable extent.[144] In this context, it would be of interest to know whether CDA from human leukemic cells deaminates DH5-AC, as CDA from HeLa cells does. If this were the case, the combination of DH5-AC with THU in human leukemias would permit a direct evaluation of the consequences of inhibiting intracellular CDA from target tumor cells without the interference from inhibiting the host's systemic and liver deaminases. This could be a biochemical difference with a potential for enhancing selective toxicity towards the tumor cell. DH5-AC is currently being evaluated in clinical phase I trials, but its use in combination with THU awaits further experimentation.

D. Antiviral Agents

Deamination of deoxycytidine (d-cytidine) appears to be a limiting factor for its incorporation into DNA in both normal and malignant tissues. In the presence of THU, 5-^{3}H-d-cytidine incorporation into DNA was increased two- to threefold in three different mouse neoplasms.[145] Interestingly, identical results were obtained when THU was administered orally or i.p. to these tumor-bearing mice.[145] With different 5-substituted d-cytidines, however, the situation changed. While THU enhanced the incorporation of 5-F-d-cytidine, it completely blocked the incorporation of 5-bromo[6-^{3}H]-d-cytidine into the DNA of these cells.[145] These results suggested that in the absence of THU, incorporation of 5-bromo-d-cytidine proceeded via its deamination to 5-bromo-d-uridine, followed by phosphorylation through the action of thymidine kinase.[146] It indicated further that while the bulky 5-halo-d-cytidine analog was readily deaminated by CDA, it resisted direct phosphorylation by deoxycytidine kinase (dCK) in these cells. In fact, the K_m values for the mouse and human dCK enzyme varied more than 200-fold depending on the size of the 5-substituent.[146] Moreover, dCK from normal human lymphoid cells was found unable to phosphorylate 5-bromo-d-cytidine.[146] By contrast, in cells infected with herpes simplex viruses (HSV) a virus-induced pyrimidine nucleoside kinase catalyzed the phosphorylation of 5-bromo-d-cytidine as readily as that of d-cytidine and thymidine.[147] This increased affinity of the virus-induced kinase for 5-Br-d-cytidine, as opposed to the relatively poor affinity shown by the mammalian cytosol dCK and d-thymidine kinase, is responsible for the selective antiherpetic activity of the 5-halogenated analog.[145,148] This difference in substrate specificity was exploited even further when used in combination with THU. Since 5-iodo and 5-bromo-d-cytidine were not phosphorylated in mammalian cells, unless previously deaminated, THU completely blocked their incorporation into the DNA of normal cells while permitting incorporation of these metabolites in virus-infected cells. On this basis, when intracranial HSV-infections in mice were treated with 5-bromo-d-cytidine, with or without THU, long-term survivors were observed only in groups that received THU.[149] Specific inhibition of 5-^{125}I-d-cytidine deamination by THU has also permitted a rapid, sensitive, and specific assay for the HSV type I thymidine kinase (or viral pyrimidine kinase) in the presence of cellular thymidine kinase.[150] HSV-infected cells also failed to incorporate d-cytidine in their DNA; however, this lack of incorporation was not due to the cell's inability to phosphorylate d-cytidine, but rather to a very rapid deamination caused by an abundant virus-specified CDA.[5] THU at 10^{-5} M produced a tenfold increase in the incorporation of d-cytidine in these HSV-infected cells. However, THU at the same dose was unable to increase the inhibitory activity of ara-C as an antiviral agent. These results indicated that ara-C is possibly not metabolized in the same manner as d-cytidine in HSV-infected cells.[151] A recently developed antiviral agent 2'-fluoro-5-iodo-1-β-D-arabinofuranosyl cytosine (FIAC)[152] is also a substrate for CDA which is deaminated at a comparable rate to ara-C.[152] However, the deaminated product, FIAU, is also an effective antiviral and antitumor agent with greater cytotoxicity than that of FIAC. The presence of the 2'-F in the ara configuration confers the compound more resistance towards the deglycosylation and dehalogenation typical of other 5-halogenated pyrimidines.[152] In addition, FIAC is at least two orders of magnitude more potent against in vitro HSV type I than either 5-I-d-cytidine or 5-I-d-uridine.[152] THU was able to completely block the deamination of FIAC and could, in principle, improve its activity in view of the fact that FIAC has a better therapeutic index than FIAU.[152] The benefits of this association await to be ascertained.

VI. CONCLUSIONS

It is clear that inhibition of CDA has been and continues to be important as a biochemical tool in the study of the mechanism of action of antitumor agents susceptible to deamination. Clinically, combinations of ara-C with the potent but rapidly excreted THU permitted a reduction of the tolerable dose of ara-C by 30-fold. This effect, however, was purely pharmacokinetic and no improved therapeutic ratio was observed as compared to ara-C alone. In primate studies, although ara-C was not rapidly deaminated in CSF fluid, dose levels of intrathecally administered drug were maintained for a longer period of time in the presence of THU without apparent sign of toxicity. Preliminary in vitro studies with the more stable reduced analog of 5-AC suggested that concomitant use of THU may have a definitive advantage in the pharmacological action of DH5-AC. On the other hand, the level of inhibition of CDA accomplished with THU has been shown to be either transient or incomplete. Therefore, combination studies with the newer and more potent inhibitors of CDA are clearly warranted. Similarly, a reevaluation of the oral route for the administration of ara-C should be conducted in the presence of the new acid-stable CDA inhibitors in an effort to determine if longer and more reliable blood levels of ara-C could be obtained by this route. In the field of antiviral chemotherapy, inhibition of the deamination of 5-halo-d-cytidines, accomplished with THU, afforded selective protection to the host's cells against the lethal action of the deamination products of the drugs. This rationale could find similar applications with the newly developed antiviral agents such as FIAC. Strong inhibition of CDA per se may prove to be advantageous in conjunction with other antimetabolites which are not substrates for CDA. For example, in cell cultures of L1210, P388, S180, etc. pyrazofurin, an inhibitor of *de novo* pyrimidine biosynthesis, imposed an absolute requirement for uridine to maintain normal cell growth. Cytidine, if deaminated to uridine, could satisfy this demand, but in the presence of THU it was unable to sustain growth.[153] Finally, a CDA inhibitor capable of being effectively phosphorylated may exert important effects at higher levels by inhibiting d-cytidilate (dCMP) deaminase. This enzyme has been shown to be elevated in rapidly growing tissue and its activity has been correlated with the rate of tumor growth.[154,155] In this context, it appears to be a critical enzyme that provides much of the dUMP necessary for thymidilate synthetase. dCMP deaminase is allosterically activated by dCTP and dCDP as well as by ara-CTP, in ara-C sensitive cells.[156] This enzyme has been considered as an enzyme capable of playing a role in the development of resistance to ara-C and suitable inhibitors of this enzyme may be worth investigating. There are no data confirming whether or not THU is phosphorylated in vivo. Most likely it is not phosphorylated at all.[56] However, its deoxy analog d-THU, after being phosphorylated by a nucleotide phosphotransferase in chick embryo, behaved as a powerful inhibitor of dCMP deaminase (K_i = 1 to 2 × 10^{-8} M).[157] The development of CDA inhibitors capable of being phosphorylated by either dCK or UCK remains a challenge to the synthetic medicinal chemist. Such compounds may likewise inhibit other enzymes in the metabolic pathway. Mechanistically, the transition states for dCMP deaminase and CTP synthetase should be structurally very similar, and activity at both of these levels should not be unexpected. The weak CDA inhibitor 3-deazauridine is a good example, since once phosphorylated it is capable of inhibiting CTP synthetase very effectively.[158]

REFERENCES

1. **Wang, T. P., Sable, H. Z., and Lampen, J. O.,** Enzymatic deamination of cytosine nucleosides, *J. Biol. Chem.,* 184, 17, 1950.
2. **Ipata, P. L., Cercignani, G., and Balestreri, E.,** Partial purification and properties of cytidine deaminase from baker's yeast, *Biochemistry,* 9, 3390, 1970.
3. **Camiener, G. W. and Smith, C. G.,** Studies on the enzymatic deamination of cytosine arabinoside. I. Enzyme distribution and species specificity, *Biochem. Pharmacol.,* 14, 1405, 1965.
4. **Ho, D. H. W.,** Distribution of kinase and deaminase of 1-β-D-arabinofuranosylcytosine in tissues of man and mouse, *Cancer Res.,* 33, 2816, 1973.
5. **Chan, T.,** Induction of deoxycytidine deaminase activity in mammalian cells by infection with herpes simplex virus type 1, *Proc. Natl. Acad. Sci. U.S.A.,* 74, 1734, 1977.
6. **Dollinger, M. R., Burchenal, J. H., Kreis, W., and Fox, J. J.,** Analogs of 1-β-D-arabinofuranosylcytosine. Studies on mechanisms of action in Burkitt's cell culture and mouse leukemia, and *in vitro* deamination studies, *Biochem. Pharmacol.,* 16, 689, 1967.
7. **Furner, R. L. and Mellet, L. B.,** Kinase and deaminase activity in a variety of subcutaneous mouse tumors, *Cancer Res.,* 35, 1799, 1975.
8. **Kreis, W., Hession, C., Soricelli, A., and Scully, K.,** Combinations of tetrahydrouridine and cytosine arabinoside in mouse tumors, *Cancer Treat. Rep.,* 61, 1355, 1977.
9. **Futterman, B., Derr, J., Beisler, J. A., Abbasi, M., and Voytek, P.,** Studies on the cytostatic action, phosphorylation and deamination of 5-azacytidine and 5,6-dihydro-5-azacytidine in HeLa cells, *Biochem. Pharmacol.,* 27, 907, 1978.
10. **Ipata, P. L. and Cercignani, G.,** Cytosine and cytidine deaminase from yeast, *Meth. Enzymol.* 51, 394, 1978.
11. **Wentworth, D. F. and Wolfenden, R.,** Cytidine deaminases (from *E. coli* and human liver), *Meth. Enzymol.,* 51, 401, 1978.
12. **Camiener, G. W.,** Studies on the enzymatic deamination of cytosine arabinoside. III. Substrate requirements and inhibitors of the deaminase of human liver, *Biochem. Pharmacol.,* 16, 1691, 1967.
13. **Schroeder, A. C., Hughes, R. G., Jr., and Bloch, A.,** Synthesis and biological effects of acyclic pyrimidin nucleoside analogs, *J. Med. Chem.,* 24, 1078, 1981.
14. **Nemec, J., Rhoades, J. M., Tinsley, P. W., and Germain, G. S.,** Abstr. 5th Int. Round Table, Nucleosides, Nucleotides and their Biological Applications, Research Triangle Park, N.C., 1982, 37.
15. **McCormack, J. J.,** personal communication.
16. **Tolman, R. L. and Robins, R. K.,** Synthesis of 1-β-L-arabinofuranosylcytosine, the enantiomer of cytosine arabinoside, *J. Med. Chem.,* 14, 1112, 1971.
17. **Brockman, R. W., Carpenter, J. W., O'Dell, C. A., Shealy, Y. F., and Bennett, L. L., Jr.,** Metabolism and mechanism of action of the carbocyclic analog of cytidine, *Fed. Proc.,* 37, 234, 1978.
18. **Kreis, W., Watanabe, K. A., and Fox, J. J.,** Structural requirements for the enzymatic deamination of cytosine nucleosides, *Helv. Chim. Acta,* 61, 1011, 1978.
19. **Krajewska, E. and Shugar, D.,** Alkylated cytosine nucleosides: substrate and inhibitor properties in enzymatic deamination, *Acta Biochim. Pol.,* 22, 185, 1975.
20. **Cheng, Y. C., Derse, D., Tan, R. S., Dutschman, G., Bobek, M., Schroeder, A., and Bloch, A.,** Biological and biochemical effects of 2'-azido-2'-deoxyarabinofuranosylcytosine on human tumor cells *in vitro, Cancer Res.,* 41, 3144, 1981.

21. **Watanabe, K. A., Reichman, V., Fox, J. J., and Chou, T. C.,** Nucleosides. CXIX. Substrate specificity and mechanism of action of cytidine deaminases of monkey plasma and mouse kidney, *Chem. Biol. Interact.,* 37, 41, 1981.

22. **Ruyle, W. V. and Shen, T. Y.,** Nucleosides. V. 2-Thio-pyrimidine β-D-arabinofuranosides, *J. Med. Chem.,* 10, 331, 1967.

23. **Bremerskov, V., Kaden, P., and Mittermayer, C.,** DNA synthesis during the life cycle of L cells: morphological histochemical and biochemical investigations with arabinofuranosylcytosine and thioarabinosylcytosine, *Eur. J. Cancer,* 6, 379, 1970.

24. **Drake, J. C., Hande, K. R., Fuller, R. W., and Chabner, B. A.,** Cytidine and deoxycytidylate deaminase inhibition by uridine analogs, *Biochem. Pharmacol.,* 29, 807, 1980.

25. **McCormack, J. J., Marquez, V. E., Liu, P. S., Vistica, D. T., and Driscoll, J. S.,** Inhibition of cytidine deaminase by 2-oxopyrimidine riboside and related compounds, *Biochem. Pharmacol.,* 29, 830, 1980.

26. **Cohen, R. M. and Wolfenden, R.,** The equilibrium of hydrolytic deamination of cytidine and N^4-methylcytidine, *J. Biol. Chem.,* 246, 7566, 1971.

27. **Leung, K. K. and Visser, D. W.,** A new deoxycytidine analog, 5-hydroxy-2′-deoxycytidine, *Biochem. Med.,* 9, 237, 1974.

28. **Chabner, B. A., Drake, J. C., and Johns, D. G.,** Deamination of 5-azacytidine by human leukemia cell cytidine deaminase, *Biochem. Pharmacol.,* 22, 2763, 1973.

29. **Schweizer, M. P., Banta, E. B., Witkowski, J. T., and Robins, R. K.,** Determination of nucleoside syn, anti conformational preference in solution by proton and carbon-13 nuclear magnetic resonance, *J. Am. Chem. Soc.,* 95, 3770, 1973.

30. **Singh, P. and Hodgson, D. J.,** Aza analogs of nucleic acid constituents. III. The molecular structure of 6-azacytidine, *J. Am. Chem. Soc.,* 96, 1239, 1974.

31. **Wentford, D. F. and Wolfenden, R.,** On the interaction of 3,4,5,6-tetrahydrouridine with human liver cytidine deaminase, *Biochemistry,* 14, 5099, 1975.

32. **Evans, B. E., Mitchell, J. N., and Wolfenden, R.,** The action of bacterial cytidine deaminase on 5,6-dihydrocytidine, *Biochemistry,* 14, 621, 1975.

33. **Voytek, P., Beisler, J. A., Abbasi, M. M., and Wolpert-DeFilippes, M. K.,** Comparative studies of the cytostatic action and metabolism of 5-aza-cytidine and 5,6-dihydro-5-azacytidine, *Cancer Res.,* 37, 1956, 1977.

34. **Cohen, R. M. and Wolfenden, R.,** Cytidine deaminase from *Escherichia coli.* Purification, properties and inhibition by the potential transition-state analog 3,4,5,6-tetrahydrouridine, *J. Biol. Chem.,* 246, 7561, 1971.

35. **Tomchick, R., Saslaw, L. D., and Waravdekar, V. S.,** Mouse kidney cytidine deaminase. Purification and properties, *J. Biol. Chem.,* 243, 2534, 1968.

36. **Sanchez, R. A. and Orgel, L. E.,** Studies in prebiotic synthesis. V. Synthesis and photoanomerization of pyrimidine nucleosides, *J. Mol. Biol.,* 47, 531, 1970.

37. **Shapiro, R. and Klein, R. S.,** Reactions of cytosine derivatives with acid buffer solutions. Studies on transamination, deamination and deuterium exchange, *Biochemistry,* 6, 3576, 1967.

38. **Notari, R. E.,** A mechanism for the hydrolytic deamination of cytosine arabinoside in aqueous buffer, *J. Pharm. Sci.,* 67, 804, 1967.

39. **Wechter, W. J.,** Nucleic acid. VII. Specific deuterium labelling of nucleosides, nucleotides, and oligonucleotides and mechanistic consequences thereof, *Coll. Czech. Chem. Commun.,* 35, 2003, 1970.

40. **Wolfenden, R.,** Analog approaches to the structure of the transition-state in enzyme reactions, *Acc. Chem. Res.,* 5, 10, 1972.

41. **Evans, B. and Wolfenden, R.,** A potential transition state analog for adenosine deaminase, *J. Am. Chem. Soc.,* 92, 4751, 1970.

42. **Slae, S. and Shapiro, R.,** Kinetics and mechanism of the deamination of 1-methyl-5,6-dihydrocytosine, *J. Org. Chem.,* 43, 1721, 1978.

43. **Stoller, R. G., Myers, C. E., and Chabner, B. A.,** Analysis of cytidine deaminase and tetrahydrouridine interactions by use of ligand techniques, *Biochem. Pharmacol.,* 27, 53, 1978.

44. **Rothman, I. K., Malathi, V. G., and Silber, R.,** Cytidine deaminase from leukemic mouse spleen, *Meth. Enzymol.,* 51, 408, 1978.

45. **Lee, S. H., Chao, D. L., Bear, J. L., and Kimball, A. P.,** Inhibition of deamination of arabinosylcytosine (NSC-63878) by rhodium (II) acetate, *Cancer Chemother. Rep.,* 59, 661, 1975.

46. **Camiener, G. W. and Tao, R. V.,** Studies of the enzymatic deamination of ara-cytidine. IV. Inhibition by an acridine analog and organic solvents, *Biochem. Pharmacol.,* 17, 1411, 1968.

47. **Hanze, A. R.,** Nucleic acids. IV. The catalytic reduction of pyrimidine nucleosides (human liver deaminase inhibitors), *J. Am. Chem. Soc.,* 89, 6720, 1967.

48. **Chabner, B. A., Johns, D. G., Coleman, N. C., Drake, J. C., and Evans, W. H.,** Purification and properties of cytidine deaminase from normal and leukemic granulocytes, *J. Clin. Invest.,* 53, 922, 1974.

49. **Furner, R. L. and Mellett, L. B.,** Inhibition of deamination of ^{14}C-cytosine arabinoside (NSC-63879): a useful biologic assay for tetrahydrouridine (NSC-112907), *Cancer Chemother. Rep.,* 59, 717, 1975.

50. **Schroeder, A. C., Srikrishnan, T., Parthasarathy, R., and Bloch, A.,** Synthesis of 4-beta-D-arabino-furanosyl-5,6-dihydro-2H-1,2,4-thiadiazin-3-one 1,1-dioxide and X-ray diffraction analysis of its 2′,3′-anhydro precursor, *J. Heterocycl. Chem.,* 18, 571, 1981.

51. **Ashley, G. W. and Bartlett, P. A.,** A phosphorus-containing pyrimidine analog as a potent inhibitor of cytidine deaminase, *Biochem. Biophys. Res. Commun.,* 108, 1467, 1982.

52. **Kreis, W. and Hession, C.,** Enzyme distribution and combination chemotherapy studies with 1-β-D-arabinofuranosylcytosine (ara-C) plus tetrahydrouridine (THU) in four animal neoplasms, *Proc. Am. Assoc. Cancer Res.,* 17, 83, 1976.

53. **El Dareer, S. M., White, V., Chen, F. P., Mellet, B. L., and Hill, D. L.,** Distribution of tetrahydrouridine in experimental animals, *Cancer Treat. Rep.,* 60, 1627, 1976.

54. **Kreis, W., Woodcock, T. M., Gordon, C. S., and Krakoff, I. H.,** Tetrahydrouridine: physiologic disposition and effect upon deamination of cytosine arabinoside in man, *Cancer Treat. Rep.,* 61, 1347, 1977.

55. **Kelley, J. A., Marquez, V. E., and Driscoll, J. S.,** The furanose-pyranose isomerization of reduced pyrimidine and 1,3-diazepin-2-one nucleosides, Pap. 107, 12th NE Reg. Meet. Am. Chem. Soc., University of Vermont, Burlington, June 1982.

56. **Ho, D. H. W., Bodey, G. P., Sr., Hall, S. W., Benjamin, R. S., Brown, N. S., Freireich, E. J., and Loo, T. L.,** Clinical pharmacology of tetrahydrouridine, *J. Clin. Pharmacol.,* 18, 259, 1978.

57. **Neil, G. L., Moxley, T., and Manak, R. C.,** Enhancement by tetrahydrouridine of 1-β-D-arabinofuranosylcytosine (cytarabine) oral activity in L1210 leukemic mice, *Cancer Res.,* 30, 2166, 1970.

58. **Katritzky, A. R., Kingsland, M., and Tee, O. S.,** Covalent hydration in simple pyrimidines: evidence from kinetics of hydrogen exchange, *Chem. Commun.,* 289, 1968.

59. **Albert, A.,** Covalent hydration in nitrogen heterocycles, *Adv. Heterocycl. Chem.,* 20, 117, 1976.

60. **Tee, O. S. and Paventi, M.,** Kinetics and mechanism of the reaction of 2(1H)-pyrimidinone with bromine. Reaction via its covalent hydrate, *J. Org. Chem.,* 45, 2072, 1980.

61. **Marquez, V. E.,** unpublished results.

62. **Furner, R. L., Mellet, L. B., and Herren, T. C.,** Influence of tetrahydrouridine on the phosphorylation of 1-β-D-arabinofuranosyl-cytosine (ara-c) by enzymes from solid tumors, *in vitro, J. Pharmacol. Exp. Ther.,* 194, 103, 1975.

63. **Goldenthal, E. I., Cookson, K. M., Geil, R. G., and Wazeter, F. X.,** Preclinical toxicologic evaluation of tetrahydrouridine (NSC-112907) in beagle dogs and rhesus monkeys, *Cancer Chemother. Rep.,* Suppl. 5, 15, 1974.

64. **Agarwal, R. P., Spector, T., and Parks, R. E., Jr.,** Tight-binding inhibitors. IV. Inhibition of adenosine deaminases by various inhibitors, *Biochem. Pharmacol.,* 26, 359, 1977.

65. **Nakamura, H., Koyama, G., Iitaka, Y., Ohno, M., Yagisawa, N., Kondo, S., Maeda, K., and Umezawa, H.,** Structure of coformycin, an unusual nucleoside of microbial origin, *J. Am. Chem. Soc.,* 96, 4327, 1974.

66. **Marquez, V. E., Liu, P. S., Kelley, J. A., Driscoll, J. S., and McCormack, J. J.,** Synthesis of 1,3-diazepin-2-one nucleosides as transition-state inhibitors of cytidine deaminase, *J. Med. Chem.,* 23, 713, 1980.

67. **Liu, P. S., Marquez, V. E., Kelley, J. A., and Driscoll, J. S.,** Synthesis of 1,3-diazepin-2-one nucleosides as transition-state inhibitors of cytidine deaminase. II, *J. Org. Chem.,* 45, 5225, 1980.

68. **Liu, P. S., Marquez, V. E., Driscoll, J. S., Fuller, R. W., and McCormack, J. J.,** Cyclic urea nucleosides. Cytidine deaminase activity as a function of ring size, *J. Med. Chem.,* 24, 662, 1981.

69. **Marquez, V. E. and McCormack, J. J.,** unpublished results.

70. **Evans, J. S., Musser, E. A., Bostwick, L., and Mengel, G. D.,** The effect of 1-β-D-arabinofuranosyl-cytosine hydrochloride on murine neoplasms, *Cancer Res.,* 24, 1285, 1964.

71. **Ellison, R. R., Holland, J. F., Weil, M., Jacquillat, C., Boiron, M., Bernard, J., Sawitsky, A., Rosner, F., Gussoff, B., Silver, R. T., Karanas, A., Cuttner, J., Spurr, C. L., Hayes, D. M., Blom, J., Leone, L. A., Haurani, F., Kyle, R., Hutchison, J. L., Forcier, R. J., and Moon, J. H.,** Arabinosyl cytosine: a useful agent in the treatment of acute leukemia in adults, *Blood,* 32, 507, 1968.

72. **Underwood, G. E.,** Activity of 1-β-D-arabinofuranosyl cytosine hydrochloride against herpes simplex keratitis, *Proc. Soc. Exp. Biol. (N.Y.),* 111, 660, 1967.

73. **Mitchell, M. S., Wade, M. E., DeConti, R. C., Bertino, J. R., and Calabresi, P.,** Immunosuppressive effects of cytosine arabinoside and methotrexate in man, *Ann. Intern. Med.,* 70, 535, 1969.

74. **Skipper, H. E., Schabel, F. M., Jr., Mellet, L. B., Montgomery, J. A., Wilkoff, L. J., Lloyd, H. H., and Brockman, R. W.,** Implications of biochemical, cytokinetic, pharmacologic, and toxicologic relationships in the design of optimal therapeutic studies, *Cancer Chemother. Rep.,* 54, 431, 1970.

75. **Bodey, G. P., Freireich, E. J., Monto, R. W., and Hewlett, J. S.,** Cytosine arabinoside (NSC 63878) therapy for acute leukemia in adults, *Cancer Chemother. Rep.,* 53, 59, 1969.

76. **Talley, R. W. and Frei, E., III,** Summary of clinical experience with cytosine arabinoside, *Arzneim. Forsch.,* 18, 93, 1968.

77. **Creasey, W. A., Papac, R. J., Markin, M. E., Calabresi, P., and Welch, A.,** Biochemical and pharmacological studies with 1-β-D-arabinofuranosylcytosine in man, *Biochem. Pharmacol.,* 15, 1417, 1966.

78. **Ho, D. H. W. and Frei, E., III,** Clinical pharmacology of 1-β-D-arabinofuranosylcytosine, *Clin. Pharmacol. Ther.,* 12, 944, 1971.

79. **Kessel, D., Hall, T. C., and Rosenthal, D.,** Uptake and phosphorylation of cytosine arabinoside by normal and leukemic human blood cells *in vitro, Cancer Res.,* 29, 459, 1969.

80. **Furth, J. J. and Cohen, S. S.,** Inhibition of mammalian DNA polymerase by the 5'-triphosphate of 1-β-D-arabinofuranosylcytosine and the 5'-triphosphate of 9-β-D-arabinofuranosyladenine, *Cancer Res.,* 28, 2061, 1968.

81. **Chu, M. Y. and Fischer, G. A.,** A proposed mechanism of action of 1-β-D-arabinofuranosylcytosine as an inhibitor of the growth of leukemic cells, *Biochem. Pharmacol.,* 11, 423, 1962.

82. **Coleman, C. N., Stoller, R. G., Drake, J. C., and Chabner, B. A.,** Deoxycytidine kinase: properties of the enzyme from human leukemic granulocytes, *Blood,* 46, 791, 1975.

83. **Harris, A. L. and Grahame-Smith, D. G.,** Cytosine arabinoside triphosphate production in human leukemic myeloblasts: interaction with deoxycytidine, *Cancer Chemother. Pharmacol.,* 5, 185, 1981.

84. **Kozai, Y. and Sugino, Y.,** Enzymatic phosphorylation of 1-β-D-arabinofuranosylcytosine, *Cancer Res.,* 31, 1376, 1971.

85. **Handke, K. R. and Chabner, B. A.,** Pyrimidine nucleoside monophosphate kinase from human leukemic blast cells, *Cancer Res.,* 35, 579, 1978.

86. **Chou, T. C., Arlin, Z., Clarkson, B. D., and Philips, F. S.,** Metabolism of 1-β-D-arabinofuranosylcytosine in human leukemic cells, *Cancer Res.,* 37, 3561, 1977.

87. **Ho, D. H. W., Carter, C. J., Brown, N. S., Hester, J., McKredie, K., Benjamin, R. S., Freireich, E. J., and Bodey, G. P.,** Effects of tetrahydrouridine on the uptake and metabolism of 1-β-arabinofuranosylcytosine in human and leukemic cells, *Cancer Res.,* 40, 2441, 1980.

88. **Harris, A. L., Grahame-Smith, D. G., Potter, C. G., and Bunch, C.,** Cytosine arabinoside deamination in human leukemic myeloblasts and resistance to cytosine arabinoside therapy, *Clin. Sci.,* 60, 191, 1981.

89. **Chu, M. Y. and Fischer, G. A.,** Comparative studies of leukemic cells sensitive and resistant to cytosine arabinoside, *Biochem. Pharmacol.,* 14, 333, 1965.

90. **Steuart, C. D. and Burke, P. J.,** Cytidine deaminase and the development of resistance to cytosine arabinoside, *Nature New Biol.,* 233, 109, 1971.

91. **Smyth, J. F., Robins, A. B., and Leese, C. L.,** The metabolism of cytosine arabinoside as a predictive test for clinical response to the drug in acute myeloid leukemia, *Eur. J. Cancer,* 12, 567, 1976.

92. **Tattersall, M. H. N., Ganeshagurn, K., and Hoffbrand, A. V.,** Mechanism of resistance of human acute leukemia cells to cytosine arabinoside, *Br. J. Haematol.,* 27, 39, 1974.

93. **Rustum, Y. M.,** Metabolism and intracellular retention of 1-β-arabinofuranosylcytosine as predictors of response to animal tumors, *Cancer Res.,* 38, 543, 1978.

94. **Kessel, D., Hall, T. C., and Rosenthal, D.,** Uptake and phosphorylation of cytosine arabinoside by normal and leukemic human blood cells in vitro, *Cancer Res.,* 29, 459, 1969.

95. **Rustum, Y. M. and Preisler, H. D.,** Correlation between leukemic cell retention of 1-β-D-arabinofuranosylcytosine 5'-triphosphate and response to therapy, *Cancer Res.,* 39, 42, 1979.

96. **de Saint Vincent, B. R. and Buttin, G.,** Studies on 1-β-D-arabinofuranosyl cytosine-resistant mutants of Chinese hamster fibroblasts. IV. Altered regulation of CTP synthetase generates arabinosylcytosine and thymidine resistance, *Biochem. Biophys. Acta,* 610, 352, 1980.

97. **Ives, D. H. and Durham, J. P.,** Deoxycytidine kinase. III. Kinetics and allosteric regulation of the calf thymus enzyme, *J. Biol. Chem.,* 245, 2285, 1970.

98. **Handke, K. R. and Chabner, B. A.,** Pyrimidine nucleoside monophosphate kinase from human leukemic blast cells, *Cancer Res.,* 38, 579, 1978.

99. **Stoller, R. G., Coleman, C. N., Chang, P., Hande, K. R., and Chabner, B. A.,** Biochemical pharmacology of cytidine analog metabolism in human leukemic cells, *Bibl. Haematol.,* 43, 531, 1976.

100. **Coleman, C. N., Johns, D. G., and Chabner, B. A.,** Studies on mechanisms of resistance of cytosine arabinoside: problems in the determination of related enzyme activities in leukemic cells, *Ann. N.Y. Acad. Sci.,* 255, 247, 1975.

101. **Harris, A. L.,** Correspondence re: D. H. W. Ho, C. J. Carter, N. S. Brown, J. Hester K. McKredie, R. S. Benjamin, E. J. Freireich, and G. P. Bodey. Effects of tetrahydrouridine on the uptake and metabolism of 1-β-D-arabinofuranosylcytosine in human normal and leukemic cells, *Cancer Res.,* 40, 2441, 1980; *Cancer Res.,* 41, 2977, 1981.

102. **Ho, D. H.,** Correspondence re: D. H. W. Ho et al., *Cancer Res.,* 40, 2441, 1981; *Cancer Res.,* 41, 2978, 1981.

103. **Ho, D. H. W.,** Potential advances in the clinical use of arabinosyl cytosine, *Cancer Treat. Rep.,* 61, 717, 1977.

104. **Theiss, J. C. and Fischer, G. A.,** Inhibition of intracellular pyrimidine ribonucleotide reductase by deoxycytidine, arabinosylcytosine and hydroxyurea, *Biochem. Pharmacol.,* 25, 73, 1976.

105. **Walsh, C. T., Craig, R. W., and Agarwal, R. P.,** Increased activation of 1-β-D-arabinofuranosylcytosine by hydroxyurea in L1210 cells, *Fed. Proc.,* 38, 370, 1979.

106. **Kinnahan, J. J., Kowal, E. P., and Grindey, G. B.,** Biochemical and antitumor effects of the combination of thymidine and 1-β-D-arabinofuranosylcytosine against leukemia L1210, *Cancer Res.,* 41, 445, 1981.

107. **Mills-Yamamoto, C., Lanzon, G. J., and Paterson, A. R.,** Toxicity of combinations of arabinosylcytosine and 3-deazauridine toward neoplastic cells in culture, *Biochem. Pharmacol.,* 27, 181, 1978.

108. **Chabner, B. A., Hande, K. R., and Drake, J. C.,** Ara-C metabolism: implications for drug resistance and drug interactions, *Bull. Cancer (Paris),* 66, 89, 1979.

109. **Barlogie, B., Plunkett, W., Raber, M., Latrielle, J., Keating, M., and McCredie, K.,** In vivo cellular kinetic and pharmacological studies of 1-β-D-arabinofuranosylcytosine and 3-deazauridine chemotherapy for relapsing acute leukemia, *Cancer Res.,* 41, 1227, 1981.

110. **Wan, C. W. and Mak, T. W.,** Effect of tetrahydrouridine on the action of 1-β-D-arabinofuranosylcytosine in synchronized cultures of normal rat kidney cells, *Cancer Res.,* 39, 3981, 1979.

111. **Camiener, G. W.,** Studies on the enzymatic deamination of ara-cytidine. V. Inhibition *in vitro* and *in vivo* by tetrahydrouridine and other reduced pyrimidine nucleosides, *Biochem. Pharmacol.,* 17, 1981, 1968.

112. **El Dareer, S. M., Mulligen, Jr., L. T., White, V., Tillery, K., Mellet, L. B., and Hill, D. L.,** Distribution of ³H-cytosine arabinoside and its products in mice, dogs, and monkeys and effect of tetrahydrouridine, *Cancer Treat. Rep.,* 61, 395, 1977.

113. **Marquez, V. E. and Vistica, D.,** unpublished results.

114. **Riccardi, R., Chabner, B., Glaubiger, D. L., Wood, J., and Poplack, D. G.,** Influence of tetrahydrouridine on the pharmacokinetics of intrathecally administered 1-β-D-arabinofuranosylcytosine, *Cancer Res.,* 42, 1736, 1982.

115. **Wong, P. P., Currie, V. E., Mackey, R. W., Krakoff, I. H., Tan, C. T. C., Burchenal, J. H., and Young, C. W.,** Phase I evaluation of tetrahydrouridine combined with cytosine arabinoside, *Cancer Treat. Rep.,* 63, 1245, 1979.

116. **Loo, T. L., Ho, D. H. W., Bodey, G. P., and Freireich, E. J.,** Pharmacological and clinical studies of some nucleoside analogs, *Ann. N.Y. Acad. Sci.,* 255, 252, 1975.

117. **Ryu, E. K., Ross, R. J., Matsushita, J., MacCoss, M., Hong, C. I., and West, C. R.,** Phospholipid-nucleoside conjugates. III. Syntheses and preliminary biological evaluation of 1-β-D-arabinofuranosylcytosine 5′-monophosphate-L-1,2-dipalmitin and selected 1-β-D-arabinofuranosylcytosine 5′-diphosphate-L-1,2-diacylglycerols, *J. Med. Chem.,* 25, 1322, 1982.

118. **Piskala, A. and Sorm, F.,** Nucleic acid components and their analogs. LI. Synthesis of 1-glycosyl derivatives of 5-azauracil and 5-azacytosine, *Coll. Czech. Chem. Commun.,* 29, 1060, 1964.

119. **Jarovicik, M., Raska, K., Sormova, C., and Sorm, F.,** Anabolic transformation of a novel metabolite, 5-azacytidine and evidence for its incorporation into nucleic acids, *Coll. Czech. Chem. Commun.,* 30, 3370, 1965.

120. **Lomen, P. L., Baker, L. H., Neil, G. L., and Samson, M. K.,** Phase I study of 5-azacytidine (NSC 102816) using 24-hour continuous infusion for 5 days, *Cancer Chemother. Rep.,* 59(1), 1121, 1975.

121. **Weiss, A. J., Metter, G. E., Nealon, T. E., Keanan, J. P., Ramirez, G., Swaminatha, A., Fletcher, W. S., Moss, S. E., and Manther, R. W.,** Phase II study of 5-azacytidine in solid tumors, *Cancer Treat. Rep.,* 61, 55, 1977.

122. **Cihak, A.,** Biological effects of 5-azacytidine in eukaryotes, *Oncology (Basel),* 30, 405, 1974.

123. **Li, L. H., Olin, E. J., Buskirk, H. H., and Reineke, L. M.,** Cytotoxicity and mode of action of 5-azacytidine on L1210 leukemia, *Cancer Res.,* 30, 2760, 1970.

124. **Reichman, M., Karlan, H., and Penman, S.,** Destructive processing of the 45S ribosomal precursor in the presence of 5-azacytidine, *Biochim. Biophys. Acta,* 299, 173, 1973.

125. **Lu, L. J. W. and Randerath, K.,** Effects of 5-azacytidine in transfer RNA methyl transferase, *Cancer Res.,* 39, 940, 1979.

126. **Glazer, R. I., Peale, A. L., Reisler, J. A., and Abbasi, M.,** The effect of 5-azacytidine and dihydro-5-azacytidine on nuclear ribosomal RNA and poly(A)RNA synthesis in L1210 cells *in vitro, Mol. Pharmacol.,* 17, 111, 1980.

127. **Vesely, J. and Cihak, A.,** 5-Azacytidine: mechanism of action and biological effects in mammalian cells, *Pharmacol. Ther.,* 2, 813, 1978.

128. **Lee, T., Karon, M., and Momparler, R.,** Kinetic studies on phosphorylation of 5-azacytidine with purified uridine-cytidine kinase from calf thymus, *Cancer Res.,* 34, 2482, 1974.

129. **Vadlamudi, S., Choudry, J. N., and Waravdekar, V. S.,** Effect of combination treatment with 5-azacytidine and cytidine on the life span and spleen and bone marrow cells of leukemic (L1210) and nonleukemic mice, *Cancer Res.,* 30, 362, 1970.

130. **Plagemann, P. G. W., Behrens, M., and Abraham, D.,** Metabolism and cytotoxicity of 5-azacytidine in cultured Novikoff rat hepatoma and P388 mouse leukemia cells and their enhancement by preincubation with pyrazofurin, *Cancer Res.,* 38, 2458, 1978.

131. **Futterman, B., Derr, J., Reisler, J. A., Abbasi, M. M., and Voytek, P.,** Studies on the cytostatic action, phosphorylation and deamination of 5-azacytidine and 5,6-dihydro-5-azacytidine in HeLa cells, *Biochem. Pharmacol.,* 27, 907, 1978.

132. **Drake, J. C., Stoller, R. G., and Chabner, B. A.,** Characteristics of the enzyme uridine-cytidine kinase isolated from a cultured human cell line, *Biochem. Pharmacol.,* 26, 64, 1977.

133. **Kelly, C. J., Gaudio, L., Yesair, D. W., Schoenemann, P. T., and Wodinsky, I.,** Pharmacokinetic considerations in evaluating the effects of tetrahydrouridine on 5-azacytidine chemotherapy in L1210 leukemic mice, *Cancer Treat. Rep.,* 62, 1025, 1978.

134. **Neil, G. L., Moxley, T. E., Kuentzel, S. L., Manak, R. C., and Hanka, L. J.,** Enhancement by tetrahydrouridine (NSC-112907) of the oral activity of 5-azacytidine (NSC-102816) in L-1210 leukemic mice, *Cancer Chemother. Rep.,* 59, 459, 1975.

135. **Beisler, J. A.,** Isolation, characterization and properties of a labile hydrolysis product of the antitumor nucleoside, 5-azacytidine, *J. Med. Chem.,* 21, 204, 1978.

136. **Grant, S., Rauscher, F. R., III, Jakubowski, A., and Cadman, E.,** Effect of *N*-(phosphonoacetyl)-L-aspartate on 5-azacytidine metabolism in P388 and L1210 cells, *Cancer Res.,* 41, 410, 1981.

137. **Grant, S. and Cadman, E.,** Altered 5-azacytidine metabolism following 3-deazauridine treatment of L5178Y cells, *Proc. Am. Fed. Clin. Res.,* 27, 385a, 1979.

138. **Beisler, J. A., Abbasi, M. M., Kelley, J. A., and Driscoll, J. S.,** Synthesis and antitumor activity of dihydro-5-azacytidine, an hydrolytically stable analog of 5-azacytidine, *J. Med. Chem.,* 20, 806, 1977.

139. **Malspeis, L. and DeSouza, J. J. V.,** Metabolism and elimination of 5,6-dihydro-5-azacytidine (NSC 264880, DHAC) by the rat, *Proc. Am. Assoc. Cancer Res.,* 22, 219, 1981.

140. **Glazer, R. I. and Hartman, K. D.,** The comparative effects of 5-aza-cytidine and dihydro-5-azacytidine on 4S and 5S nuclear RNA, *Mol. Pharmacol.,* 17, 250, 1980.

141. **Lin, H. L. and Glazer, R. I.,** The comparative effects of 5-aza-cytidine and dihydro-5-azacytidine on polysomal RNA in Erlich ascites cells *in vitro, Mol. Pharmacol.,* 20, 644, 1981.

142. **Jones, P. A. and Taylor, S. M.,** Cellular differentiation, cytidine analogs and DNA methylation, *Cell,* 20, 85, 1980.

143. **McCormack, J. J. and Mathews, L. A.,** Interaction of 5,6-dihydro-5-azacytidine with cytidine deaminase as a basis for analytical studies, *Proc. Am. Assoc. Cancer Res.,* 23, 210, 1982.

144. **McCormack, J. J.,** personal communication.

145. **Cooper, G. M. and Greer, S.,** The effect of inhibition of cytidine deaminase by tetrahydrouridine on the utilization of deoxycytidine analogs by deoxycytidine and 5-bromodeoxycytidine for deoxyribonucleic acid synthesis, *Mol. Pharmacol.,* 9, 698, 1973.

146. **Cooper, G. M. and Greer, S.,** Phosphorylation of 5-halogenated deoxycytidine kinase, *Mol. Pharmacol.,* 9, 704, 1973.

147. **Dobersen, M. J. and Greer, S.,** Herpes simplex virus type 2 induced pyrimidine nucleoside kinase: enzymatic basis for the selective antiherpetic effect of 5-halogenated analogs of deoxycytidine, *Biochemistry,* 17, 920, 1978.

148. **Lee, L. S. and Cheng, Y.,** Human deoxythymidine kinase II: substrate specificity and kinetic behavior of the cytoplasmic and mitochondrial isozymes derived from blast cells of acute myelocytic leukemia, *Biochemistry,* 15, 3686, 1976.

149. **Greer, S., Schildkraut, I., Zimmerman, T., and Kaufman, H.,** 5-Halogenated analogs of deoxycytidine as selective inhibitors of the replication of herpes simplex viruses in cell culture and related studies of intracranial herpes simplex virus infections in mice, *Ann. N.Y. Acad. Sci.,* 255, 359, 1975.

150. **Summers, W. C. and Summers, W. P.,** [^{125}I]-deoxycytidine used in a rapid, sensitive, and specific assay for herpes simplex virus type I thymidine kinase, *J. Virol.,* 24, 314, 1977.

151. **North, T. W. and Mathews, C. K.,** Tetrahydrouridine specifically facilitates deoxycytidine incorporation into herpes simplex virus DNA, *J. Virol.,* 37, 987, 1981.

152. **Chou, T. C., Feinberg, A., Grant, A. J., Vidal, P., Reichman, U., Watanabe, K. A., Fox, J. J., and Philips, F. S.,** Pharmacological disposition and metabolic fate of 2'-fluoro-5-iodo-1-β-D-arabinofuranosylcytosine in mice and rats, *Cancer Res.,* 41, 3336, 1981.

153. **Cadman, E. and Benz, C.,** Uridine and cytidine metabolism following inhibition of *de novo* pyrimidine synthesis by pyrazofurin, *Biochim. Biophys. Acta,* 609, 372, 1980.

154. **Maley, F. and Maley, G. F.,** Nucleotide interconversions. II. Elevation of deoxycytidylate deaminase and thymidylate synthetase in regenerating rat liver, *J. Biol. Chem.,* 235, 2968, 1960.

155. **Maley, F. and Maley, G. F.,** Nucleotide interconversions. IV. Activities of deoxycytidylate deaminase and thymidylate synthetase in normal rat liver and hepatomas, *Cancer Res.,* 21, 1421, 1961.

156. **George, C. B. and Cory, J. O.,** Activation of deoxycytidylate deaminase by 1-β-D-arabinofuranosylcytosine-5'-triphosphate, *Biochem. Pharmacol.,* 28, 1699, 1979.

157. **Maley, F. and Maley, G. F.,** Tetrahydrodeoxyuridylate: a potent inhibitor of deoxycytidylate deaminase, *Arch. Biochem. Biophys.,* 144, 723, 1971.
158. **McPartland, R. P., Wang, M. C., Bloch, A., and Weinfeld, H.,** Cytidine 5'-triphosphate synthetase as a target for inhibition by the antitumor agent 3-deazauridine, *Cancer Res.,* 34, 3107, 1974.

Chapter 5

METABOLIC AND MECHANISTIC STUDIES WITH TIAZOFURIN (2-β-D-RIBOFURANOSYLTHIAZOLE-4-CARBOXAMIDE)

Hiremagalur N. Jayaram and David G. Johns

TABLE OF CONTENTS

I. INTRODUCTION

In recent years an extensive search has been carried out for analogs of naturally occurring glycosyl nucleosides.[1-7] Ribavirin, 1-β-D-ribofuranosyl-1,2,4-triazole-3-carboxamide, an *N*-glycosyl nucleoside, was chemically prepared and found to exhibit potent antiviral properties.[8] An analog of ribavirin, 2-β-D-ribofuranosylthiazole-4-carboxamide (tiazofurin, TR) showed significant antiviral activity (Figure 1).[9,10] There are two unique features in the structure of TR: (1) its thiazole ring resembles neither a purine nor a pyrimidine, and (2) the thiazole base is attached to the ribose through a C–C bond which should be resistant to hydrolysis by the naturally occurring phosphorylases and transglycosidases. As part of a study of the oncolytic properties of known antiviral agents, a systematic examination of the oncolytic properties of TR was undertaken by the National Cancer Institute (NCI); it revealed that the drug possessed significant antitumor activity against the murine leukemias L1210 and P388, and curative activity against the Lewis lung carcinoma, a tumor refractory to most of the drugs tested by the program.[11] Table 1 summarizes the antitumor activity of TR. Not shown is the fact that the drug exhibited curative activity against the intravenously implanted Lewis lung carcinoma over an unusually broad range of doses (12.5 to 800 mg/kg). Most of the surviving mice were verified to be free of tumor as determined by macroscopic examination of the lungs. TR was also effective against, but not curative of, the intracranially implanted Lewis Lung carcinoma. However, unlike i.v. implanted tumor, no long-term survivors were observed. Corollary experiments were carried out in the authors' laboratory and were designed to examine the influence of TR on established Lewis lung tumor. Mice were inoculated s.c. with the tumor, but treatment (800 mg/kg, i.p., × 10 days) was not instituted until 15 days later, at which time the mean diameter of the growth was ~1 cm. In the group treated with tiazofurin, six of seven mice were cured with no macroscopic sign of the tumor, indicating the effectiveness of TR even against established tumors.

II. CYTOTOXICITY OF TIAZOFURIN

Tiazofurin exhibited a median inhibitory concentration (IC_{50}) of 2 to 5 μM against the murine tumor lines P388, L1210, and Lewis lung carcinoma in culture. Against four human lymphoid tumor lines CCRF-CEM (T-cell leukemia), HUT-78 (cutaneous T-cell lymphoma), NALM-1 (B-cell leukemia), and Molt-4 (T-cell leukemia) the drug produced an IC_{50} of 6, 7, 27 and 30 μM, respectively.[12] The drug also exhibited an IC_{50} of 10 to 100 μM against six human lung cancer cell lines[13] and an IC_{50} of 3 to 5 μM against three primary human malignant melanoma and one ovarian adenocarcinoma.[14]

A. Characterization of Cytotoxicity

To determine the cytostatic or cytocidal nature of the drug, cultures of P388 cells were exposed to an IC_{90} concentration of TR (100 μM) for 24 hr; the cells were then washed and plated in fresh, drug-free medium. The rate of replication was monitored by cell counts and cell cycle progression analysis.[15] Under these conditions, resumption of proliferation occurred within 6 hr of drug removal indicating the reversible (cytostatic) nature of the action of the drug on P388 cells. The curative activity of the drug against Lewis lung carcinoma in vivo, however, implies that TR may also be cytocidal against some cell lines.

B. Protection from Tiazofurin Toxicity

P388 cells in culture were incubated with various purine and pyrimidine precursors of nucleic acids to identify agents that might overcome the antiproliferative effect of tiazofurin and so provide an indication of its mechanism of action. None of the nucleic acid precursors were able to nullify the cytotoxicity of TR to P388 leukemia cells in vitro.[15] However, with

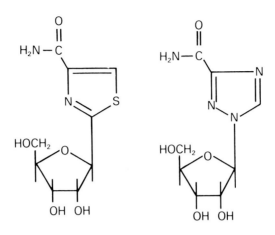

2-β-D-Ribofuranosyl-
thiazole-4-carboxamide
(NSC 286193)

1-β-D-Ribofuranosyl-
1,2,4-triazole-3-carboxamide
(Ribavirin or Virazole)

FIGURE 1.   Chemical structure of tiazofurin and ribavirin.

Table 1

SUMMARY OF ANTITUMOR ACTIVITY OF TR AGAINST
A SPECTRUM OF MURINE TUMORS AND HUMAN
TUMOR XENOGRAFTS

System	Treatment schedule	Highest dose (mg/kg)	Tumor response
Murine tumors			
i.p. B16 melanoma	I.p. Q1D, days 1—9	800	R
s.c. CD8F₁ mammary tumor	i.p. Q1D, staging day	2000	R
s.c. Colon 38 tumor	i.p. Q7D, days 2,9	1600	R
i.p. L1210 leukemia	i.p. Q1D, days 1—9	800	S
i.v. Lewis lung carcinoma	i.p. Q1D, days 1—9	800	S
i.c. Lewis lung carcinoma	i.p. Q1D, days 1—9	800	S
i.p. P388 leukemia	i.p. Q1D, days 1—9	800	S
Human tumor xenografts			
s.r.c. CX-1 colon tumor	s.c. Q4D, days 1—13	1600	R
s.r.c. LX-1 lung tumor	s.c. Q4D, days 1—9	1600	R
s.r.c. MX-1 mammary tumor	s.c. Q4D, days 1—9	1600	R

Note: R and S denote resistance or sensitivity of the tumor to TR therapy. The routes
of tumor implantations are i.p., intraperitoneal; s.c., subcutaneous; iv., intravenous; s.r.c., subrenal capsule.

Lewis lung cells in culture, it was possible to show partial reversal of cytotoxicity by
guanosine. Moreover, with human lymphoid cell lines in culture, guanosine at 50 µ*M*
afforded partial to almost complete protection from growth inhibition by 10 µ*M* TR.[12]

Despite the inability of guanosine to overcome the cytotoxicity of TR in vitro, simultaneous
daily administration of this nucleoside in vivo totally abrogated the therapeutic activity of
the drug (Table 2).[16] This result strongly suggested that tiazofurin acts by engendering a
state of guanosine (nucleotide) deprivation.

Table 2
EFFECT OF GUANOSINE ON TR TREATMENT IN MICE BEARING P388 LEUKEMIA

Treatment	Dose (mg/kg)	Survival period	%T/C[a]
Saline	—	10.8 ± 1.4	
Tiazofurin	100	14.7 ± 0.7	131
	200	17.3 ± 2.7	160
	400	20.5 ± 1.9	190
Guanosine	500	11.4 ± 1.0	105
Tiazofurin + Guanosine	200 500	13.1 ± 1.7	121
Tiazofurin + Guanosine	400 500	13.8 ± 0.7	128

Note: The experimental procedure is outlined in Reference 16.

[a]   % T/C = survival of treated mice ÷ survival of control mice × 100.

III. ROUTE OF ADMINISTRATION

Although the i.p. route has been used most widely for the administration of TR, notable improvements in the therapeutic activity of the drug vs. transplantable murine tumors can be achieved with different routes of administration and different schedules of treatment. For example, sustained oral administration of TR as a 0.125% (w/v) solution in the drinking water of mice bearing s.c. transplanted P388 leukemia achieves a T/C of 260%, which is nearly double that realized by daily i.p. injections of equivalent net doses.[17] The use of implantable Alzet osmotic pumps to deliver the drug into the peritoneal cavity over a 7- or 14-day period achieved similar results.[17] Although the exact reasons for such enhanced potency are yet unclear, it is tempting to speculate that schedules of prolonged administration of TR promote its metabolism by providing sustained blood levels of the drug.

IV. TOXICOLOGIC STUDIES

Toxicologic studies in mice and dogs were performed under the direction of the Toxicology Branch, NCI, at Battelle Columbus Laboratories. In mice, the single dose LD_{50} of TR was 10.4 g/m^2 (3.5 g/kg) while the LD_{10} and LD_{90} doses were 9.6 g/m^2 (2.9 g/kg) and 12.6 g/m^2 (4.2 g/kg), respectively. When the drug was administered i.p. daily for 5 days, the lethal doses decreased to an LD_{50} of 6.7 g/m^2 (2.2 g/kg), LD_{10} of 5.5 g/m^2 (1.8 g/kg) and an LD_{90} of 8.3 g/m^2 (2.7 g/kg), but the slope of the dose-response curve indicated the possibility that the drug can be used with a substantial margin of safety. The most obvious clinical signs seen in mice and dogs were lethargy, prostration and hypothermia which resembled anesthesia at the highest doses. The i.v. injection of TR in dogs resulted in toxicity to the hematopoietic, gastrointestinal, hepatic, renal, and endocrine systems. Sex-related toxicity was not obvious in these species, but there was a definite difference in the sensitivity between mice and dogs, with the mouse being the more sensitive species.

V. PHARMACOLOGIC STUDIES

Inasmuch as many important therapeutic and toxicologic studies with TR have been carried out in mice and dogs, it is relevant to recapitulate certain aspects of the fate and distribution of the drug in these species. Following the i.v. administration of tiazofurin (500 to 750 mg/ m^2) to mice, rats, and dogs, the drug was removed from circulation in three apparent phases with α-, β-, and γ-phase half-lives of 0.5 to 5.2, 5.1 to 17.4, and 170 to 459 min, respectively.[18] The principal route of excretion of TR in all three species was via the kidneys, since greater than 80% of the drug was recoverable in the urine within 24 hr of administration.

Although little metabolism of the drug was demonstrable in the plasma of mice, rats, and dogs,[18] significant accumulation and biotransformation of tiazofurin were found in several tissues. The highest concentration of TR was found in the spleen in the three species examined within 24 hr after drug administration. In mice and rats, extensive metabolism of TR to phosphorylated forms was observed in liver, kidney, and striated muscle. Since a sizable fraction of the body mass is accounted for as striated muscle, the latter could function as a storage depot, capable of releasing the parent drug back into the circulation as hydrolysis of the phosphate ester occurs. Such a mechanism would account for the protracted terminal half-life of tiazofurin described earlier.

VI. MECHANISM OF ACTION, IN VITRO AND IN VIVO

Since TR was synthesized as an analog of ribavirin, a potent inhibitor of guanosine nucleotide biosynthesis,[19] it was felt that these two compounds might share a similar mechanism of action.[9,20] Thus, preliminary studies with Ehrlich ascites cells in culture showed that the incorporation of labeled hypoxanthine into purine nucleotides was inhibited by TR to a similar extent as that observed with ribavirin.[9,20]

A. Influence on Macromolecular Synthesis

The influence of TR on the incorporation of metabolic precursors into DNA, RNA, and protein was examined using P388 cells in culture. Treatment for 2 hr with 100 μM TR caused only a modest inhibition of the incorporation of valine into protein (22%), but strongly restricted the incorporation of thymidine (85%) and uridine (78%) into nucleic acids.[15] In corollary studies, cells were incubated with TR for 2 hr and sampled at various times to examine the onset of inhibition of DNA synthesis; approximately 30 min elapsed before the process began to be curtailed.[15]

The influence of TR on the incorporation of labeled precursors into nucleic acids was also determined.[15] Drug treatment prevented the incorporation of all bases and nucleosides examined, except for those belonging to the guanine family even where their incorporation was stimulated by drug treatment (Table 3). In this respect, TR resembles ribavirin which also acts as a specific inhibitor of guanosine nucleotide biosynthesis.[20]

B. Influence on Nucleotide Pools

Since earlier studies suggested that tiazofurin produced a state of guanosine nucleotide depletion, the influence of the drug on ribonucleotide levels was examined. When mice bearing P388 leukemia were injected with various doses of TR and nucleoside triphosphate pools were examined, there was a pronounced dose-responsive decrease in GTP concentrations (Table 4), a modest decrease in ATP concentration (at doses larger than 100 mg/kg), and an elevation of pyrimidine nucleotides, most marked at the intermediate doses used (25 and 100 mg/kg). Such increases in pyrimidine nucleotide concentrations have also been observed with other agents such as 2-amino-1,3,4-thiadiazole, mycophenolic acid, and ribavirin.[21,22]

Table 3
THE INFLUENCE OF TR ON THE INCORPORATION OF PURINE NUCLEOSIDES INTO MACROMOLECULES OF P388 CELLS IN CULTURE

Precursor	Percent change in the incorporation of precursors by 5 μM TR
[8-^{14}C]Adenosine	-37
[8-^{3}H]Deoxyadenosine	-49
[8-^{14}C]Inosine	-64
[8-^{14}C]Hypoxanthine	-54
[U-^{14}C]Guanosine	$+130$
[8-^{14}C]Deoxyguanosine	$+140$

Note: Experimental conditions are outlined in Reference 15.

Table 4
INFLUENCE OF TR TREATMENT ON NUCLEOSIDE TRIPHOSPHATE CONCENTRATIONS IN VIVO

Dose of TR (mg/kg)	Nucleoside triphosphate levels (% of control)			
	CTP	UTP	ATP	GTP
10	93	110	90	50
25	150	190	95	45
100	135	170	80	35
250	85	105	58	18

Note: Groups of five male BDF$_1$ mice were inoculated s.c. with 10^6 P388 cells; 7 to 9 days later, mice were injected i.p. with TR or saline. Tumors were removed 2 hr later, immediately frozen on dry ice, and perchloric acid extracts were prepared. An aliquot of the neutralized extract was analyzed by HPLC as detailed earlier.[15]

To further probe the inhibitory effect of TR on GTP synthesis, the concentration of purine nucleoside monophosphates was examined (Table 5). There was a dramatic decrease in GMP levels with a concomitant increase in IMP concentration (~20-fold) following TR treatment. In separate studies, the incorporation of labeled hypoxanthine into GMP was totally inhibited (94%) following drug treatment, while its incorporation into AMP was decreased by 57%.[15] At the same time, the incorporation of hypoxanthine into IMP was potentiated tenfold.[15]

C. Enzymatic Locus of Action

Since tiazofurin produced a specific decrease in the concentration of guanine nucleotides with a substantial increase in IMP concentration, the influence of the drug on the enzymes

Table 5
PERTURBATION OF PURINE NUCLEOSIDE
MONOPHOSPHATES IN P388 CELLS IN
CULTURE FOLLOWING TR TREATMENT

| | Treatment | | | |
| | | | | |
Nucleotide	Saline (pmol/10^6 cells)	%	TR (pmol/10^6 cells)	%
AMP	104.0 ± 1.0	100	78.0 ± 3.0	75
GMP	34.0 ± 1.0	100	8.0 ± 1.5	23
IMP	1.2 ± 0.5	100	24.0 ± 2.5	2040

Note: Each value is the mean ± S.D.; data are from Reference 15.

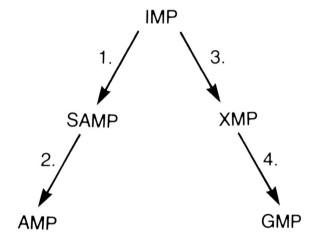

1. Adenylosuccinic Synthetase
2. Adenylosuccinic Lyase
3. IMP Dehydrogenase
4. GMP Synthetase

FIGURE 2.   Diagram of the terminal steps of purine biosynthesis.

leading to the synthesis of GMP from IMP, namely, IMP dehydrogenase (IMPD) and GMP synthetase was investigated (Figure 2). IMPD activity was strongly inhibited by the drug in vitro (78% inhibition with 12 mM TR) while only marginal inhibition of GMP synthetase activity was seen.[15] When P388 cells in culture were incubated with 5 μM TR for 2 hr, only IMPD activity was strongly inhibited (80%) and this inhibition was reversible upon dialysis.[15] In culture, 5 μM TR produced inhibition equivalent to that produced in vitro by 12 mM drug, a finding which is suggestive of metabolism to a proximate inhibitory species.[15]

The influence of TR on GTP levels and IMPD activity was measured in P388 tumors at varying times after the administration of a dose of 250 mg/kg TR (Figure 3). A temporal relationship between the two parameters was observed wherein both reached a nadir in 2 to 4 hr and substantially recovered 24 hr following drug administration.

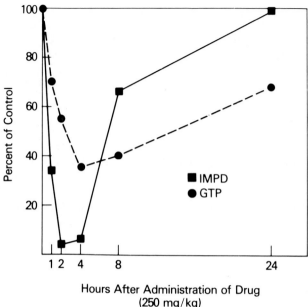

FIGURE 3.   Influence of tiazofurin on GTP pools and IMPD activity in the P388 leukemia as a function of time. BDF$_1$ mice bearing 7- to 9-day old s.c. inoculated P388 leukemia were injected i.p. with saline or tiazofurin (250 mg/kg). Groups of five mice each were sacrificed at appropriate time point and extracts analyzed for IMP dehydrogenase activity and levels of GTP as described in Reference 16.

D. Consequences of IMP Dehydrogenase Inhibition

Jackson et al.,[23] studying a spectrum of hepatomas with different growth rates, found that increased IMPD activity was associated with tumor proliferation. They also suggested that the low specific activity of IMPD in rapidly dividing tissues indicated that IMPD was one of the key rate-limiting enzymes in purine nucleotide biosynthesis. Two important biochemical consequences result from the inhibition of IMPD: accumulation of IMP and reduction in the concentration of guanine nucleotides. IMP is believed to impair the fidelity of transcription of DNA.[24] Moreover accumulation of IMP could also result in increased levels of inosine, hypoxanthine, and consequently of uric acid, resulting in hyperuricemia and hyperuricosuria.[25] Depletion of GTP could also have severe consequences on RNA synthesis and function.[26,27]

Other inhibitors of IMPD have been suggested as potential oncolytic agents.[28] Bredinin (Figure 4, No. 2), a nucleoside antibiotic bearing a close structural resemblance to ribavirin (Figure 4, No. 1), also possesses IMPD inhibitory activity[29] and is active against the murine L1210 leukemia.[30] The analogs, 3-deazaguanosine (Figure 4, No. 3) and 1-aminoguanosine (Figure 4, No. 4) were synthesized in a study aimed at finding inhibitors of IMPD.[31,32] These guanine analogs demonstrated cytotoxicity against L1210 cells in culture.[16] The inosine analogs, 6-mercaptopurine (Figure 4, No. 5) and 8-azainosine (Figure 4, No. 6), were good competitive inhibitors of IMPD and possessed antitumor activity against L1210 leukemia and adenocarcinoma 755.[33,34] 2-Amino-1,3,4-thiadiazole (Figure 4, No. 7) also inhibited IMPD and was an active antitumor agent.[35] Mycophenolic acid (Figure 4, No. 8) is one of the best-known inhibitors of IMPD and demonstrated potent antineoplastic activity against solid mouse and rat tumors.[36,37] Except for mycophenolic acid, all other agents need to be converted to their active form (as 5'-monophosphate) before exerting potent IMP dehydrogenase inhibition.

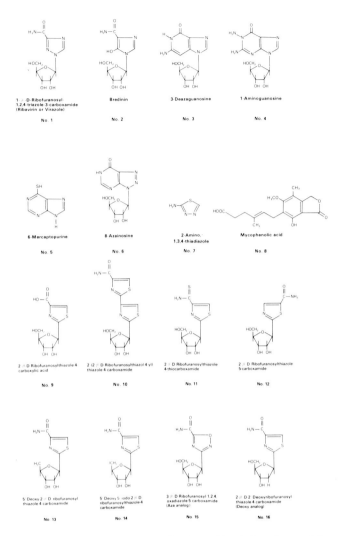

FIGURE 4. Chemical structures of analogs of tiazofurin and some of the inhibitors of IMP dehydrogenase possessing antitumor activity. Ribavirin, bredinin, 3-deazaguanosine, 1-aminoguanosine, 8-azainosine, 6-mercaptopurine, and 2-amino-1,3,4-thiadiazole need to be bioactivated (metabolized) before they exert potent IMP dehydrogenase inhibition. Mycophenolic acid directly and potently inhibits IMP dehydrogenase activity.

VII. METABOLISM OF TIAZOFURIN

Thus far, these studies have established that administration of TR powerfully inhibits IMPD resulting in depression of guanine nucleotide biosynthesis, and thereby restricting nucleic acid biosynthesis and cellular proliferation. Therefore, our attention was directed at finding the nature of the molecular species responsible for the action of the drug. The existence of a substantial lag period before inhibition of macromolecular synthesis begins to be expressed, and the large discrepancy in the doses required to produce similar inhibition in vitro and in culture, clearly indicated that the drug was being metabolized to an active enzyme-inhibitory species. Kinetic analyses of TR and its 5′-phosphate against partially purified IMPD from P388 leukemia indicated a K_i of 8.2 mM and 0.5 mM, respectively, for the two compounds. Since direct measurements of the concentration of these species in the tumors of mice treated with a large therapeutic dose (400 mg/kg) of TR yielded peak

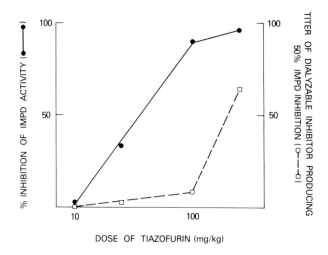

FIGURE 5. Dose-response of IMP dehydrogenase inhibition by tiazo-furin and titer of dialyzable inhibitor. Groups of five BDF$_1$ mice bearing s.c. implanted P388 leukemia were injected i.p. with saline or tiazofurin (10 to 250 mg/kg); 2 hr later tumors were excised and IMP dehydrogenase activity and titer of dialyzable inhibitor (dilution yielding 50% IMP dehydrogenase inhibition) determined according to the methodology detailed in Reference 16.

concentrations of 73 and 14 μM for the drug and its 5′-monophosphate, respectively, they were clearly not responsible for the powerful inhibition of IMPD seen after a therapeutic dose of the drug. It was soon determined that the inhibition produced by the drug was freely reversible on dialysis and that the inhibitory molecule could be recovered from the dialyzing solution. Similarly, the inhibitor was present in the acid extracts of the tumor following drug treatment and was resistant to heating at 95° for up to 2 min. Figure 5 illustrates the dose-response of the dialyzable inhibitor obtained after TR administration. The concentration of the inhibitory principle produced increased with the dose of the drug. When concentrated extracts of treated tumors were analyzed on an ion-exchange HPLC system used for nucleotides, most of the IMPD inhibitory activity eluted in the general area of nucleoside diphosphates — well separated from IMP and both the parent drug and its 5′-monophosphate.[38]

A. Characterization of the Active Principle

To characterize the active metabolite, it was exposed to a panel of enzymes capable of hydrolyzing phosphate esters, glycosides, etc. These studies revealed that the inhibitory molecule resisted hydrolysis by acid or alkaline phosphatase and other monoesterases, but was rapidly inactivated by venom phosphodiesterase and a select number of other enzymes which attack phosphodiester bonds.[39]

Since NAD is the most abundant phosphodiester metabolite in biological systems and is also an obligatory cofactor in the IMPD reaction, it was speculated that the inhibitor might be an analog of NAD in which nicotinamide was replaced by thiazole-4-carboxamide, i.e., TAD.[38]

Experiments were designed to ascertain whether the active principle incorporated both the thiazole-4-carboxamide and adenine moieties. P388 cells growing in culture were exposed to [5-^{3}H]TR or saline for 2 hr and the cell extracts subsequently analyzed by HPLC. Cells treated with [5-^{3}H]TR demonstrated a large radioactive peak corresponding to the inhibitory molecule (Figure 6A). This radioactive inhibitory peak was susceptible to phosphodiesterase treatment with the radioactivity recoverable as tiazofurin-5′-monophosphate, indicating that the inhibitor contained the thiazole ring structure.[38] Evidence for the presence of adenosine

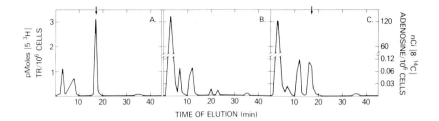

FIGURE 6. HPLC elution profile of radioactivity after exposure of P388 cells to [³H]TR or to [¹⁴C]adenosine. Experimental procedure is detailed in Reference 38. Panel A refers to the chromatographic profile of cells exposed to [5-³H]TR. Panel B and C refer to the elution profile of cells prelabeled with [¹⁴C]adenosine and then treated with saline (panel B) or with TR (1 mM) (panel C).

in the inhibitory principle was obtained by labeling P388 cells with [8-¹⁴C]adenosine for 30 min, followed by incubation with saline (Figure 6B) or with TR (Figure 6C) for 2 hr. HPLC analyses of the cell extract revealed the presence of a radioactive peak corresponding to the inhibitory molecule only in the TR-treated extract. The metabolite was susceptible to phosphodiesterase treatment and yielded labeled AMP.[38] Similar labeling studies were performed in mice bearing s.c. implanted P388 leukemia and they, too, confirmed that the inhibitory metabolite was TAD.[39]

B. Synthesis of TAD

Additional confirmation of the structure of TAD was obtained by synthesizing it by two independent routes. The first method was enzymological: when TR-MP was incubated with purified NAD pyrophosphorylase from hog liver in the presence of ATP·MgCl$_2$ substantial yields of TAD were obtained; these were purified to apparent homogeneity by column chromatography.[38] The second approach was by the classical Khorana condensation technique for dinucleotide synthesis.[38,40]

To ascertain the identity of the TAD prepared by different routes, a number of properties of the preparations were compared. All preparations exhibited a λ_{max} of 252 nm with molar extinction coefficients of $\sim$18,500 at this wavelength. Further confirmation of the structure of these preparations of TAD was obtained by NMR spectra and mass spectrometry.[38,40] TAD was a potent inhibitor of partially purified IMPD from P388 leukemia, with a K_i of $\sim$0.2 μM; with NAD as the variable substrate, the inhibition produced was noncompetitive. Thus, TAD apparently does not occupy the NAD site at the catalytic center of IMPD.

C. Synthesis of TAD Analogs

Additional dinucleotide analogs of TAD were designed and synthesized in an attempt to increase their affinity for IMPD. Three types of analogs were prepared: modification of the adenine and/or nicotinamide moiety, modification of the phosphodiester bridge, and modification of the thiazole ring.[39] The adenine moiety was altered by replacing it with guanine or hypoxanthine, or by enlargement with an etheno ring system (Table 6). In either case, the resultant dinucleotide analog exhibited a significantly lower affinity for IMPD than TAD.[39] Modification of the thiazole ring system is technically difficult and, thus, is still being investigated. For cytotoxicity, a carboxamide moiety seems to be essential since its substitution by carboxylic acid (Figure 4, No. 9), thiazole-4-carboxamide (Figure 4, No. 10), thiocarboxamide (Figure 4, No. 11), or a change of the carboxamide to the 5-position (Figure 4, No. 12), resulted in a loss of activity.[15] Substitution of the 5'-hydroxyl moiety, either with hydrogen (Figure 4, No. 13) or with iodine (Figure 4, No. 14), rendered the molecule inert. Replacement of carbon in the 5-position with oxygen and nitrogen for sulfur in the heterocyclic ring (Figure 4, No. 15) also resulted in the loss of cytotoxicity. Similarly,

Table 6
INHIBITION OF IMP DEHYDROGENASE BY DINUCLEOTIDE ANALOGS OF NAD

Compound	Median inhibitory concentration (ID_{50}) (μM)
Modification of the Nicotinamide and the Adenine Groups	
Diguanosine diphosphate	330
Thiazole guanine dinucleotide	17
Thiazole hypoxanthine dinucleotide	4.5
Thiazole adenine-N'-oxide dinucleotide	13.5
Thiazole, 1, N^6-ethenoadenine dinucleotide	720
Modification of the Nicotinamide Group	
Thiazole adenine dinucleotide	0.16
8-(6-Aminohexyl)-amino NAD$^+$	330
3-Acetylpyridine deamino NAD$^+$	25
3-Acetylpyridine NAD$^+$	330
Deamino NAD$^+$	330
Thionicotinamide adenine dinucleotide	3,300
Pyridinealdehyde NAD$^+$	3,300
Diadenosine diphosphate	330
Modification of the Phosphate Linkage	
Diadenosine pentaphosphate	330
Diguanosine tetraphosphate	330

Note: Data are from Reference 39.

substitution of deoxyribosyl moiety for the ribosyl moiety (Figure 4, No. 16) rendered the molecule nontoxic to P388 cells in culture.[15]

D. Specificity of TAD

To understand the specificity of TAD, an examination of its influence on a select number of dehydrogenases was attempted. The dinucleotide showed no coenzyme activity with IMPD, L-glutamate dehydrogenase, lactate dehydrogenase, or malate dehydrogenase. In addition, TAD was incapable of inhibiting these dehydrogenases, except for IMPD, in vitro and in vivo.[39]

VIII. MECHANISM OF RESISTANCE

A. Development of Resistant Lines

Cell lines of P388 resistant to TR were developed to examine whether the mechanism of action and metabolism of TR play a role in drug resistance. Towards this goal, over 60 generations of P388 cells in culture were exposed to step-wise increases in the concentrations (1 μM to 10 mM) of TR. The resistant variant (P388/TR) thus selected showed a 4-log lesser sensitivity to TR compared to the parent cell line (P388/S) and could be propagated without additional selection pressure.[41] The two lines exhibited similar (13 to 14 hr) doubling time. On transplantation of the resistant line into BDF$_1$ mice, stable resistance was retained without any administration of the drug. Tiazofurin exhibited no antitumor activity against P388/TR leukemia in vivo.[41]

B. Metabolism of Tiazofurin by Sensitive and Resistant Lines

Experiments were next conducted to compare the formation of TAD in the sensitive (P388/S) and resistant (P388/TR) cell lines, both in vitro and in vivo. Under these circumstances large amounts of TAD were found only in P388/S cells, clearly indicating that the resistance phenomenon in this cell line is related to an absence of TAD synthesis.[41] In addition, a two-to threefold increase in the level of TR-MP was seen in the resistant line in vitro, indicating the absence or low activity of NAD pyrophosphorylase, which presumably is responsible for the conversion of TR-MP to TAD.[41]

C. Influence on Nucleotide Concentration

Since TR treatment of P388 leukemia produced dramatic reductions in guanine nucleotide concentrations, the influence of drug administration on the nucleotide pools was examined in sensitive and resistant cells. Once again, in the resistant line there was no perturbation of the levels of GTP, while they were drastically reduced in the sensitive cell line.[41]

In another independent study aimed at understanding the mechanism of resistance, Chinese hamster ovary cells were exposed to TR and a cell line resistant to 100 μM TR was selected.[42] Like the resistant variant of P388 cells, the resistant Chinese hamster ovary cells (RO^R-1 cells) were incapable of forming TAD.[42]

D. General Applicability of the Mechanism of Resistance

To determine whether the mechanism of resistance established above had general applicability to other tumor lines, the pharmacologic effect and metabolism of the drug were examined in the six transplantable tumors comprising the NCI murine tumor panel (Table 1). Administration of TR to tumor-bearing mice resulted in significantly higher levels of TAD in the sensitive vs. resistant lines; this effect correlated well with the inhibition of IMPD and with the depression in guanine nucleotide pools.[43] Enzymologic studies revealed a similar capacity of sensitive and resistant tumors to phosphorylate TR and to TR-MP, but the pyrophosphorylase responsible for the conversion of TR-MP to TAD was significantly depressed only in the resistant lines.[43]

Studies on the metabolism of TAD by four human lymphoid tumor cell lines also indicated that the cell lines with the higher sensitivity to TR formed somewhat larger amounts of TAD compared with the less sensitive cell lines.[12]

The pharmacologic actions and metabolism of TR were examined in six human lung carcinoma cell lines, four of which were non-small-cell tumor lines sensitive to the drug and two of which were small-cell tumor lines less sensitive to TR.[13] In general, there was a positive correlation between drug sensitivity, increased formation of TAD, and reduction of guanosine nucleotide pools.[13]

IX. DISCUSSION AND CONCLUSIONS

To date, perturbation of purine and pyrimidine nucleotide synthesis is the only known biochemical effect on TR. Of these alterations, the accumulation of IMP and the depletion of guanine nucleotides would appear to be quantitatively the most significant. Furthermore, reversal of the in vivo therapeutic activity of TR was observed on administration of guanosine. Still undefined, however, is the mechanism by which guanine depletion results in growth inhibition and cell death. In the case of another IMP dehydrogenase inhibitor, mycophenolic acid, both GTP and dGTP are depleted.[22,44] The former effect (GTP depletion) appeared to be the most closely linked to DNA synthesis inhibition,[22] although the function that GTP may serve in DNA synthesis remains elusive. These considerations may also apply in the case of TR and related IMP dehydrogenase inhibitors. Other processes which may be affected by GTP depletion are 5'-cap formation in mRNA synthesis[26] and GTP-dependent initiation and elongation processes in translation.

The design of inhibitors of IMP dehydrogenase would appear, therefore, to be a promising area for antineoplastic drugs. So far, modifications of the TR structure have yielded little, although complete structure-activity relationships have not been elucidated. A promising development has been the substitution of selenium for sulfur (selenazofurin, SR).[45] Preliminary studies with SR in our laboratory indicate that this analog is fivefold more cytotoxic than TR. A threefold greater amount of selenazole-4-carboxamide adenine dinucleotide (SAD) compared to TAD was formed by P388/S cells. SAD, like TAD, was a potent inhibitor of partially purified IMP dehydrogenase from P388 cells. TR and SR seem to share similar mechanisms of resistance, since SR does not exhibit cytotoxicity against P388/TR cells. Cells resistant to TR (P388/TR) did not form TAD or SAD following incubation with TR or SR in culture. Thus, TR and SR appear to exert their action after metabolism to TAD or SAD. Other analogs of TR, namely 2-amino-1,3,4-thiadiazole,[35] ribavirin,[46] and bredinin[29] appear to work at the level of their 5'-monophosphate, which potently inhibits IMP dehydrogenase.

Among the NAD requiring enzymes, IMPD seems to be specifically inhibited by TAD. Despite the fact that TAD shows noncompetitive inhibition with respect to NAD, which would indicate that TAD does not occupy the NAD site, the orientation around the glycosidic C–C bond of TR in TAD may be as critical for IMPD inhibition as the configuration of the nicotinamide ring is in NAD to function efficiently as a coenzyme. It is known that according to their stereoselectivity pyridine nucleotide-linked enzymes are classified into two groups. The A-stereospecific enzymes (PRO-R) and the B-stereospecific enzymes (PRO-S).[47] The results appear to suggest that NAD binds A-stereospecific enzymes only in the anti orientation, whereas the syn orientation is preferred by B-stereospecific enzymes. The sulfur atom, and to a greater extent the selenium atom, by virtue of their size, may favor the syn orientation of their respective nucleotide components in TAD and SAD.[48] As such, these NAD analogs may show a stereoselective binding that would probably prefer B-type stereospecific enzymes. IMPD has been categorized as a B-type dehydrogenase,[49] and recently, in our laboratory, IMPD from P388 cells has been definitely demonstrated to be a B-type enzyme.[50] The expected preference for the syn orientation in both TR and SR may be an important factor in explaining the selectivity towards their IMPD receptor shown by the NAD analogs that contain them as nicotinamide riboside impostors. This matter is, however, by no means final since TAD, in our hands, failed to inhibit glutamate dehydrogenase which has been identified as a B-type enzyme.[39]

TR is presently being evaluated in phase I clinical trials. If it exhibits oncolytic responses in man, it will provoke further interest in the development of IMPD inhibitors, as well as affirm the importance of this enzyme in intermediary metabolism and as a chemotherapeutic target for anticancer drugs.

REFERENCES

1. **Gerzon, K., Delong, D. C., and Cline, J. C.,** C-Nucleosides: aspects of chemistry and mode of action, *Pure Appl. Chem.,* 28, 489, 1971.
2. **Koyama, G. and Umezawa, H.,** Formycin B and its relation to formycin, *J. Antibiot. Ser. A,* 18, 175, 1965.
3. **Hori, M. E., Ito, J., Takidal, G., Koyama, G., Takeuchi, T., and Umezawa, W.,** A new antibiotic, formycin, *J. Antibiot. Ser. A,* 17, 96, 1964.
4. **Sesaki, K., Kasadabe, Y., and Esumi, S.,** The structure of minimycin, a novel carbon-linked nucleoside antibiotic related to β-pseudouridine, *J. Antibiot.,* 25, 151, 1972.
5. **Nishimura, N., Mayma, M., Komatsu, Y., Kato, H., Shimaoka, N., and Tanaka, Y.,** Showdomycin, a new antibiotic from a *Streptomyces* sp., *J. Antibiot. Ser. A,* 17, 148, 1964.

6. **Srivastava, P. C., Streeter, D. G., Matthews, T. R., Allen, L. B., Sidwell, R. W., and Robins, R. K.,** Synthesis and antiviral and antimicrobial activity of certain 1-β-D-ribofuranosyl-4,5-disubstituted imidazoles, *J. Med. Chem.,* 19, 1020, 1976.

7. **Streeter, D. G. and Koyama, H. H. P.,** Inhibition of purine nucleotide biosynthesis by 3-deazaguanine, its nucleoside and 5′-nucleotide, *Biochem. Pharmacol.,* 25, 2413, 1976.

8. **Witkowski, J. T., Robins, R. K., Sidwell, R. W., and Simon, L. N.,** Design, synthesis and broad spectrum antiviral activity of 1-β-D-ribofuranosyl-1,2,4-triazole-3-carboxamide and related nucleosides, *J. Med. Chem.,* 15, 1150, 1972.

9. **Srivastava, P. C., Pickering, M. V., Allen, L. B., Streeter, D. G., Campbell, M. T., Witkowski, J. T., Sidwell, R. W., and Robins, R. K.,** Synthesis and antiviral activity of certain thiazole C-nucleosides, *J. Med. Chem.,* 20, 256, 1977.

10. **Fuertes, M., Gracia-Lopez, T., Gracia-Munoz, G., and Stud, M.,** Synthesis of C-glycosyl thiazoles, *J. Org. Chem.,* 41, 4074, 1976.

11. **Robins, R. K., Srivastava, R. C., Narayanan, V. L., Plowman, J., and Paull, K. D.,** 2-β-D-Ribofuranosylthiazole-4-carboxamide, a novel potential antitumor agent for lung tumors and metastases, *J. Med. Chem.,* 25, 107, 1982.

12. **Earle, M. F. and Glazer, R. I.,** Activity and metabolism of 2-β-D-ribofuranosylthiazole-4-carboxamide in human lymphoid tumor cells in culture, *Cancer Res.,* 43, 133, 1983.

13. **Carney, D. N., Ahluwalia, G. S., Jayaram, H. N., Cooney, D. A., Minna, J. D., and Johns, D. G.,** Biochemical correlates of clonal growth inhibition in human lung tumor cell lines by tiazofurin, *Abstr. Am. Soc. Clin. Invest.* 1983.

14. **Jayaram, H. N., Cooney, D. A., Dion, R. L., Glazer, R. I., Ardalan, B., Robins, R. K., and Johns, D. G.,** Studies on the mechanism of action of the new oncolytic thiazole nucleoside, 2-β-D-ribofuranosyl-thiazole-4-carboxamide (NSC 286193), *Proc. Am. Assoc. Cancer Res.,* 23, 217, 1982.

15. **Jayaram, H. N., Dion, R. L., Glazer, R. I., Johns, D. G., Robins, R. K., Srivastava, P. C., and Cooney, D. A.,** Initial studies on the mechanism of action of a new oncolytic thiazole nucleoside, 2-β-D-ribofuranosyl-thiazole-4-carboxamide (NSC 286193), *Biochem. Pharmacol.,* 31, 2371, 1982.

16. **Jayaram, H. N., Smith, A. I., Glazer, R. I., Johns, D. G., and Cooney, D. A.,** Studies on the mechanism of action of 2-β-D-ribofuranosylthiazole-4-carboxamide (NSC 286193). II. Relationship between dose level and biochemical effects in P388 leukemia *in vivo, Biochem. Pharmacol.,* 31, 3839, 1982.

17. **Wilson, Y. A., Vistica, B., Vistica, D., Jayaram, H. N., and Cooney, D. A.,** Improvement in the therapeutic efficacy of tiazofurin by sustained peritoneal administration, manuscript in preparation.

18. **Arnold, A., Jayaram, H. N., Harper, G., Ahluwalia, G. S., Malspies, L., Cooney, D. A., and Johns, D. G.,** Studies with tiazofurin, 2-β-D-ribofuranosylthiazole-4-carboxamide. V. The disposition and metabolism of tiazofurin in rodents and dogs, manuscript in preparation, 1983.

19. **Smith, C. M., Fontenelle, L. J., Muzik, H., Paterson, A. R. P., Unger, H., Brox, L. W., and Henderson, J. F.,** Inhibitors of inosinate dehydrogenase activity in Ehrlich ascites tumor cells *in vitro, Biochem. Pharmacol.,* 23, 2727, 1974.

20. **Streeter, D. G. and Miller, J. P.,** The *in vitro* inhibition of purine nucleotide biosynthesis by 2-β-D-ribofuranosylthiazole-4-carboxamide, *Biochem. Biophys. Res. Commun.,* 103, 1409, 1981.

21. **Nelson, J. A., Rose, L. M., and Bennett, Jr., L. L.,** Effects of 2-amino-1,3,4-thiadiazole on ribonucleotide pools of leukemia L1210 cells, *Cancer Res.,* 36, 1375, 1976.

22. **Lowe, J. K., Brox, L., and Henderson, J. F.,** Consequences of inhibition of guanine nucleotide synthesis by mycophenolic acid and virazole, *Cancer Res.,* 37, 736, 1977.

23. **Jackson, R. C., Weber, G., and Morris, H. P.,** IMP dehydrogenase, an enzyme linked with proliferation and malignancy, *Nature (London),* 256, 331, 1975.

24. **Derse, D. and Cheng, Y. C.,** Herpes simplex virus Type I DNA polymerase, *J. Biol. Chem.,* 256, 8525, 1981.

25. **Krakoff, I. H. and Balis, M. E.,** Studies of the uricogenic effect of 2-substituted thiadiazoles in man, *J. Clin. Ivest.,* 38, 907, 1959.

26. **Shatkin, A. J.,** Capping of eucaryotic mRNAs, *Cell,* 9, 645, 1976.

27. **Zieve, G. W.,** Two groups of small stable RNAs, *Cell,* 25, 296, 1981.

28. **Weber, G.,** Enzymology of cancer cells, *N. Engl. J. Med.,* 296, 486, 541, 1977.

29. **Robins, R. K.,** Nucleoside and nucleotide inhibitors of inosine monophosphate (IMP) dehydrogenase as potential antitumor inhibitors, *Nucleosides Nucleotides,* 1, 35, 1982.

30. **Sakaguchi, K., Tsujino, M., Yoshizawa, M., Mizuno, K., and Hayano, K.,** Action of bredinin on mammalian cells, *Cancer Res.,* 35, 1643, 1975.

31. **Cook, P. D., Rousseau, R. J., Mian, A. M., Meyer, R. B., Jr., Dea, P., Ivanovics, G., Streeter, D. G., Witkowski, J. T., Stout, M. G., Simon, L. N., Sidwell, R. W., and Robins, R. K.,** A new class of potent guanine antimetabolites. Synthesis of 3-deazaguanine, 3-deazaguanosine, and 3-deazaguanylic acid by a novel ring closure of imidazole precursors, *J. Am. Chem. Soc.,* 97, 2916, 1974.

32. **Cook, P. D., Rousseau, R. J., Mian, A. M., Dea, P., Meyer, R. B., Jr., and Robins, R. K.,** Synthesis of 3-deazaguanine, 3-deazaguanosine, and 3-deazaguanylic acid by a novel ring closure of imidazole precursors, *J. Am. Chem. Soc.,* 98, 1492, 1976.

33. **Hampton, A.,** Reactions of ribonucleotide derivatives of purine analogues at the catalytic site of inosine 5'-phosphate dehydrogenase, *J. Biol. Chem.,* 238, 3068, 1963.

34. **Hutzenlaub, W., Tolman, R. L., and Robins, R. K.,** Azapurine nucleosides. I. Synthesis and antitumor activity of certain 3-β-D-ribofuranosyl- and 2'-deoxy-D-ribofuranosyl-V-triazolo[4,5-d]pyrimidines, *J. Med. Chem.,* 15, 879, 1972.

35. **Hill, D. L.,** Aminothiadiazoles, *Cancer Chemother. Pharmacol.,* 4, 215, 1980.

36. **Sweeney, M. J., Gerzon, K., Harris, P. N., Holes, R. E., Poore, G. A., and Williams, R. H.,** Experimental antitumor activity and preclinical toxicity of mycophenolic acid, *Cancer Res.,* 32, 1795, 1972.

37. **Sweeney, M. J., Hoffman, D. H., and Esterman, M. A.,** Metabolism and biochemistry of mycophenolic acid, *Cancer Res.,* 32, 1803, 1972.

38. **Cooney, D. A., Jayaram, H. N., Gebeyehu, G., Betts, C. R., Kelley, J. A., Marquez, V. E., and Johns, D. G.,** The conversion of 2-β-D-ribofuranosylthiazole-4-carboxamide to an analogue of NAD with potent IMP dehydrogenase-inhibitory properties, *Biochem. Pharmacol.,* 31, 2133, 1982.

39. **Cooney, D. A., Jayaram, H. N., Glazer, R. I., Kelley, J. A., Marquez, V. E., Gebeyehu, G., Van Cott, A. C., Zwelling, L. A., and Johns, D. G.,** Studies on the mechanism of action of tiazofurin. Metabolism to an analog of NAD with potent IMP dehydrogenase-inhibitory activity, in *Advances in Enzyme Regulation,* Weber, G., Ed., Pergamon Press, New York, 1983.

40. **Gebeyehu, G., Marquez, V. E., Kelley, J. A., Cooney, D. A., Jayaram, H. N., and Johns, D. G.,** Synthesis of thiazole-4-carboxamide-adenine dinucleotide (TAD). A powerful inhibitor of IMP dehydrogenase, *J. Med. Chem.,* in press, 1983.

41. **Jayaram, H. N., Cooney, D. A., Glazer, R. I., Dion, R. L., and Johns, D. G.,** Mechanism of resistance to the oncolytic C-nucleoside, 2-β-D-ribofuranosylthiazole-4-carboxamide (NSC 286193), *Biochem. Pharmacol.,* 31, 2557, 1982.

42. **Kuttan, R., Robins, R. K., and Sanders, P. P.,** Inhibition of inosinate dehydrogenase by metabolites of 2-β-D-ribofuranosylthiazole-4-carboxamide, *Biochem. Biophys. Res. Commun.,* 107, 862, 1982.

43. **Ahluwalia, G. S., Jayaram, H. N., Cooney, D. A., and Johns, D. G.,** Factors governing the response of murine tumors to tiazofurin, manuscript in preparation, 1983.

44. **Cohen, M. B., Maybaum, J., and Sadee, W.,** Guanine nucleotide depletion and toxicity in mouse T lymphoma (S-49) cells, *J. Biol. Chem.,* 256, 8713, 1981.

45. **Robins, R. K., Revankar, G. R., Srivastava, P. C., Kirsi, J., North, J. A., Murray, B., McKernan, P. A., and Canonico, P. B.,** New nucleosides with broad spectrum antiviral activity, Am. Chem. Soc. Natl. Meet.

46. **Streeter, D. G., Witkowski, J. T., Khare, G. P., Sidwell, R. W., Bauer, R. J., Robins, R. K., and Siman, L. N.,** Mechanism of 1-β-D-ribofuranosyl-1,2,4-triazole-3-carboxamide (Virazole), a new broad spectrum antiviral agent, *Proc. Natl. Acad. Sci. U.S.A.,* 70, 1174, 1973.

47. **Shugar, D., Stolarski, R., and Dudycz, L.,** Confirmation of nucleosides and nucleotides, role in some enzymatic reactions, and relevance to design of antitumor and antiviral agents, *Excerpta Med. Int. Congr. Ser.,* 571, 74, 1982.

48. **Marquez, V. E.,** personal communication.

49. **You, K., Arnold, L. J., Jr., Allison, W. S., and Kaplan, N. O.,** Enzyme stereospecificities for nicotinamide nucleotides, *TIBS,* 265, 1978.

50. **Cooney, D. A.,** personal communication.

Chapter 6

ANTIMITOTIC DRUGS AND TUBULIN-NUCLEOTIDE INTERACTIONS

Ernest Hamel

TABLE OF CONTENTS

I. INTRODUCTION

Most clinically useful antineoplastic drugs appear to interact specifically with DNA. There are, however, several exceptions to this generalization, including the antimitotic agents. This group of drugs inhibits the functions of the cellular microtubule system, which includes the mitotic spindle, through specific interactions with its major constituent, the protein tubulin.[1]

The most important mitotic inhibitors, particularly from a clinical point of view, are the vinca alkaloids vincristine and vinblastine.[1] Two highly promising newer agents, VP-16-213 and VM-26, are semisynthetic derivatives of another antitubulin agent, podophyllotoxin. The modifications introduced into the basic structure of podophyllotoxin, studied most extensively with VP-16-213, abolished its antimitotic activity and produced an activity leading to single-strand breaks in DNA.[2] VP-16-213 and VM-26, thus, differ markedly from the parent drug in their mechanism of action. A third antimitotic drug, maytansine, has undergone clinical trials recently, but has thus far had limited activity against human tumors.[3-5] The newest agent in this class to reach preclinical testing is taxol, with initial clinical studies anticipated in the near future.

It has been known since 1967 that tubulin contains two molar equivalents of guanine nucleotide,[6,7] and, since 1972, that GTP is required for tubulin polymerization.[8] Studies on the effects of antimitotic agents on tubulin-nucleotide interactions are more recent. In this article the author will briefly summarize the essential biochemical features of tubulin, including a description of its properties in high concentrations of glutamate, and discuss aspects and implications of the effects of antimitotic drugs on tubulin-nucleotide interactions and tubulin-dependent GTP hydrolysis.

II. TUBULIN AND MICROTUBULE-ASSOCIATED PROTEINS (MAPs)

A. Temperature-Dependent Assembly and Disassembly of Microtubules

After Weisenberg's discovery that even small amounts of Ca^{2+} inhibited microtubule formation in vitro[8] and the report of Shelanski et al.[9] that glycerol markedly enhanced polymerization, cycles of temperature-dependent assembly and disassembly became the favored method for preparing these cellular organelles and the initial step in the purification of tubulin. Microtubules will form at 37°C in the presence of GTP and disassemble again at 0°C. Thus, after warming an appropriately prepared cell or tissue homogenate, particularly brain tissue, microtubules can be harvested by centrifugation and subsequently dispersed in the cold. Variations in this procedure result in protein preparations containing 75 to 95% tubulin, together with a substantial number of minor protein components referred to as microtubule-associated proteins (MAPs).

Tubulin can be separated from virtually all MAPs by ion-exchange chromatography on either DEAE- or phosphocellulose.[10,11] These experiments demonstrated that the MAPs markedly enhance tubulin polymerization at low ionic strengths and low divalent cation concentrations in an aqueous environment. A number of reaction conditions have been reported, however, in which electrophoretically homogeneous tubulin will polymerize in the absence of MAPs.[12-17]

Cycle-prepared microtubule protein and both tubulin and MAPs prepared by ion-exchange chromatography have been reported by many workers to contain multiple enzymatic activities which would complicate the study of tubulin-nucleotide interactions.[16,18-31] The most important of these are nucleoside diphosphate kinase and nonspecific phosphatase(s). Elimination of these activities will be discussed below.

B. Tubulin: Structure and Nucleotide Interactions

Tubulin is an acidic protein of molecular weight 110,000 and is composed of two similar but nonidentical subunits, α- and β-tubulin.[32,33] The subunits are both of molecular weight 55,000 and have similar isoelectric points (5.3 and 5.4)[34,35] and amino acid compositions.[32,36-38] They have only been separated preparatively after denaturation and alkylation.[38,39] There are no covalent bonds between the subunits, and in dilute solution in vitro there is a partial, reversible dissociation of the dimer.[40] Based on evidence from protein cross-linking experiments, it is believed that tubulin exists as an α-β heterodimer rather than as a mixture of α-α and β-β homodimers.[41] Detailed analysis of microtubules by optical diffraction of negatively stained electron micrographs indicate that the α and β subunits are largely distinct and in globular conformations in the polymer. They alternate both longitudinally in individual fibers, termed protofilaments, and laterally between protofilaments, although the lateral contacts are staggered.[42]

On electrofocusing gels, both the α and β subunits have been resolved into multiple bands.[33,34,38,43-45] This has been termed microheterogeneity, and it appears to be due, at least in part, to a variable primary structure at a few amino acid residues in both α- and β-tubulin.[46,47] Additional factors, such as posttranslational modifications or tubulins derived from different cell types, have not yet been adequately explored.

Tubulin contains 2 mol of tightly bound GTP per mole of protein.[6,7,16,18,19,21,48,49] Half this nucleotide cannot be removed from the protein without its denaturation, or even exchanged with free nucleotide.[7,21,49] Even in cells grown in culture, the turnover time of the nonexchangeable nucleotide is very slow and comparable to that of tubulin itself.[50]

The other half of the bound nucleotide can be rapidly exchanged with free GDP or GTP.[7,18,19,21,49,51] Ths exchangeable GTP can be removed from tubulin, at least partially, by treatment with charcoal[25,52] or alkaline phosphatase[53] or by displacement with guanosine 5'-[β,γ-methylene]triphosphate and gel filtration.[54] Generally, tubulin polymerization is associated with hydrolysis of exchangeably bound GTP to GDP.[23-25,55-57] Consequently, microtubules contain 1 mol each of GDP and GTP per mole of tubulin. In the microtubule, the GDP bound in the exchangeable site is no longer rapidly exchangeable with free nucleotide, but exchangeability is restored when the polymer is disassembled.[24,55,56] The microtubule does display slow exchange of nucleotide, but this has been interpreted to represent flux of tubulin subunits through the tubule (''treadmilling'') rather than exchange of free and bound nucleotide.[58]

Studies with GTP analogs have provided additional insights into tubulin-nucleotide interactions. Microtubule assembly can be induced with nonhydrolyzable GTP analogs (guanosine 5'-[β,γ-methylene]triphosphate and guanosine 5'-[β,γ-imido]-triphosphate)[24,25,59,60] as well as with GTP, clearly indicating that GTP hydrolysis per se is not required for tubulin polymerization. Tubulin polymerization can also be induced with a photoaffinity analog of GTP, 8-azidoguanosine 5'-triphosphate. When analog bound to tubulin was photoactivated, a covalent bond formed between the nucleotide and the β subunit.[61] Finally, studies with ribose-modified GTP analogs have demonstrated that analogs with a substituted or open ribose ring are deficient relative to GTP in supporting tubulin polymerization, while several deoxyGTP analogs are more active than GTP. These findings strongly suggest a reduced affinty on a steric basis of the former group of analogs for the exchangeable site, implying that the ribose ring may be directed toward its interior.[62-64]

Some of the preceding features of the tubulin molecule are incorporated into the diagram presented in Figure 1.

GDP has substantial inhibitory effects on tubulin polymerization.[16,24,55,57,62,63,65-67] The diphosphate has variable effects on polymer, however, depending on the system being studied.[24,67-69] Some workers have reported that polymerized tubulin is stable even in high concentrations of GDP, while others have observed depolymerization when excess GDP was added to microtubules.

C. Properties of Tubulin in High Concentrations of Glutamate

Since there had been many reports that both microtubule protein and electrophoretically

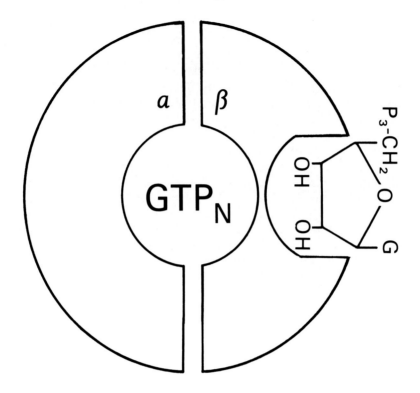

FIGURE 1.   Schematic diagram of the basic protein subunit of microtubules, the tubulin dimer. The binding site of the nonexchangeable GTP is unknown, but the exchangeable GTP has been localized to the β subunit.[61]

homogeneous tubulin prepared by ion-exchange chromatography contained nonspecific phosphatase and nucleoside diphosphate kinase activities,[20,21,24-29] we first directed our attention to the preparation of tubulin free of these contaminants. Since tubulin is a relatively labile protein,[70] we were initially frustrated by rapid loss of activity in our tissue extracts. In a search for conditions which would stabilize tubulin, as defined by its colchicine-binding activity, we found that a number of organic anions were very effective, particularly at concentrations over 0.5 M.[71] In addition, synergistic effects were observed in several cases if the reaction mixture contained either GDP or GTP with the anion.[71] Although not the most effective of these anions on a molar basis, glutamate was by far the cheapest and, thereby, deemed the most suitable for use in the purification of tubulin. Figure 2 demonstrates the effectiveness of glutamate alone and glutamate + GTP in preserving the colchicine-binding activity of tubulin during a 3-hr preincubation at 37°C.

We next found that, in the presence of GTP, high concentrations of glutamate and most of the other stabilizing anions induced tubulin to polymerize at temperatures above 20 to 25°C.[16,17] The reactions were all characterized by minimal requirements: tubulin at concentrations of at least 0.1 to 0.2 mg/mℓ together with threshold concentrations of GTP and the organic anion. These properties of glutamate-induced polymerization are illustrated in Figures 3 and 4. In these and subsequent experiments, polymerization was followed turbidimetrically as an increase in absorbance at 350 nm.

The combination of stabilization and induction of polymerization by glutamate allowed us to work out a relatively rapid, large-scale purification of tubulin.[16] A high-speed supernatant of calf brain was adsorbed to DEAE-cellulose (DEAE-Sephacel®) in 0.8 M glutamate, the maximum concentration at which tubulin would stick to the resin. Under these conditions, most other proteins did not bind. A fairly pure tubulin preparation was then eluted from the

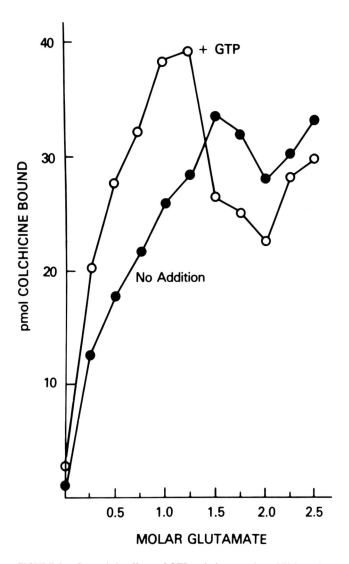

FIGURE 2. Synergistic effects of GTP and glutamate in stabilizing tubulin.[71] Reaction mixtures contained 1 mg/mℓ of tubulin and GTP and glutamate as indicated. They were preincubated for 3 hr at 37°C and then chilled. After 500 pmol of colchicine was added, the reaction mixtures were incubated for an additional hour at 37°C.

DEAE-Sephacel® with 1 M glutamate-1 M NaCl. The tubulin in the eluate was then induced to polymerize simply by adding GTP and warming. The polymerized protein was harvested by centrifugation, dispersed by homogenization on ice, and clarified by centrifugation in the cold. This cycle was repeated four times. As the polyacrylamide gels presented in Figure 5 demonstrate, all detectable contaminants remained in the warm supernatants. The final cold supernatant contained electrophoretically pure tubulin, even on overloaded gels. The warm polymerizations became decreasingly effective in purifying tubulin. Progressively smaller amounts of protein of increasing specific activity remained in the warm supernatants (Table 1). In this procedure, 4.6 g of purified tubulin was obtained from 20 calf brains, representing 60% of the colchicine-binding activity of the initial high-speed supernatant (Table 1).

The last step in our purification consists of gel filtration chromatography to separate

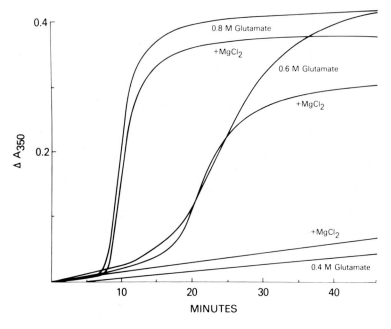

FIGURE 3.   Glutamate threshold for tubulin polymerization.[16] Reaction mixtures contained 1 mg/mℓ of tubulin, 1 mM GTP, and glutamate and 20 mM MgCl$_2$ as indicated. In this and all other experiments in which polymerization was studied, the temperature in the spectrophotometer was regulated with a thermostatically-controlled circulating water bath. Baselines were established with the samples at 0°C, and then the thermostat setting was changed to 37°C. Zero time was arbitrarily defined as the point at which the circulating water bath reached 37°C.

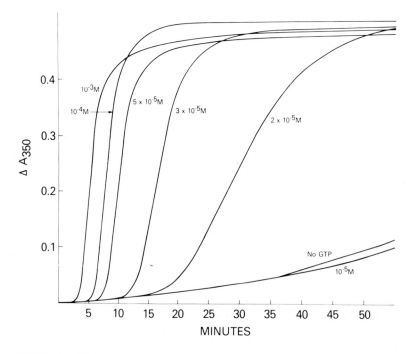

FIGURE 4.   GTP threshold for polymerization in 1.0 M glutamate.[16] Reaction mixtures contained 1 mg/mℓ of tubulin, 1.0 M glutamate, and GTP as indicated.

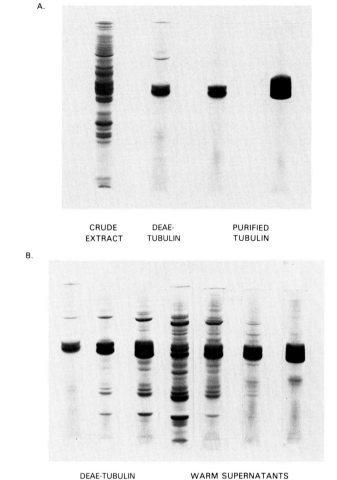

FIGURE 5. Polyacrylamide gels of purified tubulin, DEAE-tubulin, and warm supernatants.[16] The gels contained the following amounts of protein: (A) crude extract, 40 μg; DEAE-tubulin, 10 μg; purified tubulin, 10 μg; and purified tubulin, 80 μg. (B) DEAE-tubulin, 10, 20, and 40 μg; and 40 μg each of the four warm supernatants.

Table 1
PURIFICATION OF TUBULIN[16]

Preparation	Protein (g)	Colchicine bound (pmol/μg protein)	% Original colchicine-binding capacity
Crude extract	99.65	0.38	100
DEAE-tubulin	8.98	3.16	75
Purified tubulin	4.56	4.89	59
1st Warm supernatant	2.92	0.58	4.5
2nd Warm supernatant	0.35	1.33	1.2
3rd Warm supernatant	0.06	2.98	0.5
4th Warm supernatant	0.05	4.53	0.6

tubulin from residual unbound nucleotide. If the tubulin was again subjected to gel filtration chromatography, the free nucleotide peak was negligible unless 8 M urea was used in the

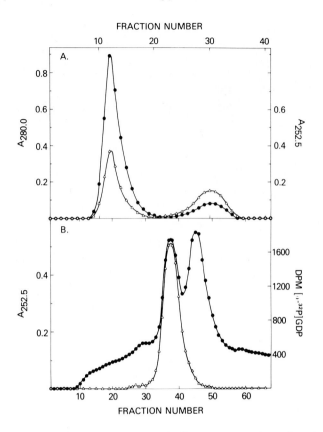

FIGURE 6. Nucleotide content of purified tubulin. (A) Separation of bound nucleotide from protein. Purified tubulin was separated from unbound nucleotide by chromatography on Sephadex® G-25 and denatured with urea. Protein and nucleotide were then separated by chromatography on Sephadex® G–100 in 8 M urea, as shown in the figure. A_{280}: ●; A_{252}: △. (B) Resolution of tubulin-bound guanine nucleotides. The nucleotide peak from the preceding column was mixed with a trace amount of [α-^{32}P]GDP, applied to DEAE-Sephadex® A-25, and resolved into GDP and GTP with a triethylammonium bicarbonate gradient. Absorbance: ●, radioactivity: △.

chromatography. Under this condition, bound nucleotide is released (Figure 6A). Assuming equal recovery of protein and nucleotide, there was 1.9 mol of guanine nucleotide per mole of tubulin in this preparation. When analyzed on DEAE-Sephadex® A-25, the nucleotide peak proved to be half GDP and half GTP (Figure 6B). (The early rise in $A_{252.5}$ represents an artifact due to the triethylammonium bicarbonate gradient used in this experiment.)

Nucleoside diphosphate kinase activity was not detectable in the purified tubulin, although abundant activity was found in both the DEAE-tubulin and the first warm supernatant (Figure 7). This was the case whether the activity was searched for with [α-^{32}P]GDP as phosphate acceptor or [γ-^{32}P]ATP as phosphate donor. Since the tubulin contained bound GDP, GTP formation was demonstrable if both nucleoside diphosphate kinase and high specific activity [γ-^{32}P]ATP, but no exogenous GDP, were mixed with tubulin (Figure 7).

Further confirmation that nucleoside diphosphate kinase activity was eliminated in this tubulin preparation was obtained in polymerization studies (Figure 8). GTP was the only ribonucleotide able to support polymerization; but polymerization could be obtained with ATP, provided exogenous nucleoside diphosphate kinase was also added.

The purified tubulin was also found to be almost totally lacking in ATPase activity, while there was easily detectable ATP hydrolysis with the DEAE-tubulin (Table 2).

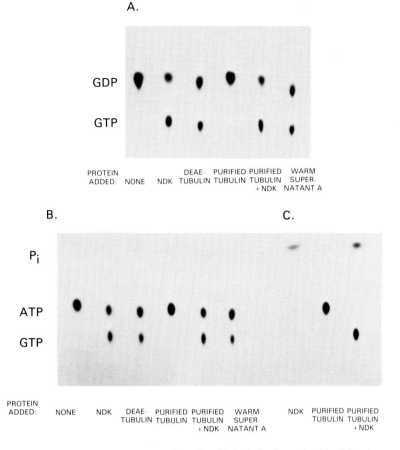

FIGURE 7. Autoradiographic examination of purified tubulin for nucleoside diphosphate kinase activity. (A) [α-³²P]GDP as phosphate acceptor. Reaction mixtures contained 1 mM ATP, 1 mM [α-³²P]GDP, 1.0 M glutamate, 2 mM MgCl₂ and, as indicated, 40 units/mℓ of yeast nucleoside diphosphate kinase (NDK), 2.2 mg/mℓ of DEAE-tubulin, 2 mg/mℓ of purified tubulin and 0.7 mg/mℓ of protein from the first warm supernatant. Incubation was for 30 min at 37°. (B) [γ-³²P]ATP as phosphate donor. Reaction conditions were identical to those described above except that the nucleotides added were 1 mM GDP and 1 mM [γ-³²P]ATP. (C) Synthesis of GTP from tubulin-bound GDP by exogenous nucleoside diphosphate kinase. Reaction mixtures contained 35 nM [γ-³²P]ATP, 1.0 M glutamate and, as indicated 20 units/mℓ of yeast nucleoside diphosphate kinase and 2 mg/mℓ of tubulin. Incubation was for 5 min at 37°C.

Tubulin polymerization in 1 M glutamate is cold-reversible and strongly inhibited by equimolar GDP and by relatively high concentrations of Ca^{2+}.[16] Furthermore, the reaction is inhibited by all classes of mitotic inhibitors which inhibit MAP-dependent polymerization. Figure 9 demonstrates this inhibition with colchicine, podophyllotoxin, vinblastine, and maytansine. Similar inhibition with nocodazole and ethyl 5-amino-1,2-dihydro-3-[(*N*-methylanilino)methyl]pyrido-[3,4-*b*]-pyrazin-7-ylcarbamate (NSC-181928) has been described elsewhere.[72]

Taxol, rather than inhibiting microtubule formation, enhances the reaction and the structures formed are highly stable. They do not disassemble in the cold, in Ca^{2+}, or upon dilution as do conventionally formed microtubules.[73] Taxol has similar effects on tubulin polymerization in 1 M glutamate.[31]

Tubulin purified in glutamate had minimal GTPase activity at low ionic strengths, but brisk GTP hydrolysis was observed in 1 M glutamate. If tubulin polymerization and GTP

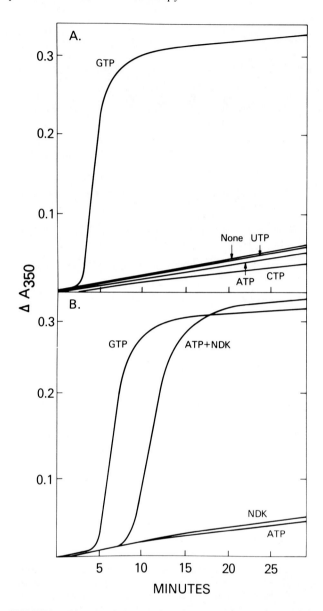

FIGURE 8.   Glutamate-induced polymerization requires GTP.[16] (A) ATP, CTP, and UTP do not support polymerization. Reaction mixtures contained 1.0 mg/mℓ of tubulin, 1.0 *M* glutamate, and the indicated nucleotide at 1 m*M*. (B) ATP and nucleoside diphosphate kinase will support polymerization. Reaction mixtures contained 1.0 mg/mℓ of tubulin, 1.0 *M* glutamate and, as indicated, 0.1 m*M* GTP, 0.1 m*M* ATP, and 25 units/mℓ of yeast nucleoside diphosphate kinase (NDK).

hydrolysis were followed together (Figure 10A), the two reactions were initially simultaneous and stoichiometric (the initial rate of GTP hydrolysis was 0.5 nmol/min/mℓ/mg tubulin). As turbidity reached its plateau, hydrolysis continued, but at a slower, linear rate (about 0.1 nmol/min/mℓ/mg tubulin).

Perhaps the major difference between the glutamate and MAPs systems is the morphology of the polymer formed. In glutamate, few microtubules are observed. Instead, open sheets or ribbons of varying width and length are the predominant product (Figures 10B and C).[17]

Table 2
LACK OF ATPASE ACTIVITY IN PURIFIED
TUBULIN[16]

Protein added	15 min at 37°C	2 hr at 37°C
Exp. I: 1 mM [γ-^{32}P]ATP	nmol P$_i$ formed	
Crude extract	4.4	14.5
DEAE-tubulin	0	2.2
Purified tubulin	0	0
Exp. II: 14 nM [γ-^{32}P]ATP	fmol P$_i$ formed	
Crude extract	412	637
DEAE-tubulin	82	216
Purified tubulin	0	8

Note: Reaction mixtures contained 1.0 M glutamate, 2 mM MgCl$_2$, and ATP and the following as indicated: 2.4 mg/mℓ of crude extract, 2.2 mg/mℓ of DEAE-tubulin, and 2.0 mg/mℓ of purified tubulin.

These sheets do display some of the fine structure of microtubules, since they also consist of parallel protofilaments (Figure 10C).

D. MAPs

It proved simple to eliminate nonspecific phosphatase and nucleoside diphosphate kinase activities from MAPs. Several workers had found that heat treatment of these proteins did not affect their ability to induce tubulin to polymerize at low ionic strengths.[74,75] David-Pfeuty et al.[26] also had reported that heat-treated MAPs no longer had GTPase activity in the absence of tubulin. We confirmed these observations with MAPs separated from tubulin on DEAE-cellulose and found, in addition, that heat treatment inactivated both nucleoside diphosphate kinase and ATPase activities found in the MAPs (Table 3).[31]

In 0.1 M glutamate, neither the tubulin nor the heat-treated MAPs alone hydrolyzed GTP or polymerized. In combination (Figure 11A), hydrolysis and polymerization were initially simultaneous and stoichiometric (the initial rate of hydrolysis was 0.7 nmol/min/mℓ/mg tubulin). As in 1.0 M glutamate, hydrolysis continued at a slower, linear rate (about 0.2 nmol/min/mℓ/mg tubulin) as polymerization reached its plateau. With the heat-treated MAPs typical microtubules were formed (Figure 11B).

III. ANTIMITOTIC DRUGS

Most antimitotic drugs are complex, natural products derived from higher plants. Before discussing their effects on tubulin-nucleotide interactions, we present the structures of seven of these drugs (Figure 12) together with a few of their salient characteristics. In terms of their interfering with each other in binding to tubulin, these agents fall into three groups.

The largest group includes the natural products colchicine and podophyllotoxin[76] and the synthetic compounds nocodazole[77] and NSC-181928.[72] Nocodazole is structurally a benzimidazole, and several drugs with the same nucleus and comparable side groups are effective anthelmintics, cause mitotic arrest, and interact with tubulin.[78,79] NSC-181928 was originally synthesized as an intermediate in a synthetic route to analogs of methotrexate, a potent inhibitor of dihydrofolate reductase.[80] Podophyllotoxin, nocodazole, and NSC-181928 all

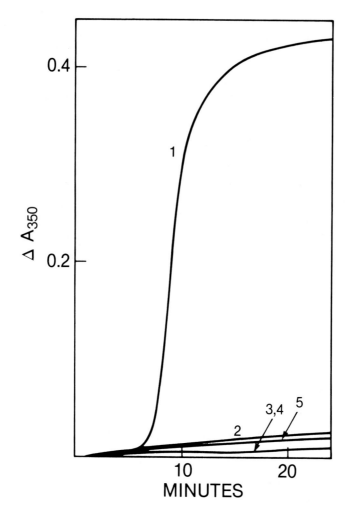

FIGURE 9.   Inhibition of glutamate-induced polymerization of tubulin by mitotic inhibitors. Reaction mixtures contained 1.0 mg/mℓ of tubulin, 1.0 *M* glutamate, 1% dimethylsulfoxide, 0.1 m*M* GTP, and drugs as follows: curve 1, none; curve 2, 10 μ*M* colchicine; curve 3, 10 μ*M* podophyllotoxin; curve 4, 10 μ*M* maytansine; and curve 5, 4 μ*M* vinblastine.

inhibit colchicine binding to tubulin.[72,76,77] All four drugs inhibit microtubule assembly and tubulin polymerization in 1 *M* glutamate.

Vinblastine and maytansine also inhibit microtubule assembly.[76,81] Although they do not affect the binding of colchicine to tubulin, they mutually inhibit each other in binding to the protein.[76,82,83]

As noted above, taxol induces rather than inhibits microtubule assembly.[73] It inhibits neither colchicine[84] nor vinblastine[97] binding to tubulin. Both podophyllotoxin and vinblastine, however, inhibit the binding of radiolabeled taxol to microtubules.[85] It is believed that taxol does not bind to the tubulin dimer, but rather to oligomers or polymer.[84,85]

IV. EFFECTS OF ANTIMITOTIC DRUGS ON TUBULIN-DEPENDENT GTP HYDROLYSIS

A. Studies in 0.1 *M* 2-(*N*-morpholino)ethanesulfonate (Mes)-0.5 m*M* MgCl$_2$

Although Bryan had demonstrated that colchicine, vinblastine, and GTP all bound to

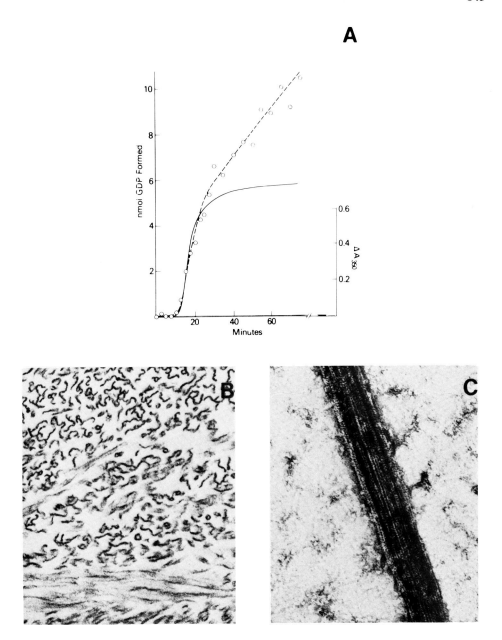

FIGURE 10. GTP hydrolysis and polymer morphology in 1.0 M glutamate.[17] Reaction mixtures contained 0.8 mg/mℓ of tubulin, 1.0 M glutamate, and 0.1 mM GTP or [α-^{32}P]GTP. (A) Time course of turbidity development and GTP hydrolysis. The line to the right of the break in the axis is the turbidity reading following cold depolymerization. (B) Thin section of tubulin polymer. (C) Negatively stained preparation of polymerized tubulin.

tubulin at independent sites without apparent cross inhibition,[48] the effects of these drugs on tubulin-dependent GTP hydrolysis were first studied by Pantaloni and collaborators.[56,86-88] Most of their experiments were performed in 0.1 M Mes-0.5 mM MgCl$_2$, a reaction condition in which tubulin will neither polymerize nor hydrolyze GTP without MAPs or other agents which stimulate polymerization. Without such agents, Pantaloni and colleagues found that colchicine induced a significant GTPase activity in tubulin.[56]

With MAPs and other inducers of polymerization, these workers observed a burst of GTP hydrolysis followed by a slower, linear hydrolytic reaction — [56,86] results qualitatively similar

Table 3
EFFECT OF HEAT-TREATMENT ON THE
NUCLEOSIDE DIPHOSPHATE KINASE, ATPASE, AND
GTPASE ACTIVITIES OF MAPS

Activity	Preparation added[31]	
Nucleoside diphosphate kinase		nmol GTP formed
	DEAE-purified MAPs	21.0
	Heat-treated MAPs	0.2
ATPase		nmol P_i formed
	DEAE-purified MAPs	21.1
	Heat-treated MAPs	0.4
GTPase		nmol GDP formed
	DEAE-purified MAPs	21.4
	Heat-treated MAPs	0.5

Note: All reaction mixtures contained 0.5 mg/mℓ of protein, 0.1 *M* Mes (pH
6.4), 1 m*M* MgCl$_2$, and 30 m*M* glutamate. In the nucleoside diphosphate
kinase experiment, reaction mixtures contained 0.1 m*M* [γ-^{32}P]ATP and
0.2 m*M* GDP, and incubation was for 30 min at 37°C. In the ATPase
experiment, reaction mixtures contained 0.1 m*M* [γ-^{32}P]ATP, and incubation was for 60 min at 37°C. In the GTPase experiment, reaction mixtures contained 0.1 m*M* [α-^{32}P]GTP, and incubation was for 60 min at
37°C.

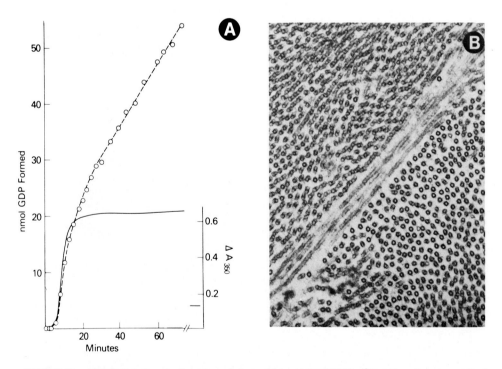

FIGURE 11.   GTP hydrolysis and polymer morphology with heat-treated MAPs.[17] Reaction mixtures contained
3.0 mg/mℓ of tubulin, 1.0 mg/mℓ of heat-treated MAPs, 0.1 *M* glutamate, and 0.3 m*M* GTP or [α-^{32}P]GTP.
(A) Time course of turbidity development and GTP hydrolysis. The line to the right of the break in the axis
is the turbidity reading following cold depolymerization. (B) Thin section of tubulin polymer.

to those described above from our laboratory (Figures 10 and 11). With colchicine, when
polymerization was inhibited there was only a linear hydrolytic reaction.[56,86] The rate of this

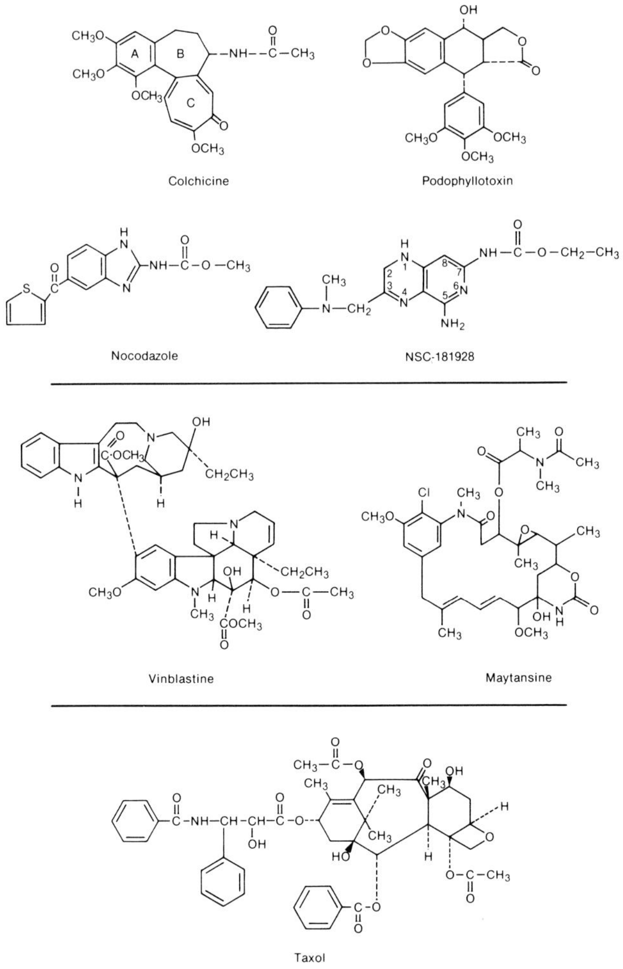

FIGURE 12. Molecular formulas of antimitotic drugs.

reaction was less than half the maximum rate obtained with MAPs, but five- to sixfold faster than the final linear rate with MAPs.[86] Although, initially, these workers felt that colchicine-dependent GTP hydrolysis was a linear function of tubulin concentration,[86] more recent experiments have demonstrated that hydrolysis is a sigmoidal function of tubulin concentration.[87] We have observed similar cooperative effects on GTP hydrolysis with either colchicine or MAPs,[97] as well as with several organic anions[17] which induce both tubulin polymerization and GTP hydrolysis. Under all these conditions, then — including colchicine-induced hydrolysis — it seems likely that tubulin-tubulin interactions are required for nucleotide hydrolysis to occur.

Even more surprising than the stimulation of tubulin-dependent GTP hydrolysis by colchicine was the finding of Pantaloni's group that podophyllotoxin inhibited GTP hydrolysis.[86] The two drugs, thus, have opposite effects on GTP hydrolysis despite their competitive binding to tubulin and similar inhibitory effects on polymerization. These workers also reported that vinblastine inhibited MAP-dependent GTP hydrolysis by tubulin, although polymerization was more sensitive to the drug than was hydrolysis.[56,86]

B. Studies in 1 *M* Glutamate

We initially began to study the effects of antimitotic agents on tubulin-dependent GTP hydrolysis in an attempt to understand the structural basis for the opposite effects of colchicine

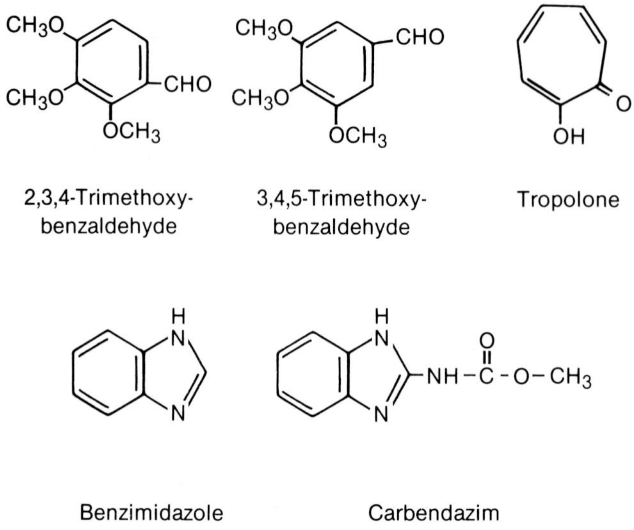

2,3,4-Trimethoxy-
benzaldehyde

3,4,5-Trimethoxy-
benzaldehyde

Tropolone

Benzimidazole

Carbendazim

FIGURE 13.   Molecular formulas of simpler analogs of colchicine and nocodazole.

and podophyllotoxin.[89] These studies have included the seven antimitotic compounds presented in Figure 12 and a number of simpler compounds presented in Figure 13.[31,72,89] Most of our experiments have been performed in 1 M glutamate, since this reaction condition permits simultaneous examination of both stimulatory and inhibitory effects. In addition, unlike with MAPs, this reaction condition permits unambiguous study of interactions of drugs with tubulin itself.

Figure 14 presents a comparison of the effects on tubulin-dependent GTP hydrolysis of colchicine, vinblastine, podophyllotoxin, nocodazole, and maytansine, while Figure 15A presents a similar study with colchicine, nocodazole, NSC-181928, and taxol. These studies confirmed the essential observations of Pantaloni's group: colchicine stimulated GTP hydrolysis, while vinblastine and higher concentrations of podophyllotoxin were inhibitory. At lower concentrations, podophyllotoxin showed mild but reproducible stimulatory effects. Maytansine, the inhibitor of vinblastine binding to tubulin, was also strongly inhibitory; but the other inhibitors of colchicine binding, nocodazole and NSC-181928, were strongly stimulatory, apparently far surpassing colchicine in stimulating GTP hydrolysis (but see below). In the experiment of Figure 15A, taxol inhibited net GTP hydrolysis.

Suspecting that the apparent superiority of nocodazole and NSC-181928 to colchicine in stimulating hydrolysis might be due to the relatively slow binding to tubulin of the latter drug,[76] we examined the effect of preincubating tubulin and the drug prior to adding GTP (Figure 15B). This preincubation enhanced only the effect of colchicine, and with a preincubation its activity was similar to that of NSC-181928. Preincubation also enhanced the inhibitory effects of taxol (Figure 15B), vinblastine,[89] and maytansine,[89] but had little effect with podophyllotoxin.[89]

In the previous experiments we examined net hydrolysis after a 20-min incubation. Somewhat different results were obtained if the time course of hydrolysis was followed with drugs at 10 μM (Figure 16A) or 100 μM (Figure 16B). Taxol was stimulatory at early times (enhancing the initial burst of hydrolysis), and mildly inhibitory at later time points (inhibiting the slower, linear reaction). Colchicine, nocodazole, and NSC-181928 all inhibited the initial burst of hydrolysis, but were stimulatory at later time points. They thus appear to stimulate the slower, linear reaction as noted by Pantaloni's group with colchicine.[56] The net inhibitory effect of podophyllotoxin, however, seems to derive entirely from inhibition of the initial burst of hydrolysis (Figure 16B). The linear reaction appears little affected by the drug.

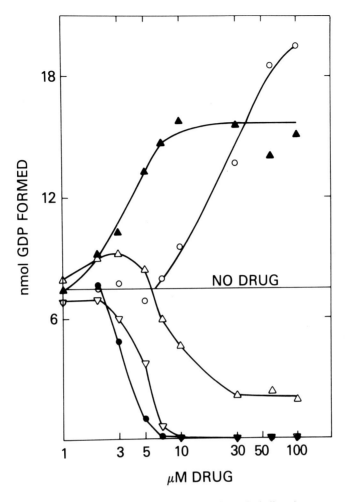

FIGURE 14. Effects of colchicine, nocodazole, podophyllotoxin, maytansine, and vinblastine on tubulin-dependent GTP hydrolysis.[89] Reaction mixtures contained 1.0 mg/mℓ of tubulin, 1.0 M glutamate, 10% dimethylsulfoxide, 50 μM [α-^{32}P]GTP, and drugs as follows: o, colchicine; ▲, nocodazole; △, podophyllotoxin; ●, vinblastine; and ▽, maytansine. The line drawn across the figure represents the reaction occurring without added drug. Incubation was for 20 min at 37°C.

The differing effects of podophyllotoxin and colchicine remained puzzling. One could have attributed the stimulatory effect of colchicine to its tropolone group, with the trimethoxybenzene ring common to both drugs being inert in its effect on GTP hydrolysis. Yet nocodazole, in particular, appeared to be most analogous to colchicine in the trimethoxybenzene ring, part of the B ring, and the acetylamino group (see Figure 12).

This postulated analogy was supported by studies with the simpler compounds whose structures were presented above in Figure 13 (Table 4). Most trimethoxybenzene structures which we examined had little effect on tubulin-dependent GTP hydrolysis, but significant stimulation of the reaction was observed with 2,3,4-trimethoxybenzaldehyde and especially 3,4,5-trimethoxybenzaldehyde.[89] Tropolone, on the other hand, had no effect on GTP hydrolysis.[89] We were, however, unable to reproduce the reported inhibition of tropolone on colchicine binding to tubulin,[90] while inhibition with 3,4,5-trimethoxybenzaldehyde was easily demonstrable. We also found little activity with benzimidazole, but addition of the methylcarbamate side chain to the benzimidazole nucleus (in the antifungal agent carben-

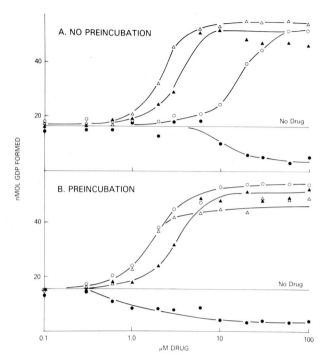

FIGURE 15.   Effects of NSC-181928, taxol, colchicine, and nocodazole on tubulin-dependent GTP hydrolysis in 1.0 M glutamate.[72] Reaction mixtures contained 1.0 mg/mℓ of tubulin, 1.0 M glutamate, 10% dimethylsulfoxide, 100 μM [α-^{32}P]GTP, and drugs as follows: $\triangle$, NSC-181928; $\blacktriangle$, nocodacole; o, colchicine; and $\bullet$, taxol. The lines drawn across the figures represent the reactions occurring without added drug. Incubation was for 20 min at 37°C. (A) No preincubation. (B) Drug and tubulin preincubated. All components except GTP were preincubated for 2 hr at 37°C prior to the addition of GTP.

dazim) resulted in a compound able to stimulate GTP hydrolysis at relatively high concentrations.

On the other hand, while the structural analogy of NSC-181928 to nocodazole is clear, its relationship to colchicine is not obvious. Furthermore, removal of the acetyl group from colchicine did not affect the stimulation of GTP hydrolysis, by the drug. Both *N*-deacetylcolchicine[91] and *N*-deacetyl-*N*-methylcolchicine had activity comparable to colchicine itself (Figure 17). Ray et al.[92] have also recently reported that an analog of colchicine lacking the B ring entirely binds rapidly to tubulin, in contrast to the slow binding of colchicine.

Assuming that occupancy of a single site on tubulin is responsible for the stimulation of GTP hydrolysis by these agents, the effects of nocodazole and NSC-181928 must represent an interaction at the same site as colchicine and 3,4,5-trimethoxybenzaldehyde. The trimethoxybenzene ring of colchicine may then be structurally analogous to the alkylcarbamate side chain and the imidazole or pyridine ring. The thiophene and methylanilinomethyl groups of nocodazole and NSC-181928 respectively, might then have functions comparable to the tropolone group of colchicine, including substantially enhancing binding of the drug to tubulin. The mild stimulation of GTP hydrolysis observed at low podophyllotoxin concentrations may indicate an initial binding of this drug to tubulin via its trimethoxybenzene ring. The decreased hydrolysis observed at higher podophyllotoxin levels probably represents a predominating effect of the tetrahydronaphthol moiety. Thus far, however, we have been unable to demonstrate any effect on tubulin-dependent GTP hydrolysis with simpler analogs of this structure, such as safrole or tetrahydronaphthol itself.

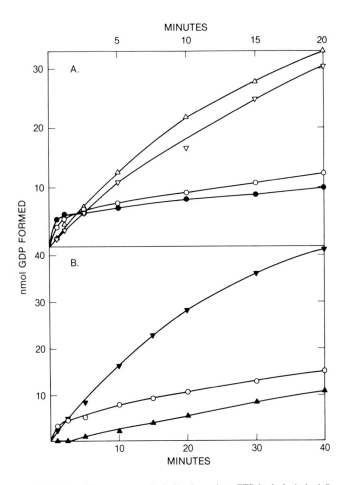

FIGURE 16. Time course of tubulin-dependent GTP hydrolysis in 1.0 M glutamate with nododazole, NSC-181928, taxol, colchicine, and podophyllotoxin. Reaction mixtures were incubated at 37°C and contained 1.0 mg/mℓ of tubulin, 1.0 M glutamate, 10% dimethylsulfoxide, 50 μM [α-^{32}P]GTP, and drugs as follows: o, none (both panels); ●, 10 μM taxol; ▽, 10 μM nocodazole; △, 10 μM NSC-181928; ▼, 100 μM colchicine; and ▲, 100 μM podophyllotoxin.

Table 4
EFFECTS OF PARTIAL ANALOGS OF COLCHICINE AND NOCODAZOLE ON TUBULIN-DEPENDENT GTP HYDROLYSIS[89]

Drug added	GDP formed (% control)
None	100
1 mM 3,4,5-trimethoxybenzaldehyde	243
1 mM 2,3,4-trimethoxybenzaldehyde	156
1 mM tropolone	107
0.1 mM benzimidazole	93
0.1 M carbendazim	180

Note: Reaction mixtures contained 1.0 mg/mℓ of tubulin, 1.0 M glutamate, 10% dimethylsulfoxide, 50 μM [α-^{32}P]GTP, and drugs as indicated. Incubation was for 30 min at 37°C.

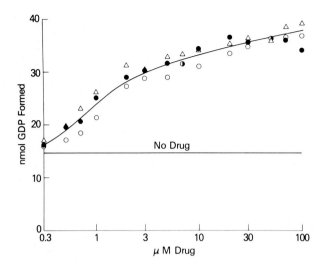

FIGURE 17. Effects of colchicine analogs on tubulin-dependent GTP hydrolysis in 1.0 M glutamate.[89] Reaction mixtures contained 1.0 mg/mℓ of tubulin, 1.0 M glutamate, 10% dimethylsulfoxide, 50 μM [α-^{32}P]GTP, and drugs as follows: ●, colchicine; △, N-deacetylcolchicine; and o, N-deacetyl-N-methylcolchicine. In this experiment tubulin and drug were preincubated for 2 hr at 37°C before the addition of GTP. Incubation was for 20 min at 37°C. The line drawn across the figure represents the reaction occurring without added drug.

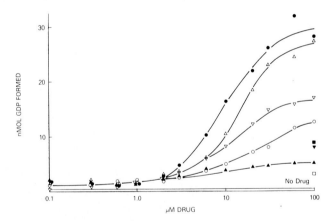

FIGURE 18. Effects of NSC-181928, nocodazole, taxol, and colchicine on tubulin-dependent GTP hydrolysis in 0.1 M glutamate.[72] Reaction mixtures contained 1.0 mg/mℓ of tubulin, 0.1M glutamate, 10% dimethylsulfoxide, 50 μM [α-^{32}P]GTP, and drugs as follows, with a 2-hr– drug– tubulin preincubation at 37°C as indicated: △, NSC-181928; ■, NSC-181928, preincubated; ▲, nocodazole; □, nocodazole, preincubated; o, colchicine; ▽, colchicine, preincubated; ●, taxol; and ▼, taxol, prein-cubated. Incubation was for 20 min at 37°C. The line drawn across the figures represents the reaction occurring without added drug.

C. Studies in 0.1 M Glutamate

In 0.1 M glutamate, tubulin neither polymerizes nor hydrolyzes GTP. Under this reaction condition, taxol potently stimulated GTP hydrolysis,[31] while NSC-181928 had almost comparable activity (Figure 18).[72] The effects of colchicine and particularly nocodazole were much weaker. Preincubation led to only moderate enhancement of the reaction with colchicine, while the reactions stimulated by taxol, NSC-181928, and nocodazole were all reduced. These preincubation effects probably are caused by the lability of tubulin in low concentrations of glutamate.[71] Since colchicine also stabilizes the protein,[93] it seems likely that the other drugs have little stabilizing effect on tubulin.

The stimulation of GTP hydrolysis observed with taxol is attributable, at least in part, to the enhanced polymerization caused by the drug (see Section VI.). We have observed no similar polymerization with NSC-181928. Like nocodazole and colchicine, the drug primarily appears to inhibit polymerization.[72]

V. GTP HYDROLYSIS AS A SCREENING TEST FOR NEW ANTIMITOTIC DRUGS

From the studies summarized above, it is clear that most, if not all, classes of antimitotic agents either inhibit or stimulate tubulin-dependent GTP hydrolysis. Technically this assay is significantly more facile than polymerization or drug binding assays or measurement of mitotic indexes, particularly if many samples are being processed. Examination of antineoplastic agents of unknown mechanism of action for effects on tubulin-dependent GTP hydrolysis should, therefore, prove to be useful as a screening test for antimitotic activity. In fact, our initial observations with NSC-181928 were its dramatic effects on GTP hydrolysis, although Wheeler et al.[94] had previously noted its antimitotic activity.

Figure 19 presents autoradiograms which demonstrate the effects of the antimitotic drugs at 0.1 mM on tubulin-dependent GTP hydrolysis in 1.0 M and 0.1 M glutamate. They are compared to several drugs which have no known interaction with tubulin and are inert as well in this assay. The effects of the antimitotic drugs are obvious by mere inspection of the autoradiograms when both reaction conditions are examined. We are currently using this method in an effort to identify new antimitotic agents.

VI. EFFECTS OF TAXOL ON TUBULIN-NUCLEOTIDE INTERACTIONS

The effect of taxol on tubulin-dependent GTP hydrolysis obviously varies greatly with reaction conditions (see above). Our initial studies, however, were limited to 0.1 M glutamate. The potent stimulation of hydrolysis (Figure 18) observed was puzzling in view of reports that taxol-induced polymerization of both microtubule protein[84] and purified tubulin[95] did not require GTP. We therefore decided to examine in detail nucleotide effects on taxol-induced polymerization with taxol. Substantial variation was observed in the polymerization reaction depending, in particular, on reaction temperature and whether or not MAPs were present.[31]

Figure 20 demonstrates that with purified tubulin, and without MAPs, there was no polymerization even at 37°C unless both taxol and GTP were added. In addition, GDP completely inhibited the taxol-dependent polymerization reaction. Finally, in contrast to the results reported with microtubule protein,[73,84] taxol- and GTP-dependent polymerization of purified tubulin was substantially, although slowly, cold-reversible.

From the experiment of Figure 21, it is clear that the GTP hydrolysis dependent on taxol in 0.1 M glutamate is closely associated with polymerization. As in 1.0 M glutamate (Figure 10) or in 0.1 M glutamate with MAPS (Figure 11), hydrolysis and polymerization were initially simultaneous and stoichiometric, with a slower hydrolytic reaction (about 0.25 nmol/min/mℓ/mg tubulin) occurring at the polymerization plateau. This GTP hydrolysis, like the polymerization reaction, could be completely inhibited with GDP.[31]

A much more complicated pattern was observed in the presence of MAPs (Figure 22). At 0°C a reaction beginning within 5 sec of the addition of taxol was observed only if both the drug and GTP were present (curve 1). This 0°C polymerization reaction was completely

1.0 M GLUTAMATE

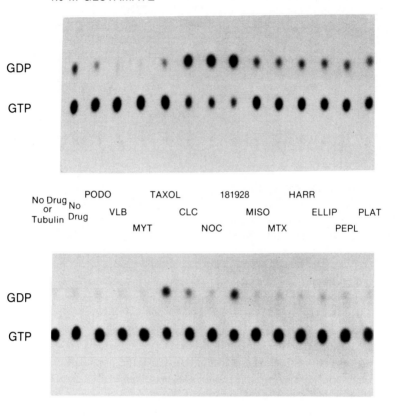

FIGURE 19.   Tubulin-dependent GTP hydrolysis as a screening test for antimitotic drugs. Each reaction mixture contained 1.0 mg/mℓ of tubulin unless indicated, glutamate as indicated, 10% dimethylsulfoxide, 50 μM [α-^{32}P]GTP, and the following drugs at 0.1 mM as indicated: podophyllotoxin (PODO), vinblastine (VLB), maytansine (MYT), taxol, colchicine (CLC), nocodazole (NOC), NSC-181928, misonidazole (MISO), methotrexate (MTX), harringtonine (HARR), ellipticine (ELLIP), pepleomycin (PEPL), and *cis*-diaminedichloroplatinum (PLAT). Incubation was for 20 min at 37°C.

inhibited by GDP (curve 1a). Warming the reaction mixture resulted in a second wave of polymerization which was much less affected by GDP. In the presence of MAPs, GTP was no longer required for polymerization at 37°C (curve 2) as a brisk reaction occurred in the absence of added nucleotide. GDP still exerted a mild inhibitory effect on this GTP-independent reaction (curve 2a). In agreement with the findings of Schiff et al. with microtubule protein, the reactions occurring with taxol and MAPs were largely cold-irreversible.[73,84] Without taxol, but with GTP, a typical cold-reversible reaction occurred at 37°C (curve 3), and it was inhibited by GDP (curve 3a). There was sluggish turbidity development at 37°C without GTP or taxol (curve 4) in the presence of MAPs. This probably represents aggregation or ring formation rather than polymerization,[10,11] as it was not cold-reversible.

When GTP hydrolysis and polymerization were followed simultaneously with taxol + MAPs (Figure 23), we found that at 0°C the two reactions again initially coincided with about a 1:1 stoichiometry. The rate of GTP hydrolysis slowed to a linear rate of about 0.12 nmol/min/mℓ/mg tubulin as polymerization reached its 0°C plateau. As the reaction mixture was warmed, the temperature-dependent phase of polymerization began. About 5 min later, when this second phase of polymerization was about 50% complete, GTP hydrolysis suddenly

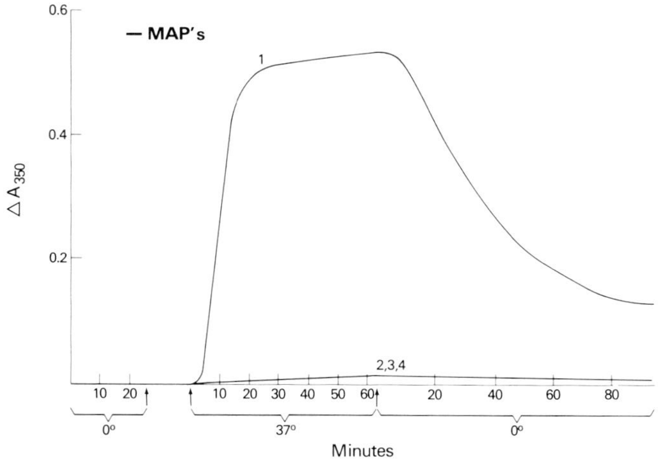

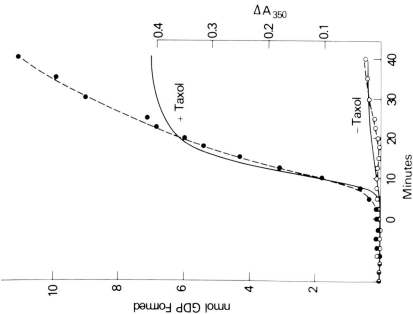

FIGURE 20. Requirements for the polymerization of purified tubulin in the presence of taxol in 0.1 *M* glutamate.[31] Reaction mixtures contained 1.0 mg/mℓ of tubulin, 0.1 *M* glutamate and the following: curve 1, 50 μ*M* GTP and 10 μ*M* taxol; curve 2, 10 μ*M* taxol; curve 3, 50 μ*M* GTP; and curve 4, 50 μ*M* GTP, 500 μ*M* GDP and 10 μ*M* taxol. At the first arrow, the thermostat setting of the water bath was raised to 37°C. The second arrow notes the point at which the water bath reached 37°C. At the third arrow, the temperature of the water bath was lowered to 0°C by the addition of ice.

FIGURE 21. Simultaneous examination of tubulin polymerization and GTP hydrolysis in the presence of taxol without MAPs.[31] Reaction mixtures contained 1.0 mg/mℓ of tubulin, 0.1 *M* glutamate, 50 μ*M* [α-³²P]GTP, and, if indicated, 10 μ*M* taxol.

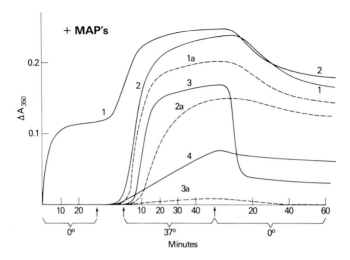

FIGURE 22. Requirements for the polymerization of purified tubulin with MAPs in the presence of taxol.[31] Reaction mixtures contained 1.0 mg/mℓ of tubulin, 0.33 mg/mℓ of heat-treated MAPs, 0.1 *M* glutamate, and the following: curve 1, 50 μ*M* GTP and 10 μ*M* taxol; curve 1a, 50 μ*M* GTP, 500 μ*M* GDP and 10 μ*M* taxol; curve 2, 10 μ*M* taxol; curve 2a, 10 μ*M* taxol and 500 μ*M* GDP; curve 3, 50 μ*M* GTP; curve 3a, 50 μ*M* GTP and 500 μ*M* GDP; and curve 4, no addition. Arrows as in Figure 20.

accelerated about 2.5-fold to 0.3 nmol/min/mℓ/mg tubulin. Figure 23 also demonstrates that GDP completely inhibited both polymerization and GTP hydrolysis at 0°C, as well as reduced the rate of temperature-dependent hydrolysis by sixfold to 0.05 nmol/min/mℓ/mg tubulin. In the presence of GDP, polymerization occurring at 37°C substantially exceeded the amount of GTP hydrolyzed.

When the glutamate concentration was raised to 0.2 *M,* the absolute requirement for GTP disappeared in taxol-induced polymerization of purified tubulin (Figure 24A). When the glutamate concentration was raised to 1.0 *M* (Figure 24B) the temperature requirement for taxol-induced polymerization disappeared. The pattern observed with 1.0 *M* glutamate was similar to that with MAPs at 0.1 *M* glutamate: a 0°C reaction dependent on GTP, a reaction occurring at higher temperatures independent of nucleotide. As with MAPs, there was a taxol-dependent hydrolysis of GTP at 0°C in 1.0 *M* glutamate.[97]

There were differences in the effect of taxol on GTP hydrolysis with MAPs as opposed to 1.0 *M* glutamate at 37°C. Under the latter reaction condition, taxol was stimulatory at earlier times and inhibitory at later times (Figure 16). With MAPs, however, taxol was stimulatory throughout the reaction (Figure 25), although the major stimulatory effect was also on the initial burst of hydrolysis associated with polymerization. Moreover, at 37°C in the presence of taxol, the MAPs themselves lost their stimulatory effect on tubulin-dependent GTP hydrolysis (Figure 25). There was essentially no difference between the complete system of MAPs + tubulin + taxol and that with only tubulin + taxol.

When the morphology of taxol-induced polymer was examined, we found predominantly microtubules when MAPs were present, regardless of reaction temperature or whether GTP was included in the reaction. In 0.1 *M* glutamate with GTP, the predominant structures were sheets of parallel protofilaments with occasional microtubules. In 1.0 *M* glutamate only sheets were observed, as without taxol.[31]

Our studies clearly demonstrate that the interaction of taxol and tubulin is profoundly influenced by other components of the reaction system. Even though taxol can cause tubulin to polymerize in the absence of GTP under some reaction conditions, it is clear that under

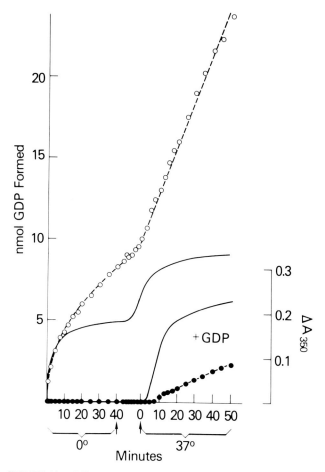

FIGURE 23.   Effect of taxol and MAPs on tubulin polymerization and GTP hydrolysis with sequential 0°C and 37°C incubations.[31] Reaction mixtures contained 1.0 mg/mℓ of tubulin, 0.33 mg/mℓ of heat-treated MAPs, 10 μM taxol, 0.1 M glutamate, 50 μM [α-^{32}P]GTP and, if indicated, 500 μM GDP. Arrows as in Figure 20.

other conditions tubulin polymerization with taxol is absolutely dependent on GTP and, conversely, that GTP hydrolysis by tubulin requires taxol. If GTP is required, GDP is an effective inhibitor of both taxol-dependent polymerization and GTP hydrolysis. Under conditions in which GTP is not required for taxol-induced polymerization, the polymerization and GTPase reactions seem to occur independently. In these reactions, GDP inhibits GTP hydrolysis to a much greater extent than it does polymerization.

Excluding solvent conditions and tubulin itself, the 0.1 M glutamate system we have examined in greatest detail has four components: taxol, GTP, MAPs, and heat (0°C being considered negative, 37°C positive for heat). Rapid tubulin polymerization occurred if any three of these components were present. Of particular note is the extremely rapid polymerization at 0°C in the presence of GTP, MAPs, and taxol. Under this condition, nucleation must be virtually instantaneous.

We have also observed no reduction in the bound GTP associated with polymerized tubulin after polymerization with taxol in the absence of exogenous GTP.[97] This indicates that the nonexchangeable GTP remains unaltered in polymerization reactions with taxol.

VII. TUBULIN-DEPENDENT GTP HYDROLYSIS AS AN ASSAY FOR ANTIMITOTIC DRUGS

In many cases, it has been difficult to develop clinical assays for antimitotic agents.

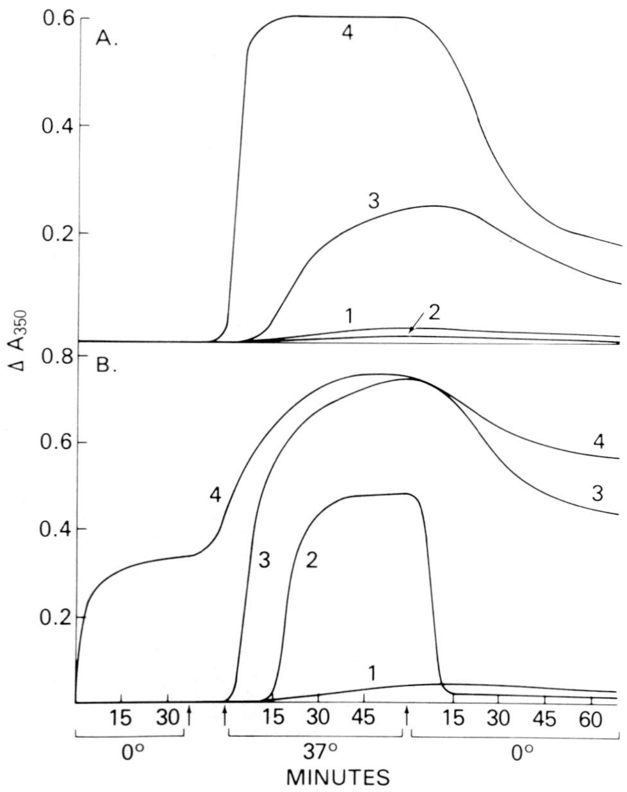

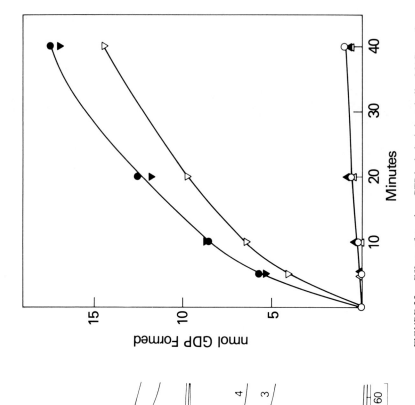

FIGURE 24.   Effects of higher concentrations of glutamate on taxol-induced tubulin polymerization.[31] (A) 0.2 *M* glutamate. (B) 1.0 *M* glutamate. Reaction mixtures contained glutamate as described above, 1.0 mg/mℓ of tubulin and the following: curves 1, no addition; curves 2, 50 *μM* GTP; curves 3, 10 *μM* taxol; and curves 4, 50 *μM* GTP and 10 *μM* taxol. Arrows as in Figure 20.

FIGURE 25.   Effects of taxol on GTP hydrolysis by tubulin, MAPs, and tubulin + MAPs at 37°C.[31] Reaction mixtures contained 50 *μM* [α-³²P]GTP, 0.1 *M* glutamate and, if indicated, 1.0 mg/mℓ of tubulin. 0.33 mg/mℓ of heat-treated MAPs and 10 *μM* taxol: o, tubulin; ●, tubulin and taxol; △, MAPs; ▲, MAPs and taxol; ▽, tubulin and MAPs; and ▼, tubulin, MAPs and taxol.

Although no attempt was made in the preceding studies to choose reaction conditions for GTP hydrolysis with maximal sensitivity for the antimitotic agents, the effects of several compounds were clear-cut at concentrations lower than 1 μM (Figures 15 and 17). Tubulin-dependent GTP hydrolysis, therefore, may have general utility as the basis for assays for this class of agent.

A. An Assay for Taxol

Since taxol is nearing clinical trials and there was no available clinical assay for the drug, we decided to explore its effects on tubulin-dependent GTP hydrolysis as a potential assay.[96] Since assay reliability would be greater with a minimal baseline, we directed our attention to conditions in which hydrolysis was dependent on taxol and searched for conditions which would maximize sensitivity for the drug. The best results were obtained using 1.0 M glutamate, 1 mM MgCl$_2$, 0.2 mg/mℓ of tubulin, 0.01 to 0.1 μM GTP, and a 0°C incubation.[96]

Taxol stimulation of tubulin-dependent GTP hydrolysis under these conditions was significantly enhanced by preincubating taxol and tubulin at 37°C in the absence of GTP (Table 5). Since this probably results in the formation of stable polymerization products prior to the addition of GTP (see Fig. 24B), it is most likely these tubulin polymers that are responsible for most of the hydrolytic reaction.

Figure 26 demonstrates the reproducibility of the assay in three separate experiments, with all experimental points representing an average of nine values. As the inset shows, sensitivity was at least as low as 0.1 μM taxol in two of these experiments and 0.2 μM in the third.

Clinical use of this assay would be complicated by substantial phosphatase activity in serum (Figure 27A). Methods of treating serum were evaluated for effectiveness in eliminating these enzyme(s) while preserving the taxol content of serum. Heat and perchlorate treatment destroyed both phosphatase activity and taxol.[97] Similar results were obtained with ultrafiltration of serum (Figure 27B), suggesting that taxol is largely bound by serum proteins. We were, however, able to recover 75 to 85% of exogenously added taxol from serum and simultaneously precipitate the phosphatase activity by adding four parts dimethylsulfoxide to serum (Figure 27C).[96]

To demonstrate the usefulness of this assay for the determination of taxol levels in clinical specimens, the serum extraction method was used to follow the pharmacokinetics of taxol in the rabbit (Figure 28). To minimize the effect of incomplete extraction of taxol, the standard curve was generated from samples of baseline rabbit serum containing known amounts of the drug (Figure 28, inset) which were extracted in the same way as the serum samples obtained after injection of taxol. Figure 28 demonstrates that taxol, after intravenous injection at a dose of 8.5 mg/kg, was rapidly cleared from the serum of this experimental animal. Assuming a two-compartment open model, its apparent α-phase half-life was 2.7 min and its β-phase half-life was 42 min. An ultrafiltrate was also prepared from the serum sample obtained 5 min after drug injection. This contained about 8% of the taxol found in the serum extract, comparable to the results obtained with exogenously added taxol. In initial studies in the rhesus monkey, a similar rapid clearance of taxol from the serum has been observed.[97]

VIII. CONCLUSION

It is clear from the studies presented above that the apparent effects of antimitotic agents on tubulin-nucleotide interactions can vary markedly with reaction conditions. From studies published thus far, it appears that the initial burst of GTP hydrolysis is associated with tubulin polymerization. All drugs except taxol inhibit this burst of hydrolysis, consistent with observations that all drugs except taxol function primarily by inhibiting microtubule

Table 5
EFFECT OF PREINCUBATING TAXOL
AND TUBULIN AT 37°C ON
SUBSEQUENT GTP HYDROLYSIS AT
0°C[96]

	% GTP hydrolyzed	
	Not preincubated	**Preincubated**
No taxol	3.7	3.6
+ 1 μM taxol	16.9	42.7

Note: Reaction mixtures of 45 μℓ contained 10 μg of
tubulin, 50 μmol of glutamate, the indicated amount
of taxol in 5 μℓ of dimethylsulfoxide, and 50 nmol
of MgCl$_2$. If indicated, reaction mixtures were
preincubated for 1 hr at 37°C and then chilled on
ice, then 5 μℓ of 0.1 μM [α-^{32}P]GTP was added
to each reaction mixture. Incubation was for 18 hr
at 0°C.

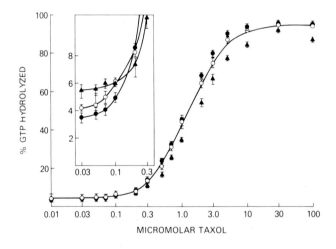

FIGURE 26.   Experimental reproducibility of taxol-dependent stimulation
of GTP hydrolysis by tubulin.[96] Reaction mixtures contained tubulin, glutamate, MgCl$_2$, [α-^{32}P]GTP, and dimethylsulfoxide as described in Table
5, and the indicated amounts of taxol. Incubations as in Table 5. Inset
presents data from 0.03 to 0.3 μM taxol on an expanded scale.

formation. The significance of the sustained hydrolytic reaction occurring at the turbidity
plateau with both MAPs and glutamate is unclear. In the absence of antimitotic drugs, this
reaction appears to require polymer[56] and may occur at microtubule ends.[26] If this reaction
indeed requires polymer, then the GTP hydrolysis occurring at colchicine, nocodazole, NSC-
181928, and even podophyllotoxin concentrations which totally inhibit polymerization must
represent a fundamentally different reaction. On the other hand, GTP hydrolysis in the
presence of these drugs may indicate the existence of oligomers undetectable by turbidimetry
which are unable to sustain polymerization but are able to hydrolyze nucleotide.

Despite the uncertain nature of tubulin-dependent GTP hydrolysis evoked by many antimitotic agents, careful study of the reaction may indicate otherwise unapparent drug anal-

RECOVERY OF EXOGENOUSLY ADDED TAXOL FROM HUMAN SERUM

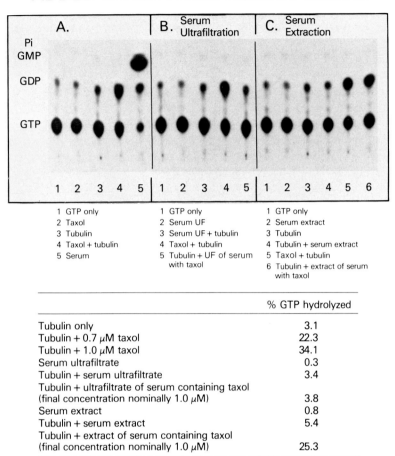

		% GTP hydrolyzed
Tubulin only		3.1
Tubulin + 0.7 μM taxol		22.3
Tubulin + 1.0 μM taxol		34.1
Serum ultrafiltrate		0.3
Tubulin + serum ultrafiltrate		3.4
Tubulin + ultrafiltrate of serum containing taxol (final concentration nominally 1.0 μM)		3.8
Serum extract		0.8
Tubulin + serum extract		5.4
Tubulin + extract of serum containing taxol (final concentration nominally 1.0 μM)		25.3

FIGURE 27. Autoradiograms of reaction mixtures used to study effects of taxol on the GTPase activity of tubulin.[96] Reaction mixtures contained glutamate, $MgCl_2$, dimethylsulfoxide, and [α-^{32}P]GTP as described in Table 5, and the following, as indicated: 10 μg of tubulin, 1 μM taxol, 5 $\mu\ell$ of human serum, 5 $\mu\ell$ of serum ultrafiltrate, 5 $\mu\ell$ of an ultrafiltrate of serum containing 10 μM taxol; 5 $\mu\ell$ of serum extracted with dimethylsulfoxide; and 5 $\mu\ell$ of an extract of serum containing 10 μM taxol with extract having the same volume as the original serum. Incubations as in Table 5.

ogies. The reaction also has definite practical applications, both as a screening test for new antimitotic drugs and as a potential clinical assay for agents with significant antineoplastic activity.

ACKNOWLEDGMENTS

The author would like to thank Dr. D. G. Johns for his encouragement and valuable discussions; A. A. del Campo for the electron microscopy; C. M. Lin for able technical assistance; and B. Singer for her help in preparing the manuscript.

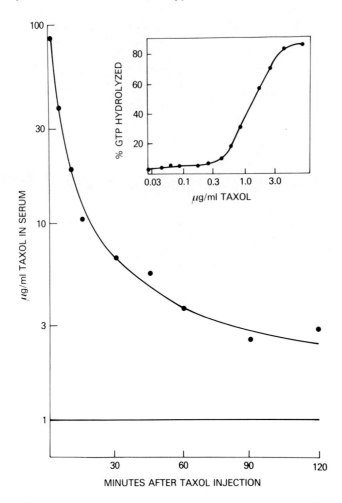

FIGURE 28.   Taxol pharmacokinetics following bolus intravenous injection in a rabbit.[96] Reaction mixtures contained glutamate, tubulin, $MgCl_2$, and $[\alpha\text{-}^{32}P]GTP$ as described in Table 5, and 5 $\mu\ell$ of either a dimethylsulfoxide extract of serum drawn at the indicated times or an extract of serum containing a known amount of taxol (inset). Incubation as in Table 5. A taxol concentration of 0.85 $\mu g/m\ell$ is equivalent to 1 μM.

REFERENCES

1. **Creasey, W. A.,** Plant alkaloids, in *Cancer, A Comprehensive Treatise,* Vol. 5, Becker, F. F., Ed., Plenum Press, New York, 1977, 379.
2. **Horwitz, S. B. and Loike, J. D.,** A comparison of the mechanism of action of VP-16-213 and podophyllotoxin, *Lloydia,* 40, 83, 1977.
3. **Cabanillas, F., Bodey, G. P., Burgess, M. A., and Freireich, E. J.,** Results of a Phase II study of maytansine in patients with breast carcinoma and melanoma, *Cancer Treat. Rep.,* 63, 507, 1979.
4. **Rosenthal, S., Harris, D. T., Horton, J., and Glick, J. H.,** Phase II study of maytansine in patients with advanced lymphomas: an Eastern Cooperative Oncology Group study, *Cancer Treat. Rep.,* 64, 1115, 1980.
5. **Franklin, R., Samson, M. K., Fraile, R. J., Abu-zahra, H., O'Bryan, R., and Baker, L. H.,** A Phase I-II study of maytansine utilizing a weekly schedule, *Cancer,* 46, 1104, 1980.
6. **Stephens, R. E., Renaud, F. L., and Gibbons, I. R.,** Guanine nucleotide associated with protein of the outer fibers of flagella and cilia, *Science,* 156, 1606, 1967.

7. **Weisenberg, R. C., Borisy, G. G., and Taylor, E. W.,** The colchicine-binding protein of mammalian brain and its relation to microtubules, *Biochemistry,* 7, 4466, 1968.

8. **Weisenberg, R. C.,** Microtubule formation in solutions containing low calcium concentrations, *Science,* 177, 1104, 1972.

9. **Shelanski, M. L., Gaskin, F., and Cantor, C. R.,** Microtubule assembly in the absence of added nucleotides, *Proc. Natl. Acad. Sci., U.S.A.,* 70, 765, 1973.

10. **Weingarten, M. D., Lockwood, A. H., Hwo, S.-Y., and Kirschner, M. W.,** A protein factor essential for microtubule assembly, *Proc. Natl. Acad. Sci. U.S.A.,* 72, 1858, 1975.

11. **Murphy, D. B. and Borisy, G. G.,** Association of high-molecular-weight proteins with microtubules and their role in microtubule assembly in vitro, *Proc. Natl. Acad. Sci. U.S.A.,* 72, 2696, 1975.

12. **Lee, J. C. and Timasheff, S. N.,** The reconstitution of microtubules from purified calf brain tubulin, *Biochemistry,* 14, 5183, 1975.

13. **Erickson, H. P. and Voter, W. A.,** Polycation-induced assembly of purified tubulin, *Proc. Natl. Acad. Sci, U.S.A.,* 73, 2813, 1976.

14. **Himes, R. H., Burton, P. R., Kersey, R. N., and Pierson, G. B.,** Brain tubulin polymerization in the absence of "microtubule-associated proteins", *Proc. Natl. Acad. Sci. U.S.A.,* 73, 4397, 1976.

15. **Herzog, W. and Weber, K.,** In vitro assembly of pure tubulin into microtubules in the absence of microtubule-associated proteins and glycerol, *Proc. Natl. Acad. Sci. U.S.A.,* 74, 1860, 1977.

16. **Hamel, E. and Lin, C. M.,** Glutamate-induced polymerization of tubulin: characteristics of the reaction and application to the large scale purification of tubulin, *Arch. Biochem. Biophys.,* 209, 29, 1981.

17. **Hamel, E., del Campo, A. A., Lowe, M. C., Waxman, P. G., and Lin, C. M.,** Effects of organic acids on tubulin polymerization and associated guanosine 5'-triphosphate hydrolysis, *Biochemistry,* 21, 503, 1982.

18. **Berry, R. W. and Shelanski, M. L.,** Interactions of tubulin with vinblastine and guanosine triphosphate, *J. Mol. Biol.,* 71, 71, 1972.

19. **Jacobs, M., Smith, H., and Taylor, E. W.,** Tubulin: nucleotide binding and enzymic activity, *J. Mol. Biol.,* 89, 455, 1974.

20. **Gaskin, F., Cantor, C. R., and Shelanski, M. L.,** Turbidimetric studies of the in vitro assembly and disassembly of porcine neurotubules, *J. Mol. Biol.,* 89, 737, 1974.

21. **Kobayashi, T.,** Nucleotides bound to brain tubulin and reconstituted microtubules, *J. Biochem. (Tokyo),* 76, 201, 1974.

22. **Piras, M. M. and Piras, R.,** Phosporylation of vinblastine-isolated microtubules from chick-embryonic muscles, *Eur. J. Biochem.,* 47, 443, 1974.

23. **Kobayashi, T.,** Dephosphorylation of tubulin-bound guanosine triphosphate during microtubule assembly, *J. Biochem. (Tokyo),* 77, 1193, 1975.

24. **Weisenberg, R. C., Deery, W. J., and Dickinson, P. J.,** Tubulin-nucleotide interactions during the polymerization and depolymerization of microtubules, *Biochemistry,* 15, 4248, 1976.

25. **Penningroth, S. M. and Kirschner, M. W.,** Nucleotide binding and phosphorylation in microtubule assembly in vitro, *J. Mol. Biol.,* 115, 643, 1977.

26. **David-Pfeuty, T., Laporte, J., and Pantaloni, D.,** GTPase activity at ends of microtubules, *Nature (London),* 272, 282, 1978.

27. **Zeeberg, B. and Caplow, M.,** Reactions of tubulin-associated guanine nucleotides, *J. Biol. Chem.,* 253, 1984, 1978.

28. **Jacobs, M. and Huitorel, P.,** Tubulin-associated nucleoside diphosphokinase, *Eur. J. Biochem.,* 99, 613, 1979.

29. **Terry, B. J. and Purich, D. L.,** Nucleotide release from tubulin and nucleoside-5'-diphosphate kinase action in microtubule assembly, *J. Biol. Chem.,* 254, 9469, 1979.

30. **Ikeda, Y. and Steiner, M.,** Phosphorylation and protein kinase activity of platelet tubulin, *J. Biol. Chem.,* 254, 66, 1979.

31. **Hamel, E., del Campo, A. A., Lowe, M. C., and Lin, C. M.,** Interactions of taxol, microtubule-associated proteins, and guanine nucleotides in tubulin polymerization, *J. Biol. Chem.,* 256, 11887, 1981.

32. **Bryan, J. and Wilson, L.,** Are cytoplasmic microtubules heteropolymers? *Proc. Natl. Acad. Sci. U.S.A.,* 68, 1762, 1971.

33. **Feit, H., Slusarek, L., and Shelanski, M. L.,** Heterogeneity of tubulin subunits, *Proc. Natl. Acad. Sci. U.S.A.,* 68, 2028, 1971.

34. **Feit, H., Neudeck, U., and Baskin, F.,** Comparison of the isoelectric and molecular weight properties of tubulin subunits, *J. Neurochem.,* 28, 697, 1977.

35. **Berkowitz, S. A., Katagiri, J., Binder, H. K., and Williams, R. C., Jr.,** Separation and characterization of microtubule proteins from calf brain, *Biochemistry,* 16, 5610, 1977.

36. **Eipper, B. A.,** Rat brain microtubule protein: purification and determination of covalently bound phosphate and carbohydrate, *Proc. Natl. Acad. Sci. U.S.A.,* 69, 2283, 1972.

37. **Luduena, R. F. and Woodward, D. O.,** Isolation and partial characterization of α- and β-tubulin from outer doublets of sea-urchin sperm and microtubules of chick-embryo brain, *Proc. Natl. Acad. Sci. U.S.A.,* 70, 3594, 1973.

38. **Lu, R. C. and Elzinga, M.,** Chromatographic resolution of the subunits of calf brain tubulin, *Anal. Biochem.,* 77, 243, 1977.

39. **Stephens, R. E.,** High resolution preparative SDS-polyacrylamide gel electrophoresis: fluorescent visualization and electrophoretic elution-concentration of protein bands, *Anal. Biochem.,* 65, 369, 1975.

40. **Detrich, H. W., III, and Williams, R. C., Jr.,** Reversible dissociation of the αβ dimer of tubulin from bovine brain, *Biochemistry,* 17, 3900, 1978.

41. **Luduena, R. F., Shooter, E. M., and Wilson, L.,** Structure of the tubulin dimer, *J. Biol. Chem.,* 252, 7006, 1977.

42. **Amos, L. A. and Klug, A.,** Arrangement of subunits in flagellar microtubules, *J. Cell Sci.,* 14, 523, 1974.

43. **Bibring, T., Baxandall, J., Denslow, S., and Walker, B.,** Heterogeneity of the alpha subunit of tubulin and the variability of tubulin within a single organism, *J. Cell Biol.,* 69, 301, 1976.

44. **Piperno, G. and Luck, D. J.,** Phosphorylation of axonemal proteins in *Chlamydomonas reinhardtii, J. Biol. Chem.,* 251, 2161, 1976.

45. **George, H. J., Misra, L., Field, D. J., and Lee, J. C.,** Polymorphism of brain tubulin, *Biochemistry,* 20, 2402, 1981.

46. **Ponstingl, H., Krauhs, E., Little, M., and Kempf, T.,** Complete amino acid sequence of α-tubulin from porcine brain, *Proc. Natl. Acad. Sci. U.S.A.,* 78, 2757, 1981.

47. **Krauhs, E., Little, M., Kempf, T., Hofer-Warbinek, R., Ade, W., and Ponstingl, H.,** Complete amino acid sequence of β-tubulin from porcine brain, *Proc. Natl. Acad. Sci. U.S.A.,* 78, 4156, 1981.

48. **Bryan, J.,** Definition of three classes of binding sites in isolated microtubule crystals, *Biochemistry,* 11, 2611, 1972.

49. **Levi, A., Cimino, M., Mercanti, D., and Calissano, P.,** Studies on the binding of GTP to the microtubule protein, *Biochim. Biophys. Acta,* 365, 450, 1974.

50. **Spiegelman, B. M., Penningroth, S. M., and Kirschner, M. W.,** Turnover of tubulin and the N site GTP in Chinese hamster ovary cells, *Cell,* 12, 587, 1977.

51. **Caplow, M. and Zeeberg, B.,** Stoichiometry for guanine nucleotide binding to tubulin under polymerizing and nonpolymerizing conditions, *Arch. Biochem. Biophys.,* 203, 404, 1980.

52. **Kirsch, M. and Yarbrough, L. R.,** Assembly of tubulin with nucleotide analogs, *J. Biol. Chem.,* 256, 106, 1981.

53. **Purich, D. L. and MacNeal, R. K.,** Properties of tubulin treated with alkaline phosphatase to remove guanine nucleotides from the exchangeable binding site, *FEBS Lett.,* 96, 83, 1978.

54. **Penningroth, S. M. and Kirschner, M. W.,** Nucleotide specificity in microtubule assembly in vitro, *Biochemistry,* 17, 734, 1978.

55. **Arai, T. and Kaziro, Y.,** Role of GTP in the assembly of microtubules, *J. Biochem. (Tokyo),* 82, 1063, 1977.

56. **David-Pfeuty, T., Erickson, H. P., and Pantaloni, D.,** Guanosinetriphosphatase activity of tubulin associated with microtubule assembly, *Proc. Natl. Acad. Sci. U.S.A.,* 74, 5372, 1977.

57. **MacNeal, R. K. and Purich, D. L.,** Stoichiometry and role of GTP hydrolysis in bovine neutrotubule assembly, *J. Biol. Chem.,* 253, 4683, 1978.

58. **Margolis, R. L. and Wilson, L.,** Opposite end assembly and disassembly of microtubules at steady state in vitro, *Cell,* 13, 1, 1978.

59. **Arai, T. and Kaziro, Y.,** Effect of guanine nucleotides on the assembly of brain microtubules: ability of 5'-guanylyl imidodiphosphate to replace GTP in promoting the polymerization of microtubules in vitro, *Biochem. Biophys. Res. Commun.,* 69, 369, 1976.

60. **Sutherland, J. W. H.,** Comparison of the effects of different adenosine and guanosine nucleotides on the assembly of bovine neurotubules, *Biochem. Biophys. Res. Commun.,* 72, 933, 1976.

61. **Geahlen, R. L. and Haley, B. E.,** Interactions of a photoaffinity analog of GTP with the proteins of microtubules, *Proc. Natl. Acad. Sci. U.S.A.,* 74, 4375, 1977.

62. **Hamel, E. and Lin, C. M.,** Interaction of tubulin with ribose-modified analogs of GTP and GDP: evidence for two mutually exclusive exchangeable nucleotide binding sites, *Proc. Natl. Acad. Sci U.S.A.,* 78, 3368, 1981.

63. **Lustbader, J. and Hamel, E.,** Di- and triphosphate derivatives of acyclo- and arabinosylguanine: effects on the polymerization of purified tubulin, *Biochim. Biophys. Acta,* 719, 215, 1982.

64. **Hamel, E., del Campo, A. A., Lustbader, J., and Lin, C. M.,** Modulation of tubulin-nucleotide interactions by microtubule-associated proteins: polymerization with ribose modified analogs of GTP, *Biochemistry,* 22, 1271, 1983.

65. **Carlier, M.-F. and Pantaloni, D.,** Kinetic analysis of cooperativity in tubulin polymerization in the presence of guanosine di- or triphosphate nucleotides, *Biochemistry,* 17, 1908, 1978.

66. **Zackroff, R. V., Weisenberg, R. C., and Deery, W. J.,** Equilibrium and kinetic analysis of microtubule assembly in the presence of guanosine diphosphate, *J. Mol. Biol.,* 139, 641, 1980.
67. **Jameson, L. and Caplow, M.,** Effect of guanosine diphosphate on microtubule assembly and stability, *J. Biol. Chem.,* 225, 2284, 1980.
68. **Margolis, R. L.,** Role of GTP hydrolysis in microtubule treadmilling and assembly, *Proc. Natl. Acad. Sci. U.S.A.,* 78, 1586, 1981.
69. **Lee, S.-H., Kristofferson, D., and Purich, D. L.,** Microtubule interactions with GDP provide evidence that assembly-disassembly properties depend on the method of brain microtubule protein isolation, *Biochem. Biophys. Res. Commun.,* 105, 1605, 1982.
70. **Wilson, L.,** Properties of colchicine binding protein from chick embryo brain. Interactions with vinca alkaloids and podophyllotoxin, *Biochemistry,* 9, 4999, 1970.
71. **Hamel, E. and Lin, C. M.,** Stabilization of the colchicine-binding activity of tubulin by organic acids, *Biochim. Biophys. Acta,* 675, 226, 1981.
72. **Hamel, E. and Lin, C. M.,** Interactions of a new antimitotic agent, NSC-181928, with purified tubulin, *Biochem. Biophys. Res. Commun.,* 104, 929, 1982.
73. **Schiff, P. B., Fant, J., and Horwitz, S. B.,** Promotion of microtubule assembly in vitro by taxol, *Nature (London),* 277, 665, 1979.
74. **Fellous, A., Francon, J., Lennon, A.-M., and Nunez, J.,** Microtubule assembly in vitro: purification of assembly-promoting factors, *Eur. J. Biochem.,* 78, 167, 1977.
75. **Cleveland, D. W., Hwo, S.-Y., and Kirschner, M. W.,** Purification of tau, a microtubule-associated protein that induces assembly of microtubules from purified protein, *J. Mol. Biol.,* 116, 207, 1977.
76. **Wilson, L., Bamburg, J. R., Mizel, S. B., Grisham, L. M., and Creswell, K. M.,** Interaction of drugs with microtubule proteins, *Fed. Proc.,* 33, 158, 1974.
77. **Hoebeke, J., Nijen, G. V., and DeBrabander, M.,** Interaction of nocodazole (R 17934), a new antitumoral drug, with rat brain tubulin, *Biochem. Biophys. Res. Commun.,* 69, 319, 1976.
78. **Delatour, P. and Richard, Y.,** Proprietes embryotoxiques et antimitotiques en serie benzimidazole, *Therapie,* 31, 505, 1976.
79. **Friedman, P. A. and Platzer, E. G.,** Interaction of anthelmintic benzimidazole derivatives with bovine brain tubulin, *Biochim. Biophys. Acta,* 544, 605, 1978.
80. **Elliott, R. D., Temple, C., Jr., and Montgomery, J. A.,** Potential folic acid antagonists. III. Deaza analogs of methotrexate. III. 1- and 3-deaza analogs of 2,4-diamino-6-[(N-methylanilino)methyl]pteridine, *J. Org. Chem.,* 33, 533, 1968.
81. **Remillard, S., Rebhun, L. I., Howie, G. A., and Kupchan, S. M.,** Antimitotic activity of the potent tumor inhibitor maytansine, *Science,* 189, 1002, 1975.
82. **Mandelbaum-Shavit, F., Wolpert-DeFilippes, M. K., and Johns, D. G.,** Binding of maytansine to rat brain tubulin, *Biochem. Biophys. Res. Commun.,* 72, 47, 1976.
83. **Bhattacharyya, B. and Wolff, J.,** Maytansine binding to the vinblastine sites of tubulin, *FEBS Lett.,* 75, 159, 1977.
84. **Schiff, P. B. and Horwitz, S. B.,** Taxol assembles tubulin in the absence of exogenous guanosine 5'-triphosphate or microtubule-associated proteins, *Biochemistry,* 20, 3247, 1981.
85. **Parness, J. and Horwitz, S. B.,** Taxol binds to polymerized tubulin in vitro, *J. Cell Biol.,* 91, 479, 1981.
86. **David-Pfeuty, T., Simon, C., and Pantaloni, D.,** Effect of antimitotic drugs on tubulin GTPase activity and self-assembly, *J. Biol. Chem.,* 254, 11696, 1979.
87. **Heusele, C. and Carlier, M.-F.,** GTPase activity of the tubulin-colchicine in relation with tubulin-tubulin interactions, *Biochem. Biophys. Res. Commun.,* 103, 332, 1981.
88. **Saltarelli, D. and Pantaloni, D.,** Polymerization of the tubulin-colchicine complex and guanosine 5'-triphosphate hydrolysis, *Biochemistry,* 21, 2996, 1982.
89. **Lin, C. M. and Hamel, E.,** Effects of inhibitors of tubulin polymerization on GTP hydrolysis, *J. Biol. Chem.,* 256, 9242, 1981.
90. **Cortese, F., Bhattacharyya, B., and Wolff, J.,** Podophyllotoxin as a probe for the colchicine binding site of tubulin, *J. Biol. Chem.,* 252, 1134, 1977.
91. **Rosner, M., Capraro, H.-G., Iorio, M. A., Jacobson, A. E., Atwell, L., Brossi, A., Williams, T. H., Sik, R. H., and Chignell, C. F.,** Biological effects of modified colchicines. Improved preparation of 2-demethylcolchicine, 3-demethylcolchicine, and (+)-colchicine and reassignment of the position of the double bond in dehydro-7-deacetamidocolchicines, *J. Med. Chem.,* 24, 257, 1981.
92. **Ray, K., Bhattacharyya, B., and Biswas, B. B.,** Role of B-ring of colchicine in its binding to tubulin, *J. Biol. Chem.,* 256, 6241, 1981.
93. **Bhattacharyya, B. and Wolff, J.,** Tubulin aggregation and disaggregation: mediation by two distinct vinblastine binding sites, *Proc. Natl. Acad. Sci. U.S.A.,* 73, 2375, 1976.
94. **Wheeler, G. P., Bowdon, B. J., Werline, J. A., and Temple, C., Jr.,** 1-deaza-7,8-dihydropteridines, a new class of mitotic inhibitors with anticancer activity, *Biochem. Pharmacol.,* 30, 2381, 1981.

95. **Gaskin, F.,** In vitro microtubule assembly regulation by divalent cations and nucleotides, *Biochemistry,* 20, 1318, 1981.
96. **Hamel, E., Lin, C. M., and Johns, D. G.,** Tubulin-dependent biochemical assay for the antineoplastic agent taxol and application to measurement of the drug in serum, *Cancer Treat. Rep.,* 66, 1381, 1982.
97. **Hamel, E.,** unpublished observations.

Chapter 7

CELLULAR AND MOLECULAR PHARMACOLOGY OF SUGAR AMINE-MODIFIED ANTHRACYCLINES

James B. Johnston and Robert I. Glazer

TABLE OF CONTENTS

I. INTRODUCTION

The anthracycline drugs, Adriamycin® (ADR) and daunorubicin (DAU), are useful anticancer agents wtih activities against a variety of solid tumors (ADR) and hematological malignancies (ADR, DAU).[1,2] However, their use has been limited by generalized toxicity, e.g., myelosuppression, and a dose-limiting cardiomyopathy necessitating the development of noncardiotoxic analogs with improved antitumor specificity.[1-6] Recently, several new promising sugar-amine-modified anthracylines have been developed at the Stanford Research Institute and were subsequently evaluated in our laboratory. In this chapter we shall review the background related to the development of these analogs and the preclinical data available on these compounds.

II. BACKGROUND

ADR and DAU consist of a naphthacenequinone chromophore connected by a glycosidic linkage to daunosamine (Figure 1), and recent reviews have outlined the antitumor properties of analogs produced by chemical modifications of this structure.[3-6] The C3' amine of daunosamine is particularly important for such activity, as stereochemical inversion of this group[7,8] or substitutions at the amine with urea,[9] guanidine,[10,11] peptides,[12,13] or acyl groups[10,11] are associated with loss of antitumor activity. This finding may be due to the decreased DNA affinity associated with sugar-amine modifications, either as a result of steric hindrance or because of reduced electrostatic binding.[4,7,8,11-13] Indeed, initial X-ray diffraction studies of a DAU:DNA complex by Pigram et al.[14] confirmed the importance of the sugar-amine for electrostatic binding, as the chromophore was observed to intercalate between base pairs and the sugar was located in the major groove forming stabilizing electrostatic bonds with the second phosphate from the intercalation site. However, subsequent NMR[15] and X-ray diffraction[16] studies of DAU:polynucleotide complexes have not confirmed these findings, but rather have shown the sugar-amine to lie in the minor groove and not to interact with DNA. An alternative explanation to account for the importance of the sugar-amine for antitumor activity is related to its ability to bind with cardiolipin in cell membranes. A number of investigators have stressed the importance of this interaction to explain the antitumor and cardiotoxic effects of the anthracyclines,[17-23] and as the sugar-amine is essential for such binding[22,23] any modifications at this site would be predicted to alter the activities of the anthracyclines.

The N-alkylated anthracyclines were synthesized in an attempt to alter the sugar-amine in such a fashion as to increase antitumor activity, for these substitutions would be predicted to enhance lipophilicity as well as retain the C3' amine basicity.[24-26] Indeed, the DNA affinities and the antitumor activities of the dimethyl and diethyl derivatives of ADR and DAU were equivalent to their parent compounds. However, the DNA-binding capacity of *N*-dibenzyldaunorubicin was reduced (presumably as a result of steric hindrance) although it demonstrated superior efficacy, but reduced potency, against murine P388 leukemia, colon carcinoma, and mammary carcinoma.[24,25] In addition, this analog had substantially reduced cardiotoxicity, which appeared related to its decreased ability to generate free radicals.[24,25,27] As an extension of these findings, a number of new analogs have been developed where a nitrogen-containing heterocyclic substituent replaced the C3' amine (Figure 1). The analogs to be discussed in this chapter are the 3'-(4-morpholinyl)- and 3'-(4-methoxyl-piperidinyl)-derivatives of 3'-deaminodaunorubicin, designated MD and MEO, respectively, and their 13-dihydro derivatives MD-OH and MEO-OH. In addition, preliminary data will be included on the 3'-(3-cyano-4-morpholinyl)- derivative of 3'-deaminoadriamycin.

III. ANTITUMOR ACTIVITIES

A. In Vivo Studies

Table 1 shows the cytocidal activities of the analogs against P388 leukemia in mice as

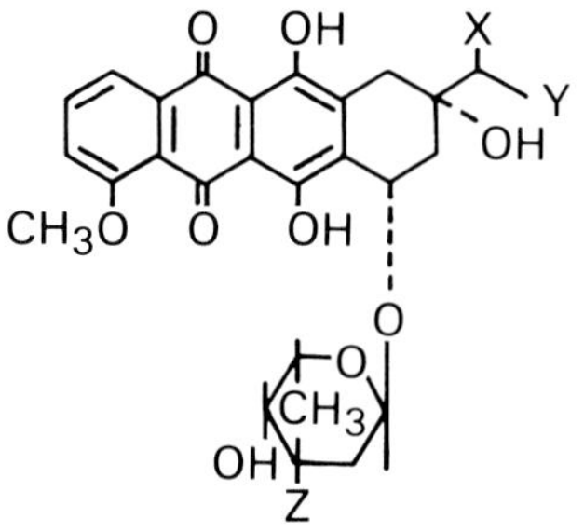

DRUG	X	Y	Z
ADR	= O	CH$_2$OH	NH$_2$
DAU	= O	CH$_3$	NH$_2$
MD	= O	CH$_3$	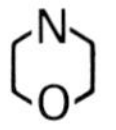 (morpholino N–O ring)
MD-OH	– OH	CH$_3$	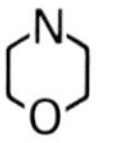 (morpholino N–O ring)
MEO	= O	CH$_3$	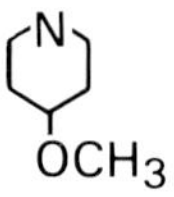 (piperidine N ring, OCH$_3$)
MEO-OH	– OH	CH$_3$	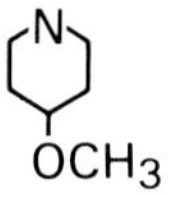 (piperidine N ring, OCH$_3$)
CMA	= O	CH$_2$OH	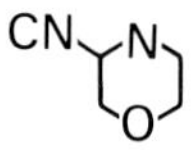 (CN–N–O ring)

FIGURE 1.   Structures of the anthracycline analogs.

carried out by the National Cancer Institute screening program.[28] MD demonstrated re-markably increased potency, producing a T/C value equivalent to that of ADR and DAU, but at 1/40 the dose. In contrast, MEO showed no increase in potency but demonstrated increased antitumor efficacy (T/C = 199%) compared to ADR (T/C = 160%) and DAU (T/C = 130%). The 13-dihydro derivatives, MD-OH and MEO-OH, had antitumor efficacies equivalent to the parent drugs, but the optimum dose was increased twofold. Most notable was the increased antitumor efficacy obtained with CMA (T/C = 187%) and its 100-fold increase in potency. This increase in potency is the greatest yet observed for any anthracycline analog.[28]

MD was also evaluated by Takahashi et al.[29] in leukemic mice, and confirmed the increased potency of this analog as well as the associated increase in general cytotoxicity. Administered on a daily i.p. dose schedule for 9 days, MD produced a T/C of 205% at an optimum dose of 0.1 mg/kg and toxicity was observed at this dosage. In contrast, at 1.25 mg/kg/day ADR

Table 1
ANTITUMOR ACTIVITY

	Activity in vivo				Activity in vitro	
	P388 leukemia in mice[28]		L1210 leukemia in mice[29]		HT-29 colon carcinoma cells[31] Drug concentration required to inhibit growth by 90%, $LC_{90}(M)$	
		Optimum dose q4d, 5,9,13		Optimum dose qd, 1—9, i.p.		
Drug	% T/C	mg/kg	%T/C	mg/kg	2 hr Treatment	24 hr Treatment
ADR	160	8.0	235	1.25	3×10^{-7}	5×10^{-8}
DAU	130	8.0	235	0.625	2×10^{-7}	3×10^{-8}
MD	166	0.2	205	0.1	1×10^{-6}	2×10^{-7}
MD-OH	153	0.4			2×10^{-6}	2×10^{-7}
MEO	199	6.25			1×10^{-6}	8×10^{-8}
MEO-OH	199	12.5			$>5 \times 10^{-6}$	2×10^{-7}
CMA	187	0.075			2×10^{-9a}	1×10^{-10a}

[a]   Unpublished results.

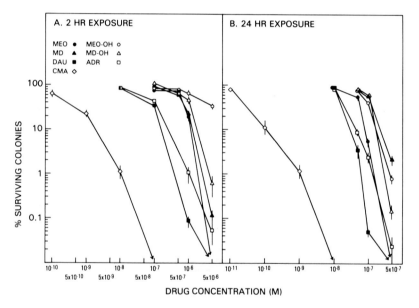

FIGURE 2.   Cell viability of HT-29 cells treated with the anthracycline analogs. Log phase cells were treated with varying concentrations of drug for either (A) 2 hr or (B) 24 hr, and cell viability assessed by soft agar cloning. Each value represents the mean ± SE of six to eight experiments.

and DAU produced a T/C of 235 and 229%, respectively, with no evidence of toxicity. MD has been evaluated against the B16 melanoma cell line in mice and again demonstrated increased potency but decreased efficacy.[28] Administered once daily, MD was active at 0.25 mg/kg with a T/C of 135% compared with ADR which had a T/C of 262% at 4 mg/kg.

B. In Vitro Studies

Figure 2 shows the activity of the analogs against a human colon carcinoma cell line (HT-29) in tissue culture, and Table 1 the drug concentration required for 90% inhibition of cell viability (LC_{90}). Cells were exposed to varying concentrations of drug for either 2 or 24 hr

Table 2
DNA BINDING AND NUCLEAR AFFINITIES

Drug	DNA binding[28] (Δ Tm of isolated helical DNA, °C)	Nuclear affinities[31] (ratio of nuclear/cell drug concentration following exposure to 1 μM drug)
ADR	13.4	0.48
DAU	11.2	0.29
MD	6.1	0.39
MD-OH	4.1	0.12
MEO	13.3	0.45
MEO-OH	9.5	0.21
CMA	5.1[a]	—[b]

[a] Unpublished results.
[b] Not determined.

and cell viability was then assessed by soft-agar cloning.[30,31] ADR and DAU were tenfold more cytocidal than MD or MEO following 2-hr drug treatment, and both 13-dihydro derivatives were less cytocidal than their parent compounds. In contrast, CMA was 100-fold more cytocidal than either ADR or DAU and showed quite a different dose-response pattern than the other analogs. Thus, a decrease in cell viability from 10 to 99% required a 1-log increase in drug concentration for ADR or DAU, but greater than a 2-log increase in drug concentration for CMA.

When drug exposure was prolonged to 24 hr the cytocidal activities of ADR and DAU increased five- to sevenfold and they were still tenfold more toxic than MD. MD and MD-OH were equitoxic, which was a result of the extensive metabolism of MD to MD-OH. Prolonging drug exposure caused a proportionally greater increase in the cytocidal activities of MEO, CMA, and particularly MEO-OH than was observed with the other analogs. Thus, the cytocidal potency of CMA was further enhanced and at 24 hr it was 500-fold more cytocidal than ADR or DAU.

It is unclear at present why differences exist between the antitumor effects in vivo of some of these analogs vs. their activities in vitro. Possible explanations include differences in drug disposition or metabolism or in the sensitivity of the cell lines investigated. However, the greatly enhanced activity of CMA against HT-29 cells is exciting in that it parallels its high potency in vivo, and further studies are warranted to determine whether it might have superior efficacy against solid tumor xenografts in vivo.

IV. DNA BINDING AND NUCLEAR AFFINITY

As previous sugar-amine modifications have been shown to profoundly affect DNA binding,[4,7,8,11-13] the affinity of the new analogs for DNA and nuclei were measured (Table 2). DNA binding was determined by the T_m of isolated helical DNA.[28,32] Nuclear affinities were assessed by exposing HT-29 cells to 1 μM drug for 2 hr and the nuclear concentrations of drug were measured and expressed as a fraction of the cellular drug concentration.[31] As previously demonstrated,[5,11,36] the DNA binding of DAU and ADR were equal, whereas the nuclear affinity of DAU was less than ADR,[26,33-35] a result presumably reflecting differences in chromatin binding.[36] Surprisingly, the nuclear affinity of DAU was less than its two derivatives, MD and MEO, whereas the DNA binding of the analogs were either equal to (MEO) or 50% less (MD) than DAU. Both MD-OH and MEO-OH had markedly reduced nuclear affinities and DNA binding compared to the parent compounds.

No correlation was apparent between the nuclear or DNA affinities of these analogs and

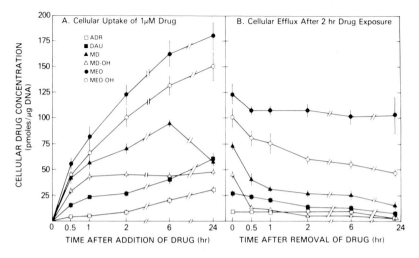

FIGURE 3. Cellular uptake and efflux of the anthracycline analogs. (A) Cells were treated with 1 μ*M* drug for varying time intervals. (B) Cells were treated for 2 hr with 1 μ*M* drug and then incubated for varying time intervals in drug-free media. Drug concentrations were determined by fluorometry and expressed as pmol/μg DNA. Each value is the mean ± SE of six experiments.

their effects on nucleic acid synthesis or cell viability. However, the rate of cellular efflux of these drugs was found to be inversely related to their nuclear affinities (see Section V).

V. PHARMACODYNAMICS

The pharmacodynamics of these analogs were assessed in HT-29 cells in tissue culture (Figure 3). Cell uptake studies were carried out by exposing log phase cells to 1 μ*M* concentrations of drug and sequentially measuring the cellular contents of the drug by fluorometry.[30,31] As previously demonstrated in other cell lines,[26,33-35,37] the uptake of DAU was threefold greater than ADR. MEO and MD accumulated five- and threefold more rapidly than DAU, respectively, whereas MD-OH and MEO-OH were taken up more slowly than their parent drugs.[37]

As the rates of cellular uptake of the different anthracyclines have been related to their lipophilicities,[37] the lipid solubilities of the analogs were assessed by measuring their retention times on a reversed-phase column (see Section VI). The relative lipophilicities of the analogs in decreasing order were MEO>MD>MEO-OH>MD-OH>Dau>ADR, demonstrating that the rate of cellular influx was dependent on the structural characteristics of the drugs in addition to their lipophilicities.[38] Over a 24-hr incubation period MEO, MEO-OH, DAU, and ADR continued to accumulate in the cells; however, the cellular concentration of MEO-OH did not increase as a result of its rapid efflux. The concentration of MD at 24 hr was 20% less than at 2 hr and this was due to its extensive metabolism to MD-OH.

The cellular efflux of the analogs was measured by incubating cells with 1 μ*M* concentrations of drug for 2 hr and then sequentially measuring the cellular concentrations of drug when cells were reincubated in drug-free medium (Figure 3B). The efflux of the anthracyclines has previously been shown to be carried out by an active cell membrane pump,[35,39] the activity of which increases with the development of drug resistance.[40-42] However, there was no correlation between the rates of efflux of these analogs and their respective cytocidal activities. Less than 10% of MEO and ADR effluxed over a 2-hr period, whereas approximately 50% of MD and DAU effluxed over the same time period. MD-OH and MEO-OH egressed more rapidly than their parent drugs and 80% of MD-OH and 40% of MEO-OH were lost from the cells in 2 hr. With the exception of MEO-OH, the rates of efflux of the

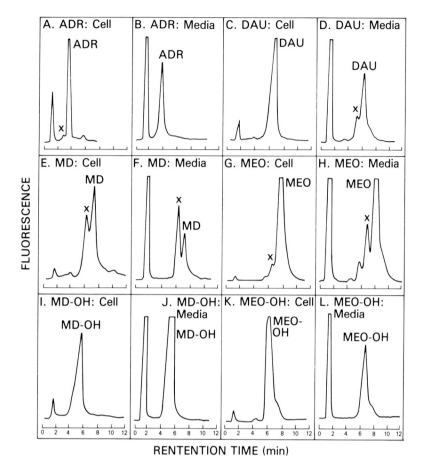

FIGURE 4. HPLC analysis of the anthracycline analogs. Cells were incubated with 1 μ*M* drug for 24 hr and the parent drug and metabolites were extracted from the cells and media and analyzed by reversed-phase HPLC. X Identifies the alcohol metabolites and the peak at 0.8 min represents endogenous fluorescent material.

analogs correlated inversely with their nuclear affinities (Table 2) demonstrating that the cellular efflux of these drugs is controlled by their release from chromatin in conjunction with the membrane pump.

VI. METABOLISM

The metabolism of the different analogs has been assessed in HT-29 cells in tissue culture.[30,31] Log phase cells were incubated with 1 μ*M* concentrations of drug, and after 2 or 24 hr the anthracyclines were extracted from the cells and media and examined by reversed-phase high performance liquid chromatography (Figure 4). The only metabolites detected were the 13-dihydro derivatives which are produced by the ubiquitous aldo-keto reductases[43-45] and are the major metabolites produced in vivo.[44-46] Neither MD-OH nor MEO-OH were further metabolized. At 2 hr, the only analog which was metabolized was MD, where 2 and 8% of the drug was found as the 13-dihydro metabolite intracellularly and in the medium, respectively. At 24 hr, the percentage of metabolite present intracellularly derived from ADR, DAU, MD, and MEO was 2,3,34, and 9%, respectively (Figure 4A,C,E,G). In each case, the percentage of metabolite in the medium was higher than its intracellular concentration and was 3, 18, 58, and 23% of the parent ADR, DAU, MD, and

Table 3
DRUG CONCENTRATIONS REQUIRED FOR 50% INHIBITION
OF DNA AND RNA SYNTHESIS (IC$_{50}$)

	HT-29 cells (IC$_{50}$, M^{31})				L1210 cells (IC$_{50}$, μM^{28})	
	2 hr Treatment		24 hr Treatment		4 hr Treatment	
Drug	DNA	RNA	DNA	RNA	DNA	RNA
ADR	7×10^{-8}	5×10^{-7}	3×10^{-8}	5×10^{-7}	2×10^{-6}	6×10^{-7}
DAU	3×10^{-7}	7×10^{-7}	3×10^{-8}	5×10^{-7}	7×10^{-7}	3×10^{-7}
MD	1×10^{-7}	2×10^{-8}	2×10^{-8}	2×10^{-8}	8×10^{-7}	1×10^{-7}
MD-OH	4×10^{-7}	5×10^{-7}	6×10^{-8}	3×10^{-7}	2×10^{-6}	5×10^{-7}
MEO	1×10^{-7}	2×10^{-8}	3×10^{-8}	3×10^{-8}	6×10^{-7}	1×10^{-7}
MEO-OH	1×10^{-7}	1×10^{-7}	6×10^{-8}	2×10^{-7}	6×10^{-7}	8×10^{-8}
CMA[a]	4×10^{-9}	1×10^{-9}	5×10^{-11}	4×10^{-10}	3×10^{-9}	5×10^{-10}

[a] Unpublished observations.

MEO, respectively (Figure 4B,D,F,H). These results reflected the decreased cellular influx and more rapid cellular efflux of the metabolite compared to the parent drugs (Figure 3).

The greater metabolism of MEO and MD vs. DAU and ADR may be related to their increased cellular uptakes and to differences in specificities and kinetics of the aldo-keto reductases.[44,45] The considerable conversion of MD to MD-OH at 24 hr explained the decreased cellular concentrations of MD at this time (Figure 3) and the equivalent cytotoxicities of MD, and MD-OH in HT-29 cells following 24 hr of drug treatment (Figure 2).

VII. EFFECTS ON NUCLEIC ACID SYNTHESIS

A. DNA and Total RNA Synthesis

The effects of the analogs on DNA and total RNA synthesis were extensively evaluated since these parameters have been proposed to be involved in their antitumor activity.[2-6,11,12] As in the cytotoxicity studies, HT-29 cells were exposed to drug for either 2 or 24 hr and DNA and RNA synthesis estimated by the incorporation of [^{14}C]Thd and [^{3}H]Urd into macromolecules during the last hour of treatment.[30,31] The concentrations of drug required for 50% inhibition of DNA and RNA synthesis (IC$_{50}$) at these times are shown in Table 3. For comparison, the IC$_{50}$ for DNA and RNA synthesis in L1210 cells in vitro (4-hr drug treatment) are also presented in Table 3, but soft-agar cloning studies have not yet been carried out in this cell line.[28,32]

When HT-29 cells were treated with ADR and DAU there was preferential inhibition of DNA synthesis vs. RNA synthesis and this was most apparent with prolonged drug exposure. In contrast, MD, MEO, and CMA preferentially inhibited RNA synthesis after 2-hr drug exposure, but this difference did not occur with 24-hr treatment. This preferential inhibition of RNA synthesis was also apparent in L1210 cells[28,29] and has previously been observed with N-alkyl derivatives[24-26] and the marcellomycin/aclacinomycin series of anthracyclines which contain a disaccharide or trisaccharide in place of daunosamine.[47-49] The increased inhibition of RNA synthesis vs. DNA synthesis by these analogs could be related to their sites of binding with DNA,[48] or to their enhanced effects on the RNA polymerase·DNA complexes.[50,51] Clearly, the reduced cytocidal activities of MD and MEO in HT-29 cells could not be related to their effects on DNA or total RNA synthesis, for they produced identical inhibition of DNA synthesis, as did ADR and DAU, but were 25-fold more potent as inhibitors of RNA synthesis. However, in keeping with its increased cytocidal activity,

CMA was also an extremely potent inhibitor of nucleic acid synthesis. Following 2-hr incubation, CMA was 100-fold more cytocidal than ADR and its IC_{50} values for DNA and RNA syntheses were 10- and 500-fold less, respectively, than the equivalent IC_{50} values of ADR. Following 24-hr incubation, CMA was 500-fold more cytocidal and 1000-fold more potent as an inhibitor of DNA and RNA synthesis than was ADR.

A surprising feature in these studies was that the analogs MD and MEO could produce such a considerable reduction in nucleic acid synthesis despite their decreased cytocidal activities. For example, 2-hr treatment with 5×10^{-8} M concentrations of these drugs decreased RNA synthesis by 50% and DNA synthesis by 35% although cell viability was reduced by less than 10%. How the tumor cells could survive such effects is at present unknown, but it could not be explained by the rapidity of drug efflux. Although MD did egress rapidly, the efflux of MEO was extremely slow (Figure 3).

B. Effects on Different RNA Species

Previous investigators have observed that DAU[52] and ADR,[49,52] and the marcellomycin series of anthracyclines[49] appeared to inhibit cytoplasmic RNA synthesis to a greater extent than nuclear RNA synthesis, suggesting that nucleocytoplasmic transport of RNA is decreased by the anthracyclines.[49] Such decreased RNA transport may be secondary to reduced transcription[53,54] or related to anthracycline-drug complexes being formed in the nuclei, thereby preventing RNA from passing out into the cytoplasm. DAU and ADR have been shown to bind to RNA in vitro[55,56] and in vivo,[57] respectively, and such binding could be due to electrostatic interaction,[55,56] covalent bonding,[58,59] or intercalation of drug into double-stranded regions of heterogeneous[60] or nucleolar RNA.[61] However, intercalation appears unlikely as the anthracyclines preferentially intercalate into helixes of type B conformation and double-stranded RNA is in the type A conformation.[8,56] Regardless of physiochemical mechanism, it would appear reasonable that more cytotoxic analogs would affect transport more profoundly that their less cytotoxic analogs. To evaluate this possibility, HT-29 cells were treated with concentrations of the analogs which decreased total RNA synthesis by 50%, and their effects on the different nuclear and cytoplasmic RNA fractions were evaluated and compared with the respective cytocidal activities of the analogs under these conditions.

Log phase HT-29 cells were treated for 2 hr with 10^{-9} M CMA, 5×10^{-8} M MD or MEO, or 5×10^{-7} M ADR or DAU. Under these conditions total RNA synthesis was decreased 50%, as evaluated by the reduction in [^{3}H]Urd incorporation during the last hour of drug treatment. Cell viability was decreased 80% by CMA, 10% by MD and MEO, and 95 to 99% by ADR and DAU. Log phase (3-day) cells were used in these experiments and were prelabeled with [^{14}C]Urd during the first 48 hr of growth. During the second hour of drug treatment the cells were pulse labeled with [^{3}H]Urd. The nucleolar, heterogeneous, and polysomal RNA fractions were isolated[62,63] and the polysomal RNA was further fractionated into poly(A)RNA and nonpoly(A)RNA using poly(U)-Sepharose.®[64] Each of the RNA fractions was then analyzed by agarose-urea gel electrophoresis.[65,66] The ^{3}H:^{14}C ratio in each RNA species in the drug-treated cells was calculated and expressed as a percentage of the ratio in the equivalent RNA fraction in control cells (Table 4).

As shown in Table 4, each analog decreased nucleolar RNA synthesis by approximately 50 to 60%. Figure 5 shows the gel electrophoretic patterns for DAU, MD, and MEO demonstrating a generalized reduction in RNA with no build-up of rRNA precursors to suggest abnormalities in processing.[52,66] As previously demonstrated with DAU,[67,68] the DAU analogs produced little inhibition of heterogeneous nuclear RNA synthesis. In contrast, ADR and CMA decreased heterogeneous nuclear RNA synthesis by 40 to 60%[69] suggesting that the presence of the C14-OH group may be an important determinant for the inhibition of this RNA species. Under these conditions, both ADR and DAU had identical antitumor activities (99% of cell kill), thus demonstrating that inhibition of heterogeneous nuclear RNA synthesis was unrelated to cytotoxicity.

Table 4
EFFECTS OF ANTHRACYCLINES ON THE SYNTHESIS OF DIFFERENT RNA SPECIES

RNA Specific Activity in Drug Treated Cells (% of Control)

| | Nuclear RNA | | Polysomal RNA | | |
| | | | | Nonpoly(A)RNA | |
Drug	Nucleolar RNA	Hetero-geneous RNA	Poly(A)RNA	18S and 28S RNA	Low-molecular-wt RNA
DAU	41 ± 3	100 ± 10	70 ± 10	15 ± 1	58 ± 6
MD	42 ± 1	87 ± 13	72 ± 14	23 ± 5	57 ± 2
MEO	46 ± 3	97 ± 3	75 ± 11	20 ± 2	47 ± 7
ADR	43 ± 6	57 ± 4	51 ± 3	N.D.	N.D.
CMA	42 ± 7	40 ± 6	33 ± 11	N.D.	N.D.

Note: HT-29 cells, prelabeled with [^{14}C]Urd, were treated for 2 hr with 1×10^{-9} M CMA, 5×10^{-8} M MD or MEO, or 5×10^{-7} M ADR and DAU, and pulse labeled during the last hour with [^{3}H]Urd. The ^{3}H:^{14}C ratios were measured in each RNA fraction and RNA synthesis in drug-treated cells expressed as a percentage of the control ratio; each value is the mean ± SE of four to eight experiments. N.D. = not derived.

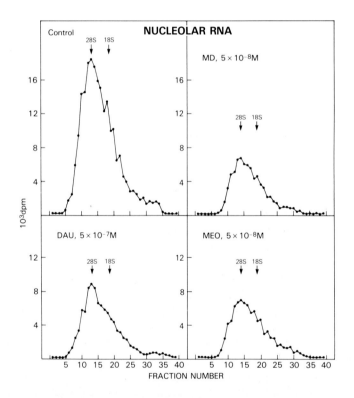

FIGURE 5. Agarose gel electrophoresis of nucleolar RNA HT-29 cells were prelabeled with [^{14}C]Urd and treated with 5×10^{-8} M MD or MED, or 5×10^{-7} M DAU for 2 hr, and pulse-labeled during the last hour with [^{3}H]Urd. Nucleolar RNA was isolated and equivalent amounts of ^{14}C dpm were run on 1.5% agarose-urea gels and the ^{3}H dpm determined in 2-mm slices.

Table 5
MICROSOMAL METABOLISM OF ANTHRACYCLINES

Drug	Augmentation of oxygen[28] consumption relative to consumption by ADR (%)	Heart microsomal lipid peroxidation by 0.1 mM drug;[a] nmoles malondialdehyde equivalents/mg protein/hr
ADR	100	
DAU	96	24.9 ± 1.9
MD	25	
MD-OH	29	
MEO	82	34.5 ± 4.3
MEO-OH	64	
CMA	29	

[a] Data from Reference 81; measured as described in Reference 76.

Although the daunorubicin analogs had little effect on heterogeneous RNA synthesis, they reduced cytoplasmic poly(A)RNA synthesis by 25 to 30%, whereas the Adriamycin® analogs inhibited this RNA fraction by 50 to 70%. All the analogs inhibited cytoplasmic non-poly(A)RNA production by approximately 50% (data not shown). To determine whether inhibition of a specific nonpoly(A)RNA fraction could explain the different cytotoxicities of DAU, MD, and MEO, this species was further examined by gel electrophoresis. However, as shown in Table 4, no differences between the analogs were found and 18S and 28S rRNA and the low-molecular-weight RNA were reduced by 80 to 85 and 40 to 45%, respectively. Thus, the considerably greater antitumor activity of DAU vs. MD and MEO was unrelated to differences in their effects on the synthesis or nucleocytoplasmic transport of RNA.

VIII. FREE RADICAL FORMATION AND CARDIOTOXICITY

The mechanism of anthracycline cardiotoxicity is unknown, but there is growing evidence to suggest that it may be related to the free radical forming potential of these drugs.[70-77] The anthracyclines may be enzymatically reduced to form semiquinones which subsequently may reduce molecular oxygen and generate reactive oxygen species (superoxide, hydrogen peroxide, and hydroxyl radicals).[70,78,79] The free radicals formed may produce cardiac damage either through lipid membrane peroxidation[73-76] or direct DNA injury,[71,72] and the heart is prone to such damage as it has a limited capacity to inactivate free radicals.[75] Support for these theories has been provided by the observation that concomitant administration of free radical scavengers may ameliorate both acute and chronic anthracycline-induced cardiotoxicity.[74,75] In addition, 5-iminodaunorubicin, which has a modified quinone ring and subsequently decreased free radical-forming potential is also less cardiotoxic.[66,77]

To predict whether the new analogs might be cardiotoxic, their potential to generate free radicals was estimated by measuring their abilities to augment oxygen consumption in a liver microsome system containing NADPH[27,28,78] (Table 5). Most striking were the decreased abilities of CMA, MD, and MD-OH, and to a lesser extent MEO and MEO-OH, to generate free radicals. These findings appear surprising, as the quinone ring is unaltered in these compounds. A similar paradox has previously been observed with *N*-dibenzyl-daunorubicin[27,72] and has been related to possible steric hindrance of cytochrome P450 reductase by the sugar-amine substituents.[72] Myocardial microsomal lipid peroxidation by MD has been assessed by Mimnaugh[81] at the National Cancer Institute, Bethesda, Md. (Table 5). This analog caused a significantly greater degree of lipid peroxidation than did DAU suggesting an *increased* potential for free radical formation. Indeed, cardiotoxicity studies in the rat appear to confirm the latter findings, for considerably more acute cardiotoxicity was observed with

MD than with ADR at equivalent cumulative doses.[80] For ADR, the cumulative doses required to prolong QRS and QT intervals by 10% were 4 and 8 mg/kg, respectively, and for MD were 0.15 to 0.2 and 0.25 to 0.4 mg/kg, respectively.[80]

IX. CONCLUSION

In this review we have discussed the cellular pharmacological effects of DAU and ADR analogs with substituents on the sugar-amine. As predicted, nuclear affinity, cellular uptake, and inhibition of nucleic acid synthesis were enhanced for the morpholinyl and methoxpi-peridinyl analogs of DAU, but their cytocidal activities in vitro were reduced compared to the parent drug. The reduced potency of these analogs could not be related to differences in their effect on different RNA species, rates of metabolism, or rates of cellular efflux. These data would suggest that other pharmacological effects, for example effects on cellular membranes,[17-23] may be involved in the antitumor activities of these analogs. Despite these in vitro findings, the new analogs had enhanced activities against murine leukemias in vivo and these data may reflect differences in drug metabolism, disposition, etc. or differences in the tumor system per se. Although, initial studies suggested that MD might have decreased potential for free radical formation, lipid peroxidation studies have demonstrated that this was not the case and, indeed, preliminary electrocardiographic studies showed MD to be highly cardiotoxic.

Substituting the sugar-amine of ADR by a cyanomorpholinyl group (CMA) produced an analog that was 100- to 500-fold greater in its potency when compared with ADR in the HT-29 colon carcinoma cell line in tissue culture. Of equal significance was the fact that CMA demonstrated increased efficacy, and was 100-fold more potent than ADR against P388 leukemia in vivo. The considerable activity against the human colon carcinoma cell line suggests that this analog may be of great value against solid tumors, and this possibility should be explored with animal xenograft studies.

REFERENCES

1. **Carter, S. K.,** The clinical evaluation of analogs. III. Anthracyclines, *Cancer Chemother. Pharmacol.,* 4, 5, 1980.
2. **Young, R. C., Ozols, R. F., and Myers, C. E.,** The anthracycline antineoplastic drugs, *N. Engl. J. Med.,* 305, 139, 1981.
3. **Brown, J. R.,** Adriamycin and related antibiotics, *Progr. Med. Chem.,* 15, 125, 1978.
4. **Di Marco, A. and Arcamone, F.,** DNA complexing antibiotics: Daunomycin, Adriamycin, and their derivatives, *Arzneim. Forsch.,* 25, 368, 1975.
5. **Arcamone, F.,** The development of new antitumor anthracyclines, *J. Med. Chem.,* 16, 1, 1980.
6. **Henry D. W.,** Structure-activity relationships among daunorubicin and Adriamycin analogs, *Cancer Treat. Rep.,* 63, 845, 1979.
7. **Zunino, F., Di Marco, A., and Velcich, A.,** Steric influence of the orientation of the primary amino group at position 3 of the sugar moiety of anthracycline antibiotics in DNA binding properties, *Cancer Lett.,* 3, 271, 1977.
8. **Plumbridge, T. W. and Brown, J. R.,** The interaction of Adriamycin and Adriamycin analogues with nucleic acids in the B and A conformations, *Biochim. Biophys. Acta,* 563, 181, 1979.
9. **Yamamato, K., Acton, E. M., and Henry, D. W.,** Antitumor activity of some derivatives of daunorubicin at the amino and methyl ketone functions, *J. Med. Chem.,* 15, 872, 1972.
10. **Chandra, P., Gericke, D., and Zunino, F.,** The relationship of chemical structure to cytostatic activity of some Daunomycin derivatives, *Pharmacol. Res. Commun.,* 4, 269, 1972.
11. **Zunino, F., Gambetta, R., Di Marco, A., and Zaccara, A.,** Interaction of Daunomycin and its derivatives with DNA, *Biochim. Biophys. Acta,* 277, 489, 1972.

12. **Gabbay, E. J., Grier, D., Fingerle, R. E., Reimer, R., Levy, R., Pearce, S. W., and Wilson, W. D.,** Interaction specificity of the anthracyclines with deoxyribonucleic acid, *Biochemistry*, 15, 4209, 1976.

13. **Wilson, D. W., Grier, D., Reimer, R., Bauman, J. D., Preston, J. F., and Gabbay, E. J.,** Structure-activity relationship of daunorubicin and its peptide derivatives, *J. Med. Chem.*, 19, 381, 1976.

14. **Pigram, W. J., Fuller, W., and Hamilton, L. D.,** Sterochemistry of intercalation: interaction of daunomycin with DNA, *Nature New. Biol.*, 235, 17, 1972.

15. **Patel, D. J., Kozlowski, S. A., and Rice, J. A.,** Hydrogen bonding, overlap geometry, and sequence specificity in anthracycline antitumor antibiotic·DNA complexes in solution, *Proc. Natl. Acad. Sci. U.S.A.*, 78, 3333, 1981.

16. **Quigley, G. J., Wang, A. H.-J., Ughetto, G., van der Marel, G., van Bloom, J. H., and Rich, A.,** Molecular structure of an anticancer drug-DNA complex: Daunomycin plus d(CpGpTpApCpG), *Proc. Natl. Acad. Sci. U.S.A.*, 77, 7204, 1980.

17. **Gosalvez, M., Pezzi, L., and Vivero, C.,** Inhibition of capping of surface immunoglobulins at fentomolar concentrations of Adriamycin, compound ICRF-159 and tetrodotoxin, *Biochem. Soc. Transact.*, 6, 659, 1978.

18. **Goldman, R., Facchinetti, T., Bach, D., Raz, A., and Shinitzky, M.,** A differential interaction of daunomycin, Adriamycin and their derivatives with human erythrocytes and phospholipid bilayers, *Biochim. Biophys. Acta*, 512, 254, 1978.

19. **Murphree, S. A., Tritton, T. R., Smith, P. L., and Sartorelli, A. C.,** Adriamycin-induced changes in the surface membrane of Sarcoma 180 ascites cells, *Biochim. Biophys. Acta*, 649, 317, 1981.

20. **Tritton, T. R., Murphree, S. A., and Sartorelli, A. C.,** Adriamycin: a proposal on the specificity of drug action, *Biochim. Biophys. Acta*, 84, 802, 1978.

21. **Schwartz, H. S., Schioppacassi, G., and Kanter, P. M.,** Mechanisms of selectivity of intercalating agents, *Antibiot. Chemother.*, 23, 247, 1978.

22. **Goormaghtigh, E., Chatelain, P., Caspers, J., and Ruysschaert, J. M.,** Evidence of a specific complex between Adriamycin and negatively-charged phospholipids, *Biochim. Biophys. Acta*, 597, 1, 1980.

23. **Goormaghtigh, E., Chatelain, P., Caspers, J., and Ruysschaert, J. M.,** Evidence of a complex between Adriamycin derivatives and cardiolipin: possible role in cardiotoxicity, *Biochem. Pharmacol.*, 29, 3003, 1980.

24. **Tong, G. L., Wu, H. Y., Smith, T. H., and Henry, D. W.,** Adriamycin analogues. III. Synthesis of N-alkylated anthracyclines with enhanced efficacy and reduced cardiotoxicity, *J. Med. Chem.*, 22, 912, 1979.

25. **Acton, E. M.,** N-alkylation of anthracyclines, in *Anthracyclines: Current Status and New Developments*, Crooke, S. T. and Reich, S. D., Eds., Academic Press, New York, 1980, 15.

26. **Egorin, M. J., Clawson, R. E., Ross, L. A., and Bachur, N. R.,** Cellular pharmacology of *N,N*-dimethyl daunorubicin and *N,N*-dimethyl Adriamycin, *Cancer Res.*, 40, 1928, 1980.

27. **Gordon, G. R. and Kashiwase, D.,** Effects of N-substitution on the stimulation of microsomal oxygen consumption by anthracyclines, *Proc. Am. Assoc. Cancer Res.*, 22, 256, 1981.

28. **Mosher, C. W., Wu, H. Y., Fujiwara, A. N., and Acton, E. M.,** Enhanced antitumor properties of 3'-(4-morpholinyl) and 3'-(4-methoxy-1-piperidinyl) derivatives of 3'-deamino-daunorubicin, *J. Med. Chem.*, 25, 18, 1982.

29. **Takahashi, Y., Kinoshita, M., Masuda, T., Tatsuta, K., Takeuchi, T., and Umezawa, H.,** 3'-Deamino-3'-morpholino derivatives of daunomycin, and Adriamycin carminomycin, *J. Antibiot.*, 35, 117, 1982.

30. **Johnston, J. B. and Glazer, R. I.,** Pharmacologic studies of 3'-(4-morpholinyl)-3'-deaminodaunorubicin in human colon carcinoma cells *in vitro*, *Cancer Res.*, 43, 1044, 1983.

31. **Johnston, J. B. and Glazer, R. I.,** The cellular pharmacology of 3'-(4-morpholinyl) and 3'-(4-methoxy-1-piperidinyl) derivatives of 3'-deamino-daunorubicin in human colon carcinoma cells *in vitro*, *Cancer Res.*, 43, 1606, 1983.

32. **Tong, G., Lee W. W., Black, D. R., and Henry, D. W.,** Adriamycin analogs. Periodate oxidation of Adriamycin, *J. Med. Chem.*, 19, 395, 1976.

33. **Peterson, C. and Trouet, A.,** Transport and storage of daunorubicin and doxorubicin in cultured fibroblasts, *Cancer Res.*, 38, 4645, 1978.

34. **Seeber, S., Loth, H., and Crooke, S. T.,** Comparative nuclear and cellular incorporation of daunorubicin, doxorubicin, carminomycin, marcellomycin, aclacinomycin, and AD32 in daunorubicin-sensitive and -resistant Ehrlich ascites *in vitro*, *J. Cancer Res. Clin. Oncol.*, 98, 109, 1980.

35. **Skovgaard, T.,** Transport and binding of daunorubicin, Adriamycin, and rubidazone in Ehrlich ascites tumor cells, *Biochem. Pharmacol.*, 26, 215, 1977.

36. **Zunino, F., Di Marco, A., Zaccara, A., and Gambetta, R. A.,** The interaction of daunorubicin and doxorubicin with DNA and chromatin, *Biochim. Biophys. Acta*, 607, 206, 1980.

37. **Bachur, N. R., Steele, M., Meriwether, W. D., and Hildebrand, R. C.,** Cellular pharmacodynamics of several anthracycline antibiotics, *J. Med. Chem.*, 19, 651, 1976.

38. **Skovgaard, T.,** Carrier-mediated transport of daunorubicin, Adriamycin, and rubidazone in Ehrlich ascites tumor cells, *Biochem. Pharmacol.,* 27, 1221, 1978.

39. **Peterson, C., Baurain, R., and Trouet, A.,** The mechanism for cellular uptake, storage and release of daunorubicin, studies on fibroblasts in culture, *Biochem. Pharmacol.,* 29, 1687, 1980.

40. **Danø, K.,** Active outward transport of daunomycin in resistant Ehrlich ascites tumor cells, *Biochim. Biophys. Acta,* 323, 466, 1973.

41. **Inaba, M., Kobayashi, H., Sakurai, Y., and Johnson, R. K.,** Active efflux of daunorubicin and Adriamycin in sensitive and resistant sublines of P388 leukemia, *Cancer Res.,* 39, 2200, 1979.

42. **Wheeler, C., Rader, R., and Kessel, D.,** Membrane alterations associated with progressive Adriamycin resistance, *Biochem. Pharmacl.,* 31, 2691, 1982.

43. **Bachur, N. R.,** Cytoplasmic aldo-keto reductases: A class of drug metabolizing enzymes, *Science,* 193, 595, 1976.

44. **Loveless, H., Arena, E., Felsted, R. L., and Bachur, N. R.,** Comparative mammalian metabolism of Adriamycin and danorubicin, *Cancer Res.,* 38, 593, 1978.

45. **Ahmed, N. K., Felsted, R. L., and Bachur, N. R.,** Heterogeneity of anthracycline antibiotic carbonyl reductases in mammalian livers, *Biochem. Pharmacol.,* 27, 2713, 1978.

46. **Pierce, R. N. and Jatlow, P. I.,** Measurement of Adriamycin (doxorubicin) and its metabolites in human plasma using reversed-phase high performance liquid chromatography and fluorescence detection, *J. Chromatogr.,* 164, 471, 1979.

47. **Crooke, S. T., DuVernay, V. H., Galvan, L., and Prestayko, A. W.,** Structure-activity relationships of anthracyclines relative to effects on macromolecular synthesis, *Mol. Pharmacol.,* 14, 290, 1978.

48. **DuVernay, V. H., Mong, S., and Crooke, S. T.,** Molecular pharmacology of anthracyclines: demonstration of multiple mechanistic classes of anthracyclines, in *Anthracyclines: Current Status and New Developments,* Crooke, S. T. and Reich, S. D., Eds., Academic Press, New York, 1980, 61.

49. **Long, B. H., Willis, C. E., Prestayko, A. W., and Crooke, S. T.,** Effect of anthracycline analogues on the appearance of newly synthesized total RNA and messenger RNA in the cytoplasm of erythroleukemia cells, *Mol. Pharmacol.,* 22, 152, 1982.

50. **Barthelemy-Clavey, V., Molinier, C., Aubel-Sadron, G., and Maral, R.,** Daunorubicin inhibition of DNA-dependent RNA polymerases from Ehrlich ascites tumor cells, *Eur. J. Biochem.,* 69, 23, 1976.

51. **Chuang, L. F., Kawahata, R. T., and Chuang, R. Y.,** Inhibition of chicken myeloblastosis RNA polymerase II activity In Vitro by *N*-trifluoroacetyladriamycin-14-valerate, *FEBS Lett.,* 117, 247, 1980.

52. **Dano, K., Frederiksen, S. and Hellung-Larsen, P.,** Inhibition of DNA and RNA synthesis by daunorubicin in sensitive and resistant Ehrlich ascites tumor cells *in vitro, Cancer Res.,* 32, 1307, 1972.

53. **Wunderlich, F.,** Nucleocytoplasmic transport of ribosomal subparticles: interplay with the nuclear envelope, in *The Cell Nucleus,* Vol. 9, Busch, H., Ed., 1981, 249.

54. **Eckert, W. A., Franke, W. W., and Scheer, U.,** Nucleocytoplasmic translocation of RNA in *Tetrahymena pyriformis* and its inhibition by actinomycin D and cycloheximide, *Exp. Cell Res.,* 94, 31, 1975.

55. **Calendi, E., Di Marco, A., Reggianni, M., Scarpinato, B., and Valentini, L.,** On physico-chemical interactions between daunomycin and nucleic acids, *Biochim. Biophys. Acta,* 103, 25, 1965.

56. **Doskocil, J. and Fric, I.,** Complex formation of daunomycin with double-stranded RNA, *FEBS Lett.,* 37, 55, 1973.

57. **Sinha, B. K. and Sik, R. H.,** Binding of [^{14}C]Adriamycin to cellular macromolecules *in vivo. Biochem. Pharmacol.,* 29, 1867, 1980.

58. **Moore, H. W.,** Bioactivation as a model for drug design bioreductive alkylation, *Science,* 197, 527, 1977.

59. **Sinha, B. K.,** Binding specificity of chemically and enzymatically activated anthracycline anticancer agents to nucleic acids, *Chem. Biol. Interact.,* 30, 67, 1980.

60. **Calvet, J. P. and Pederson, T.,** Heterogenous nuclear RNA double-stranded regions probed in living HeLa cells by crosslinking with the psoralen derivative aminomethyltrioxsalen, *Proc. Natl. Acad. Sci. U.S.A.,* 76, 755, 1979.

61. **Wollenzian, P. L., Youvan, D. C., and Hearst, J. E.,** Structure of psoralen-crosslinked ribosomal RNA from *Drosophila melangaster, Proc. Natl. Acad. Sci. U.S.A.,* 75, 1642, 1978.

62. **Kish, V. M. and Pederson, T.,** Isolation and characterization of ribonucleoprotein particles containing heterogenous nuclear RNA, *Methods Cell Biol.,* 17, 377, 1978.

63. **Palmiter, R. D.,** Magnesium precipitation of ribonucleoprotein complexes: expedient techniques for the isolation of undergraded polysomes and messenger RNA, *Biochemistry,* 13, 3606, 1974.

64. **Lindberg, U. and Persson, T.,** Isolation of mRNA from K-B cells by affinity chromatography on polyuridylic acid covalently linked to Sepharose, *Eur. J. Biochem.,* 31, 246, 1972.

65. **Locker, J.,** Analytical and preparative electrophoresis of RNA in agarose-urea, *Anal. Biochem.,* 98, 358, 1979.

66. **Glazer, R. I., Hartman, K. D., and Richardson, C. L.,** Cytokinetic and biochemical effects of 5-iminodaunorubicin in human colon carcinoma cells in culture, *Cancer Res.,* 42, 117, 1982.

67. **Crook, L. E., Rees, K. R., and Cohen, A.,** Effect of daunomycin on HeLa cell nucleic acid synthesis, *Biochem. Pharmacol.,* 21, 281, 1972.
68. **Kann, H. E. and Kohn, K. W.,** Effects of deoxyribonucleic acid-reactive drugs on ribonucleic acid synthesis in leukemia L1210 cells, *Mol. Pharmacol.,* 8, 551, 1972.
69. **Wilson, R. G., Kalonaroa, V., King, M., Lockwood, R., and McNeill, M.,** Comparative inhibition of nuclear RNA synthesis in cultured mouse leukemia L1210 cells by Adriamycin and 4-epi-Adriamycin, *Chem. Biol. Interact.,* 37, 351, 1981.
70. **Kappus, H. and Sies, H.,** Toxic drug effects associated with oxygen metabolism: redox cycling and lipid peroxidation, *Experientia,* 37, 1233, 1981.
71. **Berlin, V and Haseltine, W. A.,** Reduction for Adriamycin to a semiquinone-free radical by NADPH cytochrome P-450 reductase produces DNA cleavage in a reaction mediated by molecular oxygen, *J. Biol. Chem.,* 256, 4747, 1981.
72. **Lown, J. W., Chen, H.-H., Plambeck, J. A., and Acton, E. M.,** Further studies on the generation of reactive oxygen species from activated anthracyclines and the relationship to cytotoxic action and cardiotoxic effects, *Biochem. Pharmacol.,* 31, 575, 1982.
73. **Goodman, J. and Hochstein, P.,** Generation of free radicals and lipid peroxidation by redox cycling of Adriamycin and daunomycin, *Biochem. Biophys. Res. Commun.,* 77, 797, 1977.
74. **Myers, C. E., McGuire, W. P., Liss, R. H., Ifrim, I., Grotzinger, K., and Young, R. C.,** Adriamycin: the role of lipid peroxidation in cardiac toxicity and tumor response, *Science,* 197, 165, 1977.
75. **Doroshow, J. H., Locker, G. Y., and Myers, C. E.,** Enzymatic defenses of the mouse heart against reactive oxygen metabolites, *J. Clin. Invest.,* 65, 128, 1980.
76. **Mimnaugh, E. G., Trush, M. A., Ginsburg, E., and Gram T. E.,** Differential effects of anthracycline drugs on rat heart and liver microsomal reduced nicotinamide adenine dinucleotide phosphate-dependent lipid peroxidation, *Cancer Res.,* 42, 3574, 1982.
77. **Tong, G. L., Henry, D. W., and Acton, E. M.,** 5-Iminodaunorubicin. Reduced cardiotoxic properties in an antitumor anthracycline, *J. Med. Chem.,* 22, 36, 1979.
78. **Bachur, N. R., Gordon, S. L., Gee, M., and Kon, H.,** NADPH cytochrome P-450 reductase activation of quinone anticancer agents to free radicals, *Proc. Natl. Acad. Sci. U.S.A.,* 76, 954, 1979.
79. **Doroshow, J. H.,** Effect of anthracycline antibiotics on oxygen radical formation in rat heart, *Cancer Res.,* 43, 460, 1983.
80. **Jensen, R. A.,** Electrocardiographic effects of 3-deamino-3′-(4-morpholinyl)-daunorubicin and doxorubicin in the rat, *Proc. Am. Assoc. Cancer Res.,* 23, 174, 1982.
81. **Minnaugh, E. G.,** personal communication.

Chapter 8

INTERCALATOR-INDUCED PROTEIN-ASSOCIATED DNA STRAND BREAKS IN MAMMALIAN CELLS

Leonard A. Zwelling, Yves Pommier, Donna Kerrigan, and Michael R. Mattern

TABLE OF CONTENTS

I. INTRODUCTION

The normal functions of cellular DNA depend upon the chemical and anatomic integrity of the genome, the fidelity of its reproduction, and coordinated biochemical responses to stimuli of cell growth, differentiation, and gene regulation. Of these factors, perhaps the easiest to quantify is an interruption in the integrity of the phosphodiester backbone, i.e., a DNA strand break. Several techniques have been used to study the formation and removal of DNA breaks in whole cells in an attempt to relate DNA breakage to DNA function, dysfunction, or cell death.

DNA breakage or scission is mechanistically of two types. The first type is a direct result of exogenous physical or chemical agents. The second type arises as a cellular response to exogenous agents which produce abnormal adducts within genomic DNA. Both types result from the actions of cytotoxic agents and the DNA effects appear to reflect potentially lethal DNA damage.

Examples of the first type of scission are breaks produced by X-radiation or bleomycin. This direct DNA breakage is probably the result of locally generated free radicals in the cell nucleus producing interruptions in the DNA phosphodiester backbone.[1-3] Additionally, some breaks may arise through the elimination of damaged DNA bases, either directly or through excision of bases in the vicinity of the lesion.[4] Repair DNA synthesis then fills in the gaps in the cellular genome. The efficiency of this repair may affect cell survival following such damage.

The second type of DNA scission is indirect. Chemical or physical agents such as alkylating drugs or ultraviolet radiation produce abnormal DNA adducts without concomitant direct DNA strand breakage. The subsequent strand breakage arises primarily from cellular responses to these adducts. The backbone is incised at or near the adduct site, a section of DNA is enzymatically removed, and subsequently the patch is filled by DNA repair synthesis.[4] Thus the DNA break is actually an early step in the reconstitution of normal DNA integrity following damage rather than a component of the damage. Again, the efficiency of this repair synthesis may affect cell survival.

In both types of DNA scission, the break is a reflection of the quantity of DNA damage produced by, and the cytotoxic potency of, the exogenous agent. Not only are these DNA-breaking agents cytotoxic, but they are mutagenic. Further, they elicit cellular responses that are common to DNA-breaking agents, e.g., the synthesis of poly(adenosine diphosphoribose) (ADP-R)[5] and unscheduled DNA repair synthesis.[4]

In the Laboratory of Molecular Pharmacology, NCI, and subsequently in several other laboratories, a different sort of cellular response to a class of exogenous cytotoxic agents has been described. These agents are DNA intercalators, potent cytocidal and tumoricidal compounds which interdigitate between DNA base pairs, distorting normal helical structure and interfering with a number of DNA-dependent cellular functions. In cells treated with these agents, a heretofore undetected form of DNA scisson has been described, the protein-associated DNA strand break.[6,7] The nature of this break has been the subject of intense scrutiny in our laboratory for over 5 years. In this review we will summarize what is currently known about these breaks based on our data and those from other laboratories, and will present some hypotheses concerning the nature of these DNA breaks. The major questions have to do with (1) the novelty of the response, and (2) its relation both to the cytotoxic action of DNA intercalators and to normal cellular function, i.e., why do cells have protein-associated DNA breaks?

II. THE METHOD OF QUANTIFYING PROTEIN-ASSOCIATED DNA STRAND SCISSION: FILTER ELUTION OF CELLULAR DNA

A. DNA Single-Strand Breaks (SSB) — Alkaline Elution

The measurement of DNA single-strand break frequencies by the alkaline elution technique of Kohn[8,9] will be briefly reviewed. This technique quantifies the lengths of cellular DNA released from membrane filters in alkali. DNA of small length (high SSB frequency) will pass through filters more rapidly than DNA of longer length (low SSB frequency). The assay is calibrated relative to the independently determined efficiency for SSB production by X-radiation (by alkaline sedimentation = 0.9×10^{-9} SSB per nucleotide per rad). A given increase in alkaline elution rate produced by a drug was gauged in terms of the X-ray dose (in rads) which would give a similar increase in elution rate. Thus SSB frequency can be expressed in rad-equivalents.

This assay can be performed in the presence or absence of maneuvers aimed at minimizing protein adsorption to the membrane filters.[9] These maneuvers include (1) enzymatic proteolysis of cell lysates prior to alkaline elution, (2) the inclusion of sodium dodecylsulfate in both the cell lysis and the elution solutions, and (3) the use of nonadsorbent polycarbonate membrane filters. Regardless of the assay used, in each experiment quantifying the DNA breaking effects of drugs, the effect of X-radiation is concurrently measured and used to calibrate the DNA SSB frequency produced by the experimental agents.

B. DNA-Protein Crosslinking (DPC) — Alkaline Elution

The assay for DPC is performed similarly to that which quantifies DNA SSB, but with two critical differences. First, all the maneuvers minimizing the adsorption of proteins to filters are eliminated, thus maximizing the adsorption of protein to the filter and, likewise, any DNA bound to the protein. Second, a known distribution of DNA single-strand fragment lengths is produced by exposing the cells to a suitable dose of X-ray prior to elution, but following drug treatment. The X-radiation results in DNA fragments of two types, short pieces attached covalently to proteins, and short pieces free of protein. DNA fragments that are not bound to protein pass rapidly through the filter; DNA fragments that are bound to proteins are retained due to the adsorption of the protein(s). From the fraction of the DNA retained on the polyvinyl chloride membrane filter following alkaline elution, the DPC frequency can be calculated on the basis of simple probability theory.[7,11]

C. Double-Strand Breaks (DSB) — Elution at pH 9.6

Using a modification of the filter elution technique minimizing protein-adsorption to membrane filters, a method was developed by Bradley and Kohn to quantify DSB by eluting at pH 9.6, which is below the pH at which DNA strands denature.[12] X-radiation served to calibrate this assay, and the results of DSB measurements with drugs is expressed in DSB-rad-equivalents. However, the absolute DSB frequency per rad of X-ray has been difficult to determine because of the requirement for very high X-ray doses to avoid sedimentation anomalies. Reported values for the ratio of X-ray-induced SSB to DSB in mammalian cells, measured by sedimentation techniques, have ranged from 10 to 40.[13-16] In addition, in alkaline assays, DSB will give rise to two SSB. Thus in alkaline assays, two types of breaks could exist, true SSB (a break in one strand with no break near it in the opposite strand) or two SSBs from a true DSB. The relationship between measured and true break frequencies is described by:

$$k_{RS} [SSB] = s + 2d$$

$$k_{RD} [DSB] = d \qquad (1)$$

where [SSB] is the measured SSB frequency in SSB rad-equivalents as measured by alkaline elution; [DSB] is the measured DSB frequency in DSB rad-equivalents; s is the absolute frequency of SSB, excluding those arising from DSB; d is the absolute DSB frequency; k_{RS} is the SSB frequency produced per unit X-ray dose as measured in the alkaline assay, and k_{RD} is the DSB frequency per unit X-ray dose. The brackets denote the frequencies of SSB or DSB measured in terms of the X-ray dose producing an equivalent effect in the corresponding assay. Although both k_{RS} and k_{RD} are not known, k_{RS}/k_{RD} is between 10 and 40.

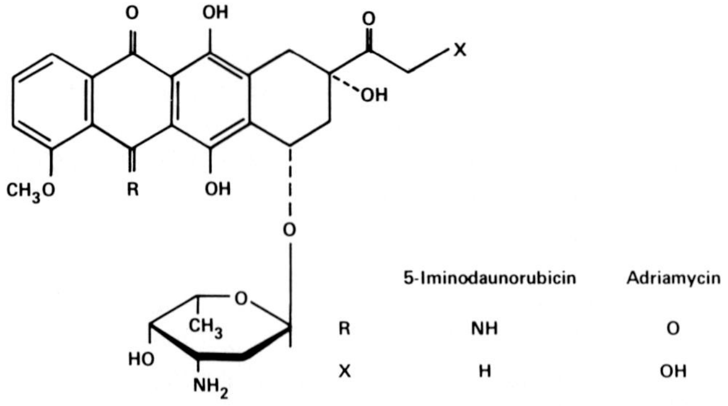

	5-Iminodaunorubicin	Adriamycin
R	NH	O
X	H	OH

FIGURE 1. Structures of Adriamycin® and 5-iminodaunorubicin.

Therefore a ratio can be computed for the actual SSB (s) to actual DSB (d) frequency produced by a given drug treatment by measuring the effects of the treatment in both assays ([SSB]/[DSB]) and relating this measurement to the effects of X-ray in the same assay. This is expressed by calculating s/d from Equation 1:

$$\frac{s}{d} = \frac{k_{RS}}{k_{RD}} \frac{[SSB]}{[DSB]} - 2 \qquad (2)$$

A range of drug-induced s/d is obtained by setting k_{RS}/k_{RD} equal to 10 or 40. If an agent produces only DSB, s/d would equal zero.

III. INTERCALATOR-INDUCED DNA SCISSION: PAST FINDINGS

Previous studies have shown that the DNA of cells treated with a number of intercalating agents including anthracyclines,[17,18] ellipticines,[19] acridines,[20,21] and actinomycin D[22] contained strand breaks. A number of mechanisms have been proposed for this DNA scission (*vide infra*), and they fall into either of the two general categories described above, i.e., direct damage through putative free radical mechanisms or the stimulation of endogenous nuclease activity.

A. Direct DNA Damage

Direct DNA damage has been studied extensively, both in chemical systems (cell free environment) and in whole cells. The intercalating agents for which free radical mechanisms are most likely to be important are the anthracycline antibiotics (Figure 1), particularly Adriamycin® and daunorubicin. It has been hypothesized by a number of investigators that the quinone moiety of the C-ring of these anthracyclines could act as a carrier of free radicals.[23-31] The drugs have been shown to form free radicals spontaneously[30] as well as be activated to free radicals by a number of naturally occurring enzymatic reduction processes in vitro.[23-25,27-29,31-33] Some of these enzymatic pathways exist in isolated nuclei.[23] Further, activated Adriamycin® can break DNA in vitro,[29,33] and this breakage may not depend upon drug intercalation. It is, therefore, possible that the DNA scission produced by Adriamycin® is free-radical mediated. However, other intercalating agents, even anthracyclines like 5-iminodaunorubicin, with a far lower potential for free radical formation, form breaks in cellular DNA to an equal or greater extent than does Adriamycin®.[34] Although the DNA-localized, site-specific generation of potentially damaging free radicals could explain the cytotoxic and/or mutagenic actions of active anthracyclines, more recent work demonstrating this DNA scission at more pharmacologic Adriamycin® concentrations, under conditions established to minimize free radical formation, mitigate against this mechanism (see Section VII.E) for all intercalator-induced DNA scission.[35,36]

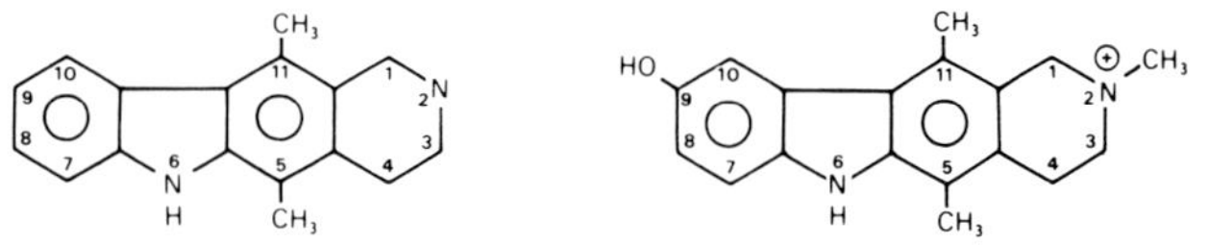

FIGURE 2. Structures of ellipticine and 2-methyl-9-hydroxyellipticinium cation (2-Me-9-OH-E$^+$).

Free radical mechanisms, however, may be critically important in the antineoplastic or cardiotoxic actions of anthracyclines,[37-42] especially if, as we shall discuss below, the cytotoxic mechanisms of intercalators can be distinguished from mechanisms which produce DNA scission (see Section VI.C).

B. Indirect DNA Damage

The alternate hypothesis for the production of DNA scission by anthracyclines as well as other intercalating agents is that these breaks result from the action of endogenous cellular nucleases which either are activated by the drug or respond to a drug-induced alteration in normal cell anatomy or physiology.[17,19-22,43-45] This conclusion arises from the finding that intercalating agents capable of producing DNA breaks in whole cells are ineffective in some subcellular (isolated nuclei) or chemical systems.[19-22]

In the case of the direct DNA damage hypothesis, the intercalating agents function as DNA site-specific delivery systems of a radiomimetic lethal event, free-radical-mediated DNA scission. In the second hypothesis, the cell becomes an obligate participant in the production of the DNA break. This second hypothesis requires further elaboration. What kind of response is this DNA-breaking response? Is it similar to other cellular responses to cytotoxic insult? Is it enzymatically mediated? Is the break damage, or a reflection of a repair response? Is the intercalator break-producing response similar to other responses to DNA damage in the elicitation of DNA repair synthesis or poly(ADP-R) synthesis? Are cells defective in DNA repair following other DNA-breaking agents also sensitive to intercalating agents? Is the whole cell required to demonstrate this response or can the DNA from isolated nuclei also be cut in response to DNA intercalators? Is this response produced by a wide variety of intercalators or limited to certain chemical classes? Can this response be related to the cytocidal actions of intercalators? Finally, if these breaks are a nucleolytic cellular response to intercalation, what is the significance of the response, for surely DNA-breaking responses to intercalating antineoplastic chemicals are not prerequisites for normal cell function. Can this artificially triggered response have a normal function within the living cell which intercalators aberrantly elicit? Will pharmacologic manipulation of cells, which result in perturbations in the response, help us understand its potential function within normal cells?

IV. THE DNA SCISSION PRODUCED BY INTERCALATING AGENTS IS ASSOCIATED WITH PROTEINS BOUND TO THE BREAK TERMINI

Although the second hypothesis regarding the origin of intercalator-induced DNA scission raises a myriad of fascinating biological questions, the first hypothesis, that of direct, drug-induced DNA scission, was the more accessible to experimental testing. A drug producing direct DNA scission, particularly free-radical-mediated scission, would be expected to produce effects similar to those produced by X-irradiation or bleomycin (*vide supra*). Adriamycin® had been shown to be a good generator of free radicals in a number of systems (see Section III.A); ellipticine (Figure 2), another DNA intercalator, was much less likely to produce free radicals. Ross et al. clearly demonstrated that *both* agents produced breaks in

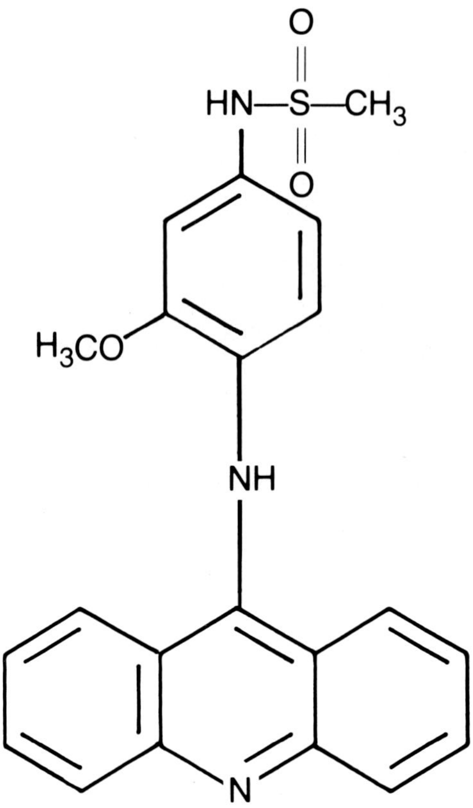

FIGURE 3. Structure of 4′(9-acridinylamino)metha-nesulfon-*m*-anisidide (*m*-AMSA).

L1210 murine leukemia cell DNA.[6,7] However, the more important findings contained within this work were about the nature of these DNA breaks.

Using alkaline elution technology (see Section II), the rapid filter elution of cellular DNA characteristic of DNA scission was detectable only when the lysates of intercalator-treated cells contained proteolytic enzymes. In the absence of proteolysis, almost no DNA eluted from the filter. This result has subsequently been reproduced for a large number of inter-calating agents, including the active, antitumor acridine *m*-AMSA (see Figures 3 and 4 and Table 1). This dependence of break detection upon proteolysis distinguishes the intercalator-induced DNA scission from that produced by X-radiation. This type of DNA scission has thus been termed "protein-concealed". In addition, when SSB and DPC were quantified (Sections II.A and B) for any given drug treatment, the number of SSB was approximately equal to the number of DPC. Not only were the SSB "protein-concealed", but they were also stoichiometrically "protein-associated".

These two findings have led to a model concerning the anatomic relationship between the DNA breakage and the DNA-bound protein. Because all breaks were concealed by protein and each break was accompanied by a protein crosslink, it was reasonable to postulate that the two phenomena (SSB and DPC) were neither independent, nor random, but that they were mechanistically and anatomically related. If the two effects had been the results of independent and/or random events within the cell genome, calculations of the elution results would have yielded more detectable breaks than crosslinks.[7] Therefore, some elution should have been discernible without proteinase treatment of lysates. As this last feature was not a description of the cellular DNA effects produced by the intercalating agents, a nonrandom,

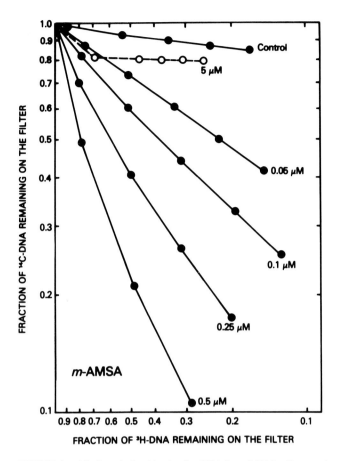

FIGURE 4. Alkaline elution kinetics for DNA from L1210 cells treated with various concentrations of *m*-AMSA for 1 hr. Assays performed without proteinase (open symbols and dashed lines). Assays performed with proteinase K (filled symbols and solid lines). Horizonal axis is essentially a corrected time scale based on elution of internal standard cells (^{3}H-labeled, 300 R irradiated). (From Zwelling, L. A., Michaels, S., Erickson, L. C., Ungerleider, R. S., Nichols, M., and Kohn, K. W., *Biochemistry*, 20, 6553, 1981. With permission.)

Table 1
INTERCALATORS WHICH PRODUCE PROTEIN-ASSOCIATED DNA SCISSION IN MAMMALIAN CELLS

Adriamycin®
Daunomycin
5-Iminodaunorubicin
N-trifluoroacetyladriamycin-14-valerate(AD 32)and
  metabolites
m-AMSA
Lucanthone
Hycanthone
Actinomycin D

Ethidium Bromide
Ellipticine
2-Me-9-OH-E$^+$
Dihydroxyanthracenedione

9,10-Anthracene dicarboxyaldehyde bis-[(4,5-dihydro-1-H-imidazol-2-yl)] hydrazone

''bound-to-one-terminus'' model (Figure 5) was developed which fit more closely the data obtained with Adriamycin® and ellipticine.[6,7,11]

From this work, it became evident that the DNA scission detected by filter elution in cells

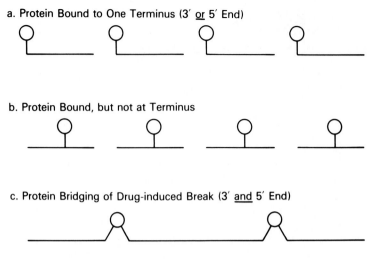

a. Protein Bound to One Terminus (3′ <u>or</u> 5′ End)

b. Protein Bound, but not at Terminus

c. Protein Bridging of Drug-induced Break (3′ <u>and</u> 5′ End)

FIGURE 5.   Hypothetical models of the structural relationship between DNA-protein crosslinking and DNA single-strand breakage produced by intercalators.

following their treatment with intercalators was to some extent unique in its relationship to DNA-bound proteins. The nature of the breaks or the bound proteins as well as their relation to other drug actions such as cytotoxicity remained unknown.

V. *m*-AMASA DNA SCISSION

The initial data obtained with Adriamycin® and ellipticine suggested an anatomic relationship between intercalator-induced DPC and SSB. The protein was most probably bound to the terminus of the strand break. Ross et al.[6,7] also suggested a mechanistic relationship between breaks and crosslinks. They speculated that the protein associated with each SSB was an endonuclease which produced the SSB and remained bound to one DNA strand terminus following enzymatic DNA cleavage.

Work with the 9-anilinoacridine intercalating derivative, 4′-(9-acridinylamino)methanesulfon-*m*-anisidide (*m*-AMSA) supported this hypothesis.[46] Like Adriamycin® and ellipticine, *m*-AMSA produced protein-associated and protein-concealed breaks in the DNA of L1210 cells. Several important new facts about this process were ascertained. *m*-AMSA produced a far greater number of SSB per molecule of added drug and at less cytotoxic doses than had been used with Adriamycin.® This greater magnitude of breakage allowed more accurate quantification of intercalator-induced DNA effects without complications from effects upon DNA produced by rapid cell lysis. *m*-AMSA-induced breakage was found to be limited; the SSB frequency showed saturation above 2 μM (Figure 6). *m*-AMSA cellular uptake was proportional to extracellular concentration up to 7.5 μM. The saturation of DNA strand breakage was not due to saturation of drug uptake.

m-AMSA breaks formed to their maximum level within 10 min of drug addition and disappeared with equal rapidity following *m*-AMSA removal (Figure 7). These processes were, however, slower than drug uptake or egress. Further *m*-AMSA-induced SSB formation and resealing were highly temperature dependent. At 25°C, the rates of these processes were reduced, while at 4°C there was no DNA breakage. *m*-AMSA cell uptake and egress were slowed slightly at 25°C and somewhat more so at 4°C, but as in the case of the saturation of SSB magnitude with dose and the case of the rate of SSB formation at 37°C, the slowing of break formation and resealing at 25°C and the blockade of these processes at 4°C were clearly dissociated from temperature effects on drug transport (Figures 8 and 9). The blockade

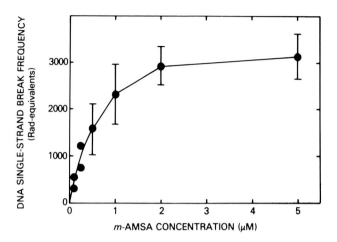

FIGURE 6. Dependence of SSB frequency on *m*-AMSA concentration following 1-hr drug exposure. (From Zwelling, L. A., Michaels, S., Erickson, L. C., Ungerleider, R. S., Nichols, M., and Kohn, K. W., *Biochemistry*, 20, 6553, 1981. With permission.)

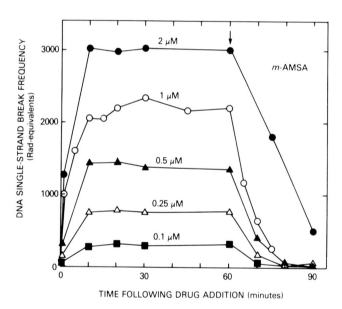

FIGURE 7. Kinetics of formation and disappearance of SSB in L1210 cells exposed to indicated concentrations of *m*-AMSA. Cells were treated for 60 min during which time aliquots were removed for SSB quantification. At 60 min (arrow), the drug was removed and samples were again taken at various times. (From Zwelling, L. A., Michaels, S., Erickson, L. C., Ungerleider, R. S., Nichols, M., and Kohn, K. W., *Biochemistry*, 20, 6553, 1981. With permission.)

of SSB formation and resealing at 4°C was not a nonspecific premorbid effect of reduced temperature on all cell function, as cells kept at 4°C for 1 hr either immediately following *m*-AMSA addition (to prevent SSB formation) or following an incubation with drug at 37°C followed by drug removal at ice temperature (to prevent SSB resealing) went on to form or reseal SSB once shifted to 37°C. Thus, the reduced temperature inhibited the function of the breaking-rejoining process reversibly, without permanently disrupting it.

Similar experiments performed with Adriamycin® showed that the breaks formed slowly

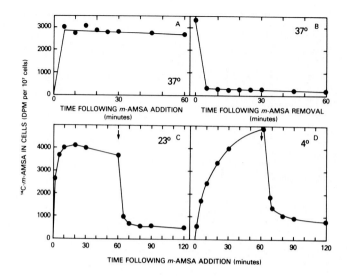

FIGURE 8.   Kinetics of uptake and egress of [^{14}C]-*m*-AMSA. Uptake (A) and egress (B) at 37°C. Uptake and egress at 23°C (C) and 4°C (D). Arrow indicates time of drug removal. (From Zwelling, L. A., Michaels, S., Erickson, L. C., Ungerleider, R. S., Nichols, M., and Kohn, K. W., *Biochemistry,* 20, 6553, 1981. With permission.)

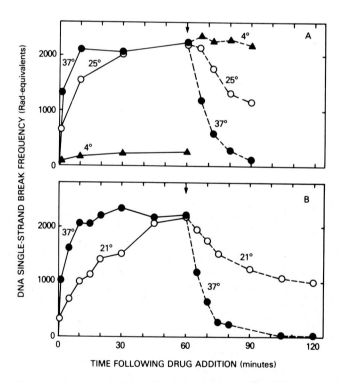

FIGURE 9.   Kinetics of formation and disappearance of SSB in L1210 cells at various temperatures following the addition of 1 μ*M m*-AMSA. (From Zwelling, L. A., Michaels, S., Erickson, L. C., Ungerleider, R. S., Nichols, M., and Kohn, K. W., *Biochemistry,* 20, 6553, 1981. With permission.)

at a constant rate and were not readily reversible. Further, the Adriamycin® SSB formation process was even more temperature dependent than that governing *m*-ASMA break formation,

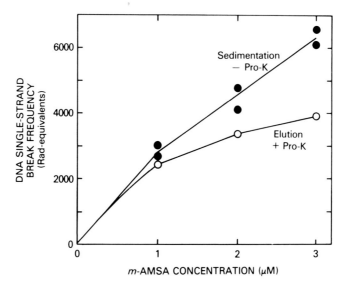

FIGURE 10. SSB frequencies following 1-hr treatment with various concentrations of *m*-AMSA quantified by alkaline sedimentation (●) or alkaline elution (○). Cell lysates were proteolytically digested in elution assays only. (From Zwelling, L. A., Michaels, S., Erickson, L. C., Ungerleider, R. S., Nichols, M., and Kohn, K. W., *Biochemistry*, 20, 6553, 1981. With permission.)

as no SSB formed at 25°C in Adriamycin®-treated cells. Transport studies were not performed with Adriamycin®, however, and some of these effects could be the result of alterations in Adriamycin® transport.

As with the other intercalators studied, *m*-AMSA produced SSB and DPC at approximately equal frequencies, and SSB and DPC formed and resealed with comparable kinetics.

The high frequency of *m*-AMSA-induced breakage allowed an independent quantification of intercalator-induced breakage by alkaline sucrose gradient sedimentation, a technique relatively insensitive to the lower break frequencies produced by pharmacologic doses of other intercalators. Agreement between the two methods was reasonable (Figure 10). Further, because *m*-AMSA SSB were detectable using gradients employing no enzymatic deproteinization of cell lysates, the proteins bound to DNA following *m*-AMSA treatment either do not bridge the strand break (which would have concealed the SSB in a gradient by functionally increasing the size of sedimenting DNA) or, if a protein bridge exists in vivo, at least one of the DNA-protein bonds is alkali-labile (see Figure 5 and Reference 47). The alkaline (pH 13.0) conditions of these gradients did not remove the protein from the DNA as the breaks remained concealed in filter elution assays unless proteinase digestion is employed, even if elution was performed with the pH 13.0 sucrose gradient solution. Hence, a protein prevented filter elution of DNA under the same conditions which showed reduced DNA sedimentation (increased breakage). Either model a or c in Figure 5 is the most likely to be correct; (it seems unlikely that a concerted DNA scission and protein-binding would be anatomically separate). If c is correct, one of the bridging protein-DNA bonds is probably not covalent.

Double-strand breaks (DSB) were also quantified using filter elution technology (see Section II.C)[12] following the treatment of cells with *m*-AMSA or Adriamycin.® DSB and SSB formed and disappeared with similar kinetics.[46] Differences were apparent, however, among the ratios of SSB to DSB produced by the different intercalators. The data acquired in our laboratory, as well as those from Ross and Bradley,[48] are included in Table 2. This will be discussed further in Section VII.A).

An attempt was made to relate these DNA effects to the cytotoxic potency of *m*-AMSA

Table 2
THE RELATIONSHIP BETWEEN DNA SINGLE-STRAND BREAKS (SSB) AND DOUBLE-STRAND BREAKS (DSB) PRODUCED BY VARIOUS INTERCALATING AGENTS IN MOUSE LEUKEMIA L1210 CELLS[a]

| | | s/d^c | | |
| | Estimated[b] | $k_{RS}/k_{RD} =$ | $k_{RS}/k_{RD} =$ | |
Drug	[SSB]/[DSB]	10	40	Ref.
Adriamycin®	0.181	−0.2	5.2	48
	0.190	−0.1	5.6	46
5-Iminodaunorubicin	0.120	−0.8	2.8	34
Ellipticine	0.076	−1.2	1.0	48
	0.100	−1.0	2.0	54
2-Me-9-OH-E⁺	0.110	−0.9	2.4	54
Actinomycin D	0.226	0.3	7.1	48
m-AMSA	0.530	3.3	19.0	46

[a] Measurements of single-strand break frequency were made by alkaline elution; measurements of double-strand break frequency were made by filter elution at pH 9.6.

[b] [SSB] = measured single-strand break frequency in single-strand break rad-equivalents; [DSB] = measured double-strand break frequency in double-strand break rad-equivalents.

[c] s/d = ratio of actual single-strand breaks (excluding those arising from double-strand breaks) to actual double-strand breaks; k_{RS}, k_{RD} are the efficiencies of single- or double-strand break production by X-irradiation, taken to be either 10 or 40 as the extreme values reported. (See Section II.C for a further discussion of these calculations.)

and Adriamycin®. A first examination by Ross et al. concluded that the breaks produced by Adriamycin® appeared to be associated with a larger magnitude of cytotoxicity (as measured by soft agar cloning) than the DNA scission produced by ellipticine.[49] Cohen et al.[50] characterized the DNA breaks produced by dihydroxyanthracenedione as also correlated with high cytotoxic potency.[50] However, the kinetic studies showing vast differences between the half-lives of the DNA SSB produced by *m*-AMSA and Adriamycin® indicated that simple comparisons between DNA effects immediately following drug treatments, and subsequent colony-forming ability in these treated cell populations may be hazardous in attempting to mechanistically relate intercalator-induced DNA scission and intercalator-induced cytotoxicity.

Intercalating agents from different chemical classes could be compared only if their DNA effects have similar half-lives. Short-lived DNA breaks would be easier to use for this comparison, as the resealing of the breaks following drug removal from cells would indicate the cellular egress of the breaking agent, giving a clear indication that the exposure of potential intracellular targets of drug action, DNA or otherwise, would be limited.

The work with *m*-AMSA strongly suggested that the intercalator-induced DNA scission was enzymatically mediated, because the scission displayed apparent saturation with increasing drug dose and temperature dependence, both clearly separable from effects of drug transport. Further, the alkaline sucrose gradient data appear to limit the potential configurations of the DNA-protein complex surrounding the intercalator-induced break site (Figure 5, *vide supra*). The markedly different kinetics of break formation and disappearance between Adriamycin® and *m*-AMSA necessitated a search for intercalators producing DNA effects with similar reversal kinetics prior to speculating on the relationship between these effects and cytocidal drug action.

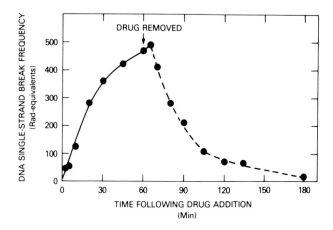

FIGURE 11. Kinetics of formation and disappearance of SSB in L1210 cells exposed to 2.5 μM 5-iminodaunorubicin. Experiment performed as described in Figure 7 legend. (From Zwelling, L. A., Kerrigan, D., and Michaels, S., *Cancer Res.*, 42, 2687, 1982. With permission.)

VI. OTHER INTERCALATORS PRODUCING REVERSIBLE, PROTEIN-ASSOCIATED DNA SCISSION

A. 5-Iminodaunorubicin

The anthracyclines are particularly potent antineoplastic intercalators. Some of their cellular actions, including DNA scission, have been attributed to their potential for free radical formation in the quinone ring (Figure 1) (see Section III.A). 5-Iminodaunorubicin is the first active antineoplastic anthracycline modified within the quinone ring.[51] This modification results in a decreased potential for free radical formation.[28,30] 5-Iminodaunorubicin breaks DNA in chemical systems with a lower efficiency than Adriamycin®[28] and may, therefore, be similarly less efficient in cells. If so, the comparative free radical potential of anthracyclines might correlate with their relative DNA-breaking potential. Additionally, if free radical potential is related to break persistence or intracellular drug persistence, the breaks produced by 5-iminodaunorubicin may be short-lived.

5-Iminodaunorubicin and Adriamycin® intercalate comparably in isolated DNA.[52] 5-Iminodaunorubicin produced more protein-associated DNA SSB than Adriamycin® per mole of drug.[34] Like Adriamycin®, it was a potent producer of DSB as well (Table 2 and Section VII.A). Most importantly, the DNA scission produced by 5-Iminodaunorubicin, unlike that produced by Adriamycin®, was rapidly reversible (Figure 11). An anthracycline with the desired property of rapidly reversible DNA kinetics was found. Further, assuming no great differences between Adriamycin® and 5-iminodaunorubicin cell uptake (in both cases breaks increased linearly with time), the agent with the lower free radical potential produced the greater frequency of DNA scission per mole of added drug, appearing to dissociate the intracellular formation of DNA breaks from free radical mechanisms (see Section III.A). Whether the greater free radical potential of Adriamycin® accounts for the persistence of DNA scission following this drug is not, at present, known.

B. 2-Methyl-9-Hydroxyellipticinium

The original work of Ross et al.[6,7] utilized ellipticine as a simple intercalator possessing activity similar to Adriamycin® in its ability to produce protein-associated scission in cellular DNA. However, like Adriamycin®, ellipticine produced breaks which barely reversed following routine cell washing (Figure 12), again complicating a comparison between cytotoxicity and intercalator-induced DNA scission.[53,54] The persistence of ellipticine-induced

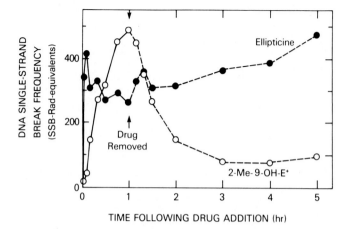

FIGURE 12.   Kinetics of formation and disappearance of SSB in L1210 cells exposed to 10 μM ellipticine (●) or 8.25 μM 2-Me-9-OH-E⁺ (○). Experiment performed as describe in Figure 7 legend. (From Zwelling, L. A., Michaels, S., Kerrigan, D., Pommier, Y., and Kohn, K. W., *Biochem. Pharmacol.*, 32, 3261, 1982. With permission.)

DNA breaks presumably arises from the lipophilicity of the compound[55,56] and its resultant close association with the cell membrane[57] which can serve as a reservoir for continued exposure of intracellular contents to the drug.

The cationic ellipticine derivative, 2-methyl-9-hydroxyellipticinium (2-Me-9-OH-E⁺), is an active analogue[58] which is always cationic in aqueous solution and is less lipophilic and more water soluble than ellipticine.[54] This compound produced reversible, protein-associated single- and double-strand breaks in L1210 cell DNA (Figure 12). Thus a third chemical class of intercalators could now be compared with acridines (*m*-AMSA) and anthracyclines (5-iminodaunorubicin) to see if a uniform relationship exists between intercalator-induced DNA scission and cytotoxicity.

C. Intercalator-Induced DNA Scission and Cytotoxicity

If the DNA scission produced by intercalators is the mechanism by which these agents kill cells, then doses of the various agents which produce comparable break frequencies would be expected to produce comparable reductions in cell survival as measured by colony-forming assays. Figure 13 displays a comparison among the agents from three chemical classes of intercalators for reductions in cell survival vs. measured single- or double-strand break frequency. Neither DNA effect uniformly predicted cytotoxic potency. The results of these experiments can be summarized as follows:

DSB/SSB ratio:	2-Me-9-OH-E⁺ > 5-iminodaunorubicin > *m*-AMSA
$t_{1/2}$ of SSB reversal:	2-Me-9-OH-E⁺ > 5-iminodaunorubicin > *m*-AMSA
Cell kill per SSB:	5-iminodaunorubicin ≥ 2-Me-9-OH-E⁺ > *m*-AMSA
Cell kill per DSB:	5-iminodaunorubicin > 2-Me-9-OH-E⁺ > *m*-AMSA

Neither slow resealing of DNA scission nor a preponderance of DSB (also see Section VII.A) indicated the most potent cytotoxic agent. No uniform relationship exists between the frequency of intercalator-induced DNA scission and cytotoxic potency for the intercalators studied.

VII. BIOLOGICAL AND BIOCHEMICAL CHARACTERISTICS OF THE INTERCALATOR-INDUCED BREAKING-REJOINING RESPONSE IN CELLULAR AND SUBCELLULAR DNA TARGETS

A. Single- to Double-Strand Break Ratios

In Section II.C we discussed the method by which measured, drug-induced SSB and DSB

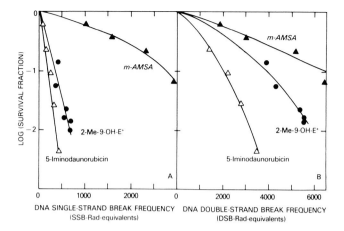

FIGURE 13. Relationship between colony formation and DNA break frequency following 1-hr treatments with various concentrations of *m*-AMSA (▲), 5-iminodaunorubicin (△) or 2-Me-9-OH-E⁺ (●). Log survival fraction vs. SSB frequency (A) or DSB frequency (B). (From Zwelling, L. A., Michaels, S., Kerrigan, D., Pommier, Y., and Kohn, K. W., *Biochem. Pharmacol.*, 32, 3261, 1982. With permission.)

frequencies can be related to one another through a comparison with the break frequencies produced by X-radiation in our assays and the published ratios of X-ray-induced SSB/DSB of between 10 and 40. Table 2 lists the results obtained with all of the compounds examined by filter elution technology thus far.

If s/d = 0 (in Equation 2), then all of the measured DNA scission is double-stranded. Clearly the breaks produced by actinomycin D and *m*-AMSA fall outside of this range, regardless of which value for k_{RS}/k_{RD} is correct. It is reasonable to assume, therefore, that these two agents produce both single- and double-strand breaks in L1210 cell DNA. However, the other agents are all potential candidates to be solely double-strand break producers as the calculated values for s/d fall on either side of zero for these agents, depending on which value of k_{RS}/k_{RD} is used. If however, we assume that the most extreme case biologically is an agent producing solely double-strand scission, we would expect that such an agent would most likely produce results in this assay giving the lowest [SSB]/[DSB]. The ellipticines most nearly fulfill these criteria. If k_{RS}/k_{RD} is actually close to 20, then the ellipticines would precisely give s/d = 0. The anthracyclines then would produce both single- and double-strand breaks, but with a greater number of DSB per SSB than actinomycin D, *m*-AMSA, or X-radiation. Note that all of the intercalators produce a higher frequency of DSB to SSB than X-radiation, suggesting that the mechanism of intercalator-induced DNA scission differs from that of X-ray-induced strand breakage, and that the intercalator-induced double-strand breakage is not solely the result of the random approximation of opposing single-strand breaks.

B. The DNA Breaking Activity Elicited by Intercalators Can Be Localized to the Cell Nucleus

The action of various intercalators, most notably the anthracyclines, may not be the same in isolated chemical systems as in whole cells. There is evidence for the free radical mechanism of anthracycline DNA scission in various isolated chemical systems (Section II.A), but not in whole cells (see Sections VI.A and VII.F). The intercalator-induced DNA scission in L1210 cells could be characterized better if a system could be found that retains the reversible, protein-associated character of the breaks produced by *m*-AMSA, 5-iminodaunorubicin, and 2-Me-9-OH-E⁺, but has a defined chemical constitution and is accessible to

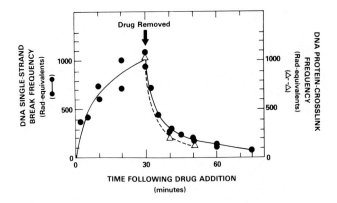

FIGURE 14.   Kinetics of formation and disappearance of SSB (●) and
DPC (△) in isolated L1210 cell nuclei exposed to 1 μ*M* *m*-AMSA. (From
Pommier, Y., Kerrigan, D., Schwartz, R., and Zwelling, L. A., *Biochem.
Biophys. Research Commun.*, 107, 576, 1982. With permission.)

manipulations aimed at defining the biochemical mechanism of this putative enzymatic DNA
breaking-rejoining process.

Filipski and Kohn had demonstrated SSB and DPC in isolated nuclei treated with ellipticine.[59] Detailed quantitation or studies of SSB or DPC reversibility were not reported.
Pommier et al. have recently demonstrated the SSB and DPC frequencies produced by *m*-
AMSA or 5-iminodaunorubicin in isolated L1210 cell nuclei were, indeed, comparable to
those seen in whole L1210 cells.[60] Further, both effects of *m*-AMSA were rapidly reversible
(Figure 14) as had been the case in cells. These findings suggest that, at least in the cases
of *m*-AMSA and 5-iminodaunorubicin, cellular metabolism is not required to produce the
breaking-rejoining response to intercalators. This response appears localized to the cell
nucleus; ATP (absent from these nuclei) is not required for this activity. This response also
occurred with no other added cofactor and *m*-ASMA breaks resealed in the salt buffer (150
m*M* NaCl; 1 m*M* KH$_2$PO$_4$; 5 m*M* M$_g$Cl$_2$; 1 m*M* EGTA; 0.1 m*M* dithiothreitol, pH 6.4) with
no added nucleotide triphosphates.

It is of interest to note that 2-Me-9-OH-E$^+$ did not produce breaks in the DNA of isolated
nuclei.[60] Nuclei buffer did not inactivate the drug, as the DNA of cells treated in this buffer
was broken. Either 2-Me-9-OH-E$^+$ requires cytoplasmic activation prior to acquiring the
chemical form which stimulates DNA scission, or cofactors are removed from nuclei which
are needed for 2-Me-9-OH-E$^+$-induced scission. Alternatively, the actual enzyme(s) which
putatively produces the 2-Me-9-OH-E$^+$-induced breaks is removed during nuclei isolation.

This system is currently being used to characterize more extensively the biochemical
parameters and required factors for the DNA breaking-rejoining response.

C. Formation and Resealing of Intercalator-Induced Scission Without the Stimulated Synthesis of Poly(ADP-Ribose)

The synthesis of poly(adenosine diphosphoribose) (ADP-R) accompanies DNA scission
produced by a variety of physical and chemical agents. Agents which directly break DNA,
like X-rays,[61,62] or indirectly by eliciting repair endonuclease-mediated scission like UV
light[63-67] stimulate poly(ADP-R) synthesis. The function of this polymer is not known,
but the stimulation of its synthesis in response to DNA damage and the enhancement
of the cytotoxicity of these damaging agents when poly(ADP-R) synthesis is specifically
inhibited[68-71] have led to the hypothesis that poly(ADP-R) synthesis is an integral part of
the DNA repair process.

In the majority of systems utilized to quantify poly(ADP-R) synthesis, a DNA break
frequency in excess of that produced by 1000 rad of X-rays is required to produce a detectable

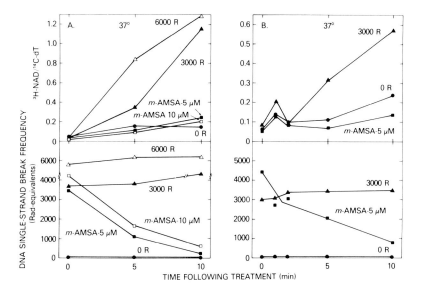

FIGURE 15. The relationship between DNA SSB and poly(ADP-ribose) synthesis in L1210 cells treated with X-ray or *m*-AMSA. Untreated (●), 3000 R (▲), 6000 R (△), *m*-AMSA, 10 µ*M* (□) or 5 µ*M* (■) for 30 min at 37°. Treatment was of whole cells prior to permeabilization. Quantification of SSB by alkaline elution (bottom panels) or poly(ADP-R) synthesis (top panels) followed permeabilization (at 4°C) and transfer to a 37°C water bath. Poly(ADP-R) synthesis is expressed as the DPM of ³H-NAD incorporation into acid-insoluble material per ¹⁴C-dT from prelabeled DNA. (From Zwelling, L. A., Kerrigan, D., Pommier, Y., Michaels, S., Steren, A., and Kohn, K. W., *J. Biol. Chem.*, 257, 8957, 1982. With permission.)

quantity of polymer synthesis. The large magnitude of DNA scission produced by *m*-AMSA allowed us to compare *m*-AMSA with X-rays for their relative abilities to stimulate poly(ADP-R) synthesis at equal break frequencies.

The permeabilized cell system of Berger et al.[5] was used to quantify poly(ADP-R) synthesis.[72] Whole cells were either drug-treated or X-irradiated, then permeabilized by cold shock and incubated with ³H-nicotinamide adenine dinucleotide (NAD) in the presence of permeabilization buffer and Triton® X-100. NAD is the obligate substrate of poly(ADP-R) polymerase and the incorporation of ³H-NAD into acid-insoluble radioactivity is taken as a measure of poly(ADP-R) synthesis.

m-AMSA did not stimulate poly(ADP-R) synthesis (Figure 15) despite producing DNA single-strand break frequencies comparable to those produced by doses of X-ray which stimulated poly(ADP-R) synthesis three to ten times that of untreated controls. *m*-AMSA did not inhibit poly(ADP-R) synthesis if co-incubated with X-irradiated permeabilized cell suspensions. Perhaps the most surprising finding was that *m*-AMSA breaks would reseal in permeabilized cells despite the absence of exogenous ATP or nucleotide triphosphates, suggesting that DNA synthesis, as well as poly(ADP-R) synthesis, was not required for intercalator-induced break resealing.

These data clearly distinguished intercalator-induced DNA scission from that produced by all other forms of DNA breakage. The protein-concealed nature of this break may preclude its access to the endogenous DNA break-detecting system which triggers poly(ADP-R) synthesis. The break site may possess chemical properties which do not stimulate poly(ADP-R) synthesis. A third possibility is that the *m*-AMSA break frequency, measured by alkaline or pH 9.6 elution or by alkaline sucrose sedimentation (Section V.), is significantly greater than that which is actually extant within the treated cells, particularly if the measured break frequency reveals all potential break sites which in actuality are constantly opening and

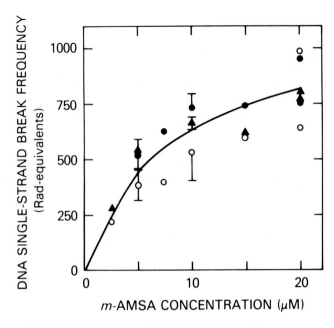

FIGURE 16.   Dependence of SSB frequency on *m*-AMSA concentration following 1-hr drug exposures in CRL 1187 (normal) (●), CRL 1160 (XP) (○) or A-T 5BI (ataxia telangiectasia) (▲) human fibroblasts. (From Zwelling, L. A. and Mattern, M. R., *Mutat. Res.*, 104, 295, 1982. With permission.)

closing in vivo making any given DNA break very transient. Finally, the break configuration within cells may not stimulate poly(ADP-R) synthesis. This latter possibility could arise if the putative break-producing enzyme remains bound to the DNA break site and prevents relaxation of supercoiling, possibly by bridging the break (Figure 5, model c). As poly(ADP-R) has been hypothesized to approximate cut strands or alter local conditions to potentiate strand rejoining,[73] an absence of helical relaxation despite strand scission may not serve to stimulate poly(ADP-R) synthesis in response to intercalator-induced DNA breakage.

D. DNA-Repair Deficiencies Do Not Affect Intercalator-Induced Cytotoxicity or DNA Scission in Human Cells

The processes by which cells repair damaged DNA have been studied using human cell strains having abnormal responses to various DNA damaging agents. *Xeroderma pigmentosum* (XP) cells are particularly sensitive to the cytotoxic actions of UV light, presumably because they are defective in excision repair of UV-induced thymine dimers.[74-76] *Ataxia telangiectasia* (A-T) cells are hypersensitive to X-ray-induced lethality.[77,78] Thus, these physical agents as well as chemical agents which produce similar damage usually resulting in cellular DNA scission, are particularly toxic to one or the other type of repair-defective cells.

A comparison between a normal diploid fibroblast line, an XP line, and an A-T line revealed no differences in the cytotoxicity, DNA scission, or cellular drug uptake following *m*-AMSA treatment[79] (Figure 16). *m*-AMSA is thus unique in its ability to produce breaks in cellular DNA that are not associated with an enhanced sensitivity in one or the other of these repair-deficient cells. Intercalator-induced, protein-associated DNA scission is thus likely to be the result of a novel cellular response which differs from that which is abnormal in XP or A-T cells, and different from responses elicited by agents like X-radiation or UV light to which these cells are hypersensitive.

E. Free Radical Scavengers Do Not Uniformly Inhibit Intercalator-Induced DNA Scission or Cytotoxicity

The contribution to intercalator-induced DNA scission by free radicals has been discussed with respect to results of experiments done in chemical systems which support a free-radical mechanism (see Section II.A) and in intact cells, which exclude such a mechanism. Recently, we have addressed this question directly by attempting to alter the DNA scission and cytotoxic potency of a variety of intercalators in L1210 cells with the free radical scavengers, dimethyl sulfoxide (DMSO) or thiourea.[35] Both agents blocked X-ray-induced DNA scission and cytotoxicity comparably. DMSO enhanced Adriamycin,® 5-iminodaunorubicin, and m-AMSA-induced DNA scission without a commensurate effect on drug-induced cytotoxicity. DMSO did not enhance Adriamycin® or m-AMSA cellular uptake. Thiourea decreased both drug-induced DNA scission and cytotoxicity, but did not do so in a collateral fashion with all of the agents. Thiourea, like DMSO, did not alter m-AMSA or adriamycin® uptake, nor did thiourea chemically inactivate the intercalating agents. These data tend to dissociate inter-calator-induced DNA break production from lethality and from the mechanism of X-ray break production, which is putatively mediated by the generation of free radicals.[2,80]

A recent report by Potmesil et al.[36] reconciles the apparently contradictory data regarding the participation of free radicals in Adriamycin®-induced DNA scission. These authors quantified DNA scission in L1210 cells treated with various concentrations of Adriamycin® under hypoxic (95% N_2/5% CO_2) or euoxic (95% air/5% CO_2) conditions. Doses ranged from those that are pharmacologically obtainable in vivo ($2.8 \times 10^{-8} M$) to the high doses often used in chemical studies ($2.8 \times 10^{-4} M$). Cellular drug uptake was monitored and found to be linear with dose and unaffected by O_2 content. At 10^{-8} to 10^{-6} Adriamycin® concentrations all DNA scission detected was protein-associated and occurred with equal frequency in hypoxic and euoxic cells. At concentrations of $2.8 \times 10^{-5} M$ or above, DNA scission, unassociated with protein, became apparent only in euoxic cells. Thus, the magnitude of protein-associated DNA scission is not sensitive to O_2 tension, whereas a second type of DNA break becomes detectable at high drug concentrations in euoxic cells only. This latter process may be free-radical-mediated and consistent with the DNA-breaking action ascribed to Adriamycin® in vitro. These breaks were detectable only at doses in excess of that usually obtained in vivo. They may be relevant, however, if local concentrations of Adriamycin® within target tissues are high secondary to selective drug accumulation, or if this type of break reflects a form of chemical damage not generally present in cellular DNA, which may be concentrated at other cell sites (e.g., membranes) due to local subcellular drug accumulations, increased target susceptibility, or the presence of chemical systems within subcellular compartments which could potentiate the generation of drug-induced radicals.[23-25]

F. Alterations in the Three-Dimensional Structure of Target DNA Correlate with Altered Target Susceptibility to Intercalator-Induced DNA Scission

Free-radical-mediated chemical reactions are unlikely to explain the majority of the scission produced in cellular DNA by representatives from these various chemical classes of inter-calators (*vide supra* Table 1). However, in our studies with DMSO and thiourea we identified an alternative to the free-radical mechanism.[35] DMSO and thiourea altered the sedimentation of nucleoids derived from L1210 cells. Nucleoids are structures consisting of double-stranded, cellular DNA constrained by nonhistone protein plus some RNA. These structures are generated by neutral nonionic detergent lysis and sedimentation in 1.9 M NaCl-15 to 30% neutral sucrose gradients.[81,82] The distance sedimented is dependent upon the degree of compaction of the sedimenting nucleoid structure. This compaction is decreased by DNA strand breakage or unwinding of supercoiled DNA. The degree of nucleoid supercoiling can be altered by including within the sucrose-salt gradient the intercalator ethidium bromide, increasing doses of which first unwind, then rewind, the sedimenting supercoiled structure.

Table 3

CHARACTERISTICS OF INTERCALATOR-INDUCED DNA SCISSION

1.   Protein-concealed.
2.   Associated with an equal frequency of DNA-protein crosslinking.
3.   Proteins are most likely bound to the termini of the break and may actually bridge the break.
4.   DNA scission can be single- and/or double-stranded and the ratio of single- to double-strand breaks varies for different classes of intercalators.
5.   The number of breaks produced per cell appears to be limited, and the breaking rejoining response is inhibitable at reduced temperature suggesting break production may in some way be mediated by an enzymatic process.
6.   There is no uniform quantitative relationship between intercalator-induced DNA scission and cytotoxicity.
7.   The DNA breaking-rejoining response is demonstrable in isolated cell nuclei.
8.   The breaks form and reseal without poly(ADP-R) or DNA synthesis.
9.   Cells hypersensitive to physical and chemical agents which result in cellular DNA scission are not hyper-sensitive to intercalators, nor is the level of DNA scission per drug dose different in these repair-deficient human cells vs. normal human cells.
10.   Free radical mechanisms are unlikely to play a role in this DNA scission.
11.   Alterations in DNA three-dimensional structure may correlate with an altered susceptibility of that cellular DNA to intercalator-induced DNA scission, suggesting that the scission itself might in some way result from drug-induced alterations in DNA topology.

The relative ability to relax nucleoids maximally is taken as a measure of the DNA supercoil density within the cells from which these nucleoids came.

The nucleoids from DMSO-treated cells were more relaxed than those from controls, whereas nucleoids from thiourea-treated cells were more compacted.[35] As neither compound broke the cellular DNA, DMSO and thiourea apparently altered the three-dimensional structure of the DNA in opposite ways. These alterations may reflect a critical change in the target for intercalators, which suggests that the topological state of the DNA target at the time of intercalator treatment may critically determine the resultant DNA scission measured within the target following intercalator addition.

G. Summary of the Characteristics of Intercalator-Induced DNA Scission and Findings from Other Investigators

Table 3 summarizes the observed characteristics of the DNA scission produced by inter-calators in whole cells. Any model developed to explain this response needs to account for all of the points listed in the table.

Since the original description of the special DNA scission produced by intercalators,[6,7] several newer agents have been added to those initially found to produce this effect. These include the acridine, anthracycline, and ellipticine derivatives described above as well as dihydroxyanthracenedione,[50] 9,10-anthracenedicarboxaldehyde bis[(4,5-dihydro-1-H-imi-dazol-2-yl)hydrazone]dihydrochloride,[83] and the *N*-trifluoro-acetyladriamycin-14-valerate (AD32) and its metabolites (AD41, AD92).[84] These last agents are reported not to bind to DNA, which makes DNA scission unexpected.[84,85] AD32 has also been reported not to compact isolated chromatin, while adriamycin and anthracenedione do.[85] Either the DNA scission produced by AD32 is unique among intercalator-induced scission (despite being protein-associated[84]), or a higher-order DNA structure than that of isolated DNA or chro-matin, but which remains intact in isolated nuclei,[60] and to which AD32 can bind, is the critical one for intercalator-induced scission.

It is clear the intercalator response is present in several mammalian cell types (including human cells) following treatment with a wide variety of DNA intercalating drugs. The potential biological significance of this observation will be discussed in the final section.

VIII. THE BIOLOGICAL SIGNIFICANCE OF INTERCALATOR-INDUCED DNA SCISSION: AN HYPOTHESIS

The characteristics of this novel, breaking-rejoining response listed in Table 3 have led us to speculate about its etiology. It would appear that the enzymatic nature of the cotemporal and stoichiometric formation of DNA-bound protein and DNA scission is best explained by a model in which the DNA breaks bear a protein linked to either the 3' and/or 5' termini of the breaks. If the protein bridges the break, then one of the bonds may not be covalent (see Section V). That DNA-bound protein could be the enzyme responsible for the break. A candidate for such a protein is a class of enzymes called topoisomerases, which bind to supercoiled DNA and alter its three-dimensional structure by breaking the phosphodiester backbone, passing intact DNA strands through the break, and resealing the break with energy stored within the DNA-protein bond.[87,88] The resultant DNA has an altered winding number. The different ratios of DSB to SSB produced by different intercalators could reside in chemical differences among the compounds, allowing more or less complete double-strand scission on the basis of local steric considerations at the intercalation site.[48] This hypothesis to explain the variable DSB to SSB ratios, however, presumes that the intercalator-induced scission is at or near the intercalation site. Alternatively, there may be both single- and double-strand specific cutting enzymes within the cell which are stimulated to varying degrees by the different drugs. If topoisomerases permanently reside at specific nuclear DNA sites,[89-91] then the intercalator-induced signal that stimulates their activity may be different for different agents, and the scission induced by a drug may be at a point quite distant from the drug-DNA binding site.

Topoisomerase activity could be stimulated by torsional strain produced by intercalation. The enzyme would then act upon the DNA to return the DNA structure to its configuration prior to drug treatment or to release intercalator-induced DNA torsion. Obviously, the normal function of topoisomerase(s) is not to respond to intercalators. The function of these enzymes within cells has been speculated to reside in the necessity for replicating or transcribing DNA to unwind efficiently and rapidly prior to strand separation and enzymatic synthesis of DNA or RNA upon the template.[88] Further, DNA unwinding may be required to allow access of repair enzymes to damaged DNA.[92] Thus, topoisomerases would be expected to be present in all cells, but their intrinsic activity may vary from cell type to cell type, and within a cell type the activity may depend on the state of the cell with regard to gene transcription or DNA replication.

Our current model has the enzyme or enzymes present constantly within the cell nucleus. The breaking-rejoining activity is stimulated by alterations in DNA torsion produced by intercalation. The change in torsion is propagated along portions of the DNA helix to the enzyme sites, where abnormal stress is perceived and the cut is made. Drug removal results in the elimination of the stimulation to break DNA, and ultimately in rejoining DNA cut ends. The model predicts that the DNA break is rejoined without base excision or replacement (repair-type synthesis). In fact, neither is observed. This type of scission may not stimulate poly(ADP-R) synthesis either, because the break is protein-concealed (bridged ?), transient in existence, or the topology of the break site is not sufficiently distorted (aberrantly supercoiled) to be detected by the poly(ADP-R) synthesis sensing system. In addition, the topoisomerase model postulates that the break would be sealed without DNA ligase action. Although a functional role for poly ADP-ribosylation has not been demonstrated rigorously, evidence has been presented that implicates ribosylation with the activation of mammalian (repair) ligase II.[93] If this in vitro property has physiological relevance, the topoisomerase mechanism of intercalator break formation would be consistent with independence of break sealing from poly(ADP-ribose) biosynthesis.

The plateau in the number of breaks as the intercalator concentration is increased might derive from a limited number of enzyme sites or molecules or from a confining of intercalator-induced strain to specific, limited areas within the cellular genome. If cellular DNA is organized into domains,[81,82,94] strain may not be able to be passed from one domain to the next. Such limits could be imposed by proteins, possibly the topoisomerases themselves, or even DNA of unusual configuration such as the newly described left-handed Z-DNA[95] which could dampen intercalator-induced DNA torsion by its alternate helical directionality as well as its probably inferiority to B-DNA as an intercalation target.

The challenge is to provide a connection between the breaks we measure following intercalator treatment and some functional endogenous protein. Work is proceeding in that investigation. If a DNA breaking and binding activity can be isolated which is stimulated in the presence of intercalators, the first step will have been taken. Its normal cellular function, its potential variability from cell type to cell type, and its relation to DNA replication and gene transcription in malignant and nonmalignant cells may provide critical answers to the questions of how normal cells work and possibly why malignant cells are abnormal.

ACKNOWLEDGMENTS

We would like to thank our collaborators and colleagues Drs. Kurt Kohn, Warren Ross, Richard Ungerleider, and Leonard Erickson as well as Messrs. Ronald Schwartz, Albert Steren, Stephen Michaels, and Ms. Margaret Nichols. We thank Ms. Madie Tyler for typing the manuscript.

REFERENCES

1. **Ormerod, M. G.,** Radiation-induced strand breaks in the DNA of mammalian cells, in *Radiation Carcinogenesis,* Yuhas, J. M., Tennant, R. W., and Regan, J. D., Eds., Raven Press, New York, 1976, 67.
2. **Repine, J. E., Pfenninger, O. W., Talmage, D. W., Berger, E. M., and Pettijohn, D. E.,** Dimethyl sulfoxide prevents DNA nicking mediated by ionizing radiation or iron/hydrogen peroxide-generated hydroxyl radical, *Proc. Natl. Acad. Sci. U.S.A.,* 78, 1001, 1981.
3. **Chabner, B. A.,** Bleomycin, in *Principles of Cancer Treatment,* Chabner, B. A., Ed., W. B. Saunders, Philadelphia, 1982, 377.
4. **Cleaver, J.,** DNA repair and its coupling to DNA replication in eukaryotic cells, *Biochim. Biophys. Acta,* 516, 489, 1978.
5. **Berger, N. A., Weber, G., and Kaichi, A. S.,** Characterization and comparison of poly(adenosine diphosphoribose) synthesis and DNA synthesis in nucleotide-permeable cells, *Biochim. Biophys. Acta,* 519, 87, 1978.
6. **Ross, W. E., Glaubiger, D. L., and Kohn, K. W.,** Protein-associated DNA breaks in cells treated with adriamycin or ellipticine, *Biochim. Biophys. Acta,* 519, 23, 1978.
7. **Ross, W. E., Glaubiger, D., and Kohn, K. W.,** Qualitative and quantitative aspects of intercalator-induced DNA strand breaks, *Biochim. Biophys. Acta,* 562, 41, 1979.
8. **Kohn, K. W.,** DNA as a target in cancer chemotherapy: measurement of macromolecular DNA damage produced in mammalian cells by anticancer agents and carcinogens, in *Methods in Cancer Research,* Busch, H. and DeVita, V., Eds., Academic Press, New York, 1979, 291.
9. **Kohn, K. W., Ewig, R. A. G., Erickson, L. C., and Zwelling, L. A.,** Measurement of strand breaks and cross-links by alkaline elution, in *DNA Repair: A Laboratory Manual of Research Procedures,* Friedberg, E. C. and Hanawalt, P. C., Eds., Marcel Dekker, New York, 1981, 379.
10. **Kohn, K. W., Erickson, L. C., Ewig, R. A. G., and Friedman, C. A.,** Fractionation of DNA from mammalian cells by alkaline elution, *Biochemistry,* 14, 4629, 1976.
11. **Kohn, K. W. and Ewig, R. A. G.,** DNA-protein crosslinking by *trans*-platinum(II) diamminedichloride in mammalian cells, a new method of analysis, *Biochim. Biophys. Acta,* 562, 32, 1979.
12. **Bradley, M. O. and Kohn, K. W.,** X-ray-induced DNA double strand break production and repair in mammalian cells as measured by neutral filter elution, *Nucl. Acids Res.,* 7, 793, 1979.
13. **Dugle, D. L., Gillespie, C. J., and Chapman, J. D.,** DNA strand breaks, repair, and survival in X-irradiated mammalian cells, *Proc. Natl. Acad. Sci. U.S.A.,* 73, 809, 1976.
14. **Lennartz, M., Coquerelle, T., Bopp, A., and Hagen, U.,** Oxygen-effect on strand breaks and specific end-groups in DNA of irradiated thymocytes, *Int. J. Radiat. Biol.,* 27, 577, 1975.
15. **Sinden, R. R. and Pettijohn, D. E.,** Chromosomes in living *Escherichia coli* cells are segregated into domains of supercoiling, *Proc. Natl. Acad. Sci. U.S.A.,* 78, 224, 1981.
16. **Veatch, W. and Okada, S.,** Radiation-induced breaks of DNA in cultured mammalian cells, *Biophys. J.,* 9, 330, 1969.

17. **Lee, Y. C. and Byfield, J. E.,** Induction of DNA degradation *in vivo* by adriamycin, *J. Natl. Cancer Inst.,* 57, 221, 1976.

18. **Schwartz, H. S.,** Alkali-labile regions and strand breaks in DNA from cells treated with daunorubicin, *J. Med.,* 7, 33, 1976.

19. **Paoletti, C., Lesca, C., Cros, S., Malvy, C., and Auclair, C.,** Ellipticine and derivatives induce breakage of L1210 cells DNA *in vitro, Biochem. Pharmacol.,* 28, 345, 1979.

20. **Burr Furlong, N., Sato, J., Brown, T., Chavez, F., and Hulbert, R. B.,** Induction of limited DNA damage by the antitumor agent Cain's acridine, *Cancer Res.,* 38, 1329, 1978.

21. **Ralph, R. K.,** On the mechanism of action of 4'-[(9-acridinyl)-amino] methanesulphon-*m*-anisidide, *Eur. J. Cancer,* 16, 595, 1980.

22. **Pater, M. M. and Mak, S.,** Actinomycin-D-induced breakage of human KB cell DNA, *Nature (London),* 250, 786, 1974.

23. **Bachur, N. R., Gee, M. Y., and Friedman, R. D.,** Nuclear catalyzed antibiotic free radical formation, *Cancer Res.,* 42, 107, 1078, 1982.

24. **Bachur, N. R., Gordon, S. L., and Gee, M. Y.,** A general mechanism for microsomal activation of quinone anticancer agents to free radicals, *Cancer Res.,* 38, 1745, 1978.

25. **Bachur, N. R., Gordon, S. L., Gee, M. V., and Kon, K.,** NADPH cytochrome P-450 reductase activation of quinone anticancer agents to free radicals, *Proc. Natl. Acad. Sci. U.S.A.,* 76, 954, 1979.

26. **Goodman, J. and Hochstein, P.,** Generation of free radicals and lipid peroxidation by redox cycling of adriamycin and daunomycin, *Biochem. Biophys. Res. Commun.,* 77, 797, 1977.

27. **Handa, K. and Sato, S.,** Generation of free radicals of quinone group-containing anticancer chemicals in NADPH-microsome system as evidenced by initiation of sulfite oxidation, *Gann,* 66, 43, 1975.

28. **Lown, J. W., Chen, H.-H., Plambeck, T. A., and Acton, E. M.,** Diminished superoxide anion generation by reduced 5-iminodaunorubicin relative to daunorubicin and the relationship to cardiotoxicity of the anthracycline antitumor agents, *Biochem. Pharmacol.,* 28, 2563, 1979.

29. **Lown, J. W., Sim, S.-K., and Majumdar, K. C., and Chana, R.-Y.,** Strand scission of DNA by bound adriamycin and daunorubicin in the presence of reducing agents, *Biochem. Biophys. Res. Commun.,* 76, 705, 1977.

30. **Pietronigro, D. D., McGinness, J. E., Koren, M. J., Crippa, R., Seligman, M. L., and Demopoulos, H. B.,** Spontaneous generation of adriamycin semiquinone radicals at physiologic pH, *Physiol. Chem. Phys.,* 11, 405, 1979.

31. **Sinha, B. K. and Chignell, C. F.,** Binding mode of chemically activated semiquinone free radicals from quinone anticancer agents to DNA, *Chem. Biol. Interact.,* 28, 301, 1979.

32. **Thayer, W. S.** Adriamycin stimulated superoxide formation in submitochondrial particles, *Chem. Biol. Interact.,* 19, 265, 1977.

33. **Berlin, V. and Haseltine, W. A.,** Reduction of adriamycin to a semiquinone-free radical by NADPH cytochrome P-450 reductase produces DNA cleavage in a reaction mediated by molecular oxygen, *J. Biol. Chem.,* 256, 4747, 1981.

34. **Zwelling, L. A., Kerrigan, D., and Michaels, S.,** Cytotoxicity and DNA strand breaks by 5-iminodaunorubicin in mouse leukemia L1210 cells: comparison with adriamycin and 4'-(9-acridinlyamino)methane sulfon-*m*-anisidide, *Cancer Res.,* 42, 2687, 1982.

35. **Pommier, Y., Kerrigan, D., and Zwelling, L. A.,** Enhancement of intercalator-induced DNA breakage in mammalian cells by dimethyl sulfoxide, *Clin. Res.,* 30, 422A, 1982.

36. **Potmesil, M., Kirschenbaum, S., Levin, M., and Silber, R.,** Relationship of adriamycin concentration to induced DNA lesions in hypoxic and euoxic L1210 cells, *Proc. Am. Assoc. Cancer Res.,* 23, 176, 1982.

37. **Doroshow, J. H., Locker, G. Y., and Myers, C. E.,** Enzymatic defenses of the mouse heart against reactive oxygen metabolites, *J. Clin. Invest.,* 65, 128, 1980.

38. **Forssen, E. A., and Tokes, Z. A.,** Use of anionic liposomes for the reduction of chronic doxorubicin-induced cardiotoxicity, *Proc. Natl. Acad. Sci. U.S.A.,* 78, 1873, 1981.

39. **Myers, C. E., Gianni, L., Simone, C. B., Klecker, R., and Greene, R.,** Oxidative destruction of erythrocyte ghost membranes catalyzed by the doxorubicin-iron complex, *Biochemistry,* 21, 1707, 1982.

40. **Myers, C. E., McGuire, W. P., Liss, R. H., Infrim, I., Grotzinger, K., and Young, R. C.,** Adriamycin: the role of lipid peroxidation in cardiac toxicity and tumor response, *Science,* 197, 165, 1977.

41. **Tokes, Z. A., Rogers, K. E., and Rembaum, A.,** Synthesis of adriamycin-coupled polyglutaraldehyde microspheres and evaluation of their cytostatic activity, *Proc. Natl. Acad. Sci. U.S.A.,* 79, 2026, 1982.

42. **Tritton, T. R. and Yee, G.,** The anticancer agent adriamycin can be actively cytotoxic without entering cells, *Science,* 217, 248, 1982.

43. **Byfield, J. E., Lee, Y. C., and Tu, L.,** Molecular interactions between adriamycin and X-ray damage in mammalian cells, *Int. J. Cancer,* 19, 186, 1977.

44. **Center, M. S.,** Induction of single-strand regions in nuclear DNA by adriamycin, *Biochem. Biophys. Res. Commun.,* 89, 1231, 1979.

45. **Schwartz, H. S., Schioppacassi, G., and Kanter, P. M.,** Mechanisms of selectivity of intercalating agents, *Antibiot. Chemother.*, 23, 247, 1978.

46. **Zwelling, L. A., Michaels, S., Erickson, L. C., Ungerleider, R. S., Nichols, M., and Kohn, K. W.,** Protein-associated deoxyribonucleic acid strand breaks in L1210 cells treated with the deoxyribonucleic acid intercalating agents 4'-(9-acridinlyamino)methanesulfon-*m*-anisidide and adriamycin, *Biochemistry*, 20, 6553, 1981.

47. **Pulleyblank, D. E. and Ellison, M. J.,** Purification and properties of a type I topoisomerase from chicken erythrocytes: mechanism of eukaryotic topoisomerase action, *Biochemistry*, 21, 1155, 1982.

48. **Ross, W. E. and Bradley, M. O.,** DNA double-strand breaks in mammalian cells after exposure to intercalating agents, *Biochem. Biophys. Acta*, 654, 129, 1981.

49. **Ross, W. E., Zwelling, L. A., and Kohn, K. W.,** Relationship between cytotoxicity and DNA strand breakage produced by adriamycin and other intercalating agents, *Int. J. Radiat. Oncol. Biol. Phys.*, 5, 1221, 1979.

50. **Cohen, L. F., Glaubiger, D. L., Kann, H. E., and Kohn, K. W.,** Protein associated DNA single strand breaks and cytotoxicity of dihydroxyanthracenedione (DHAD), NSC-301739, in mouse L1210 leukemia cells, *Proc. A. Assoc. Cancer Res.*, 21, 277, 1980.

51. **Tong, G. L., Henry, D. W., and Acton, E. M.,** 5-Iminodaunorubicin. Reduced cardiotoxic properties in an antitumor anthracycline, *J. Med. Chem.*, 22, 36, 1979.

52. **Glazer, R. I., Hartman, K. D., and Richardson, C. L.,** Cytokinetic and biochemical effects of 5-iminodaunorubicin in human colon carcinoma in culture, *Cancer Res.*, 42, 117, 1982.

53. **Ross, W. R. and Smith, M. C.,** Repair of deoxyribonucleic acid lesions caused by adriamycin and ellipticine, *Biochem. Pharmacol.*, 31, 1931, 1982.

54. **Zwelling, L. A., Michaels, S., Kerrigan, D., Pommier, Y., and Kohn, K. W.,** Protein-associated deoxyribonucleic acid strand breaks produced in mouse leukemia L1210 cells by ellipticine and 2-methyl-9-hydroxyellipticinium, *Biochem. Pharmacol.*, 32, 3261, 1982.

55. **Kohn, K. W., Ross, W. E., and Glaubiger, D.,** Ellipticine, in *Mechanism of Action of Antieukaryotic and Antiviral Compounds*, Hahn, F. F., Ed., Springer-Verlag, New York, 1979, 195.

56. **Kohn, K. W., Waring, M. J., Galubiger, D., and Friedman, C. A.,** Intercalative binding of ellipticine to DNA, *Cancer Res.*, 35, 71, 1975.

57. **Lee, I. P.,** A possible mechanism of ellipticine-induced hemolysis, *J. Pharmacol. Exp. Ther.*, 196, 525, 1976.

58. **Juret, P., Tanguy, A., Girard, A., LeTalaer, J. Y., Abbatucci, J. S., Dat-Xuong, N., LePecq, J. B., and Paoletti, C.,** Preliminary trial of 9-hydroxy-2-methyl ellipticinim (NSC 264-137) in advanced human cancers, *Eur. J. Cancer*, 14, 205, 1978.

59. **Filipski, J. and Kohn, K. W.,** Ellipticine-induced protein-associated DNA breaks in isolated L1210 nuclei, *Biochim. Biophys. Acta*, 698, 280, 1982.

60. **Pommier, Y. Kerrigan, D., Schwartz, R., and Zwelling, L.,** The formation and resealing of intercalator-induced DNA strand breaks in isolated L1210 cell nuclei, *Biochem. Biophys. Res. Commun.*, 107, 576, 1982.

61. **Benjamin, R. C. and Gill, D. M.,** ADP-ribosylation in mammalian cell ghosts. Dependence of poly(ADP-ribose) synthesis on strand breakage in DNA, *J. Biol. Chem.*, 255, 10493, 1980.

62. **Nolan, N. L. and Kidwell, W. R.,** Effect of heat shock on poly(ADP-ribose) synthesis and DNA repair in *Drosophila* cells, *Radiat. Res.*, 90, 187, 1982.

63. **Berger, N. A., Sikorski, G. W., Petzold, S. J., and Kurohara, K. K.,** Association of poly(adenosine diphosphoribose) synthesis with DNA damage and repair in normal human lymphocytes, *J. Clin. Invest.*, 63, 1164, 1979.

64. **Berger, N. A. and Sikorski, G. W.,** Poly(adenosine diphosphoribose) synthesis in ultraviolet-irradiated *Xeroderma pigmentosum* cells reconstituted with *Micrococcus luteus* UV endonuclease, *Biochemistry*, 20, 3610, 1981.

65. **Berger, N. A., Sikorski, G. W., Petzold, S. J., and Kurohara, K. K.,** Defective poly(adenosine diphosphoribose) synthesis in *Xeroderma pigmentosum*, *Biochemistry*, 19, 289, 1980.

66. **Miwa, M., Kanai, M., Kondo, T., Hoshino, H.O., Ishihara, K., and Sugimara, T.,** Inhibitors of poly(ADP-ribose) polymerase enhance unscheduled DNA synthesis in human peripheral lymphocytes, *Biochem. Biophys. Res. Commun.*, 100, 463, 1981.

67. **McCurry L. S. and Jacobson, M. K.,** Poly(ADP-ribose) synthesis following DNA damage in cells heterozygous or homozygous for *Xeroderma pigmentosum* genotype, *J. Biol. Chem.*, 256, 551, 1981.

68. **Davies, M. I., Halldorsson, H., Nduka, N., Shall, S., and Skidmore, C. J.,** The involvement of poly(adenosine diphosphate-ribose) in deoxynucleic acid repair, *Biochem. Soc. Transact.*, 6, 1056, 1978.

69. **Durkacz, B. W., Omidiji, O., Gray, D. A., and Shall, S.,** (ADP-ribose)$_n$ participates in DNA excision repair, *Nature (London)*, 283, 593, 1980.

70. **Durrant, L. G. and Boyle, J. M.,** Potentiation of cell killing by inhibitors of poly(ADP-ribose) polymerase in four rodent cell lines exposed to N-methyl-N-nitrosourea or UV light, *Chem. Biol. Interact.,* 38, 325, 1982.

71. **Nduka, N., Skidmore, C. J., and Shall, S.,** The enhancement of cytotoxicity of N-methyl-N-nitrosourea and of radiation by inhibitors of poly(ADP-ribose) polymerase, *Eur. J. Biochem.,* 105, 525, 1980.

72. **Zwelling, L. A., Kerrigan, D., Pommier, Y., Michaels, S., Steren, A., and Kohn, K. W.,** Formation and resealing of intercalator-induced DNA strand breaks in permeabilized L1210 cells without the stimulated synthesis of poly(ADP-Ribose), *J. Biol. Chem.,* 257, 8957, 1982.

73. **Benjamin, R. C. and Gill, D. M.,** PolyADP-ribose) synthesis *in vitro* programmed by damaged DNA. A comparison of DNA molecules containing different types of strand breaks, *J. Biol. Chem.,* 255, 10502, 1980

74. **Fornace, A. J., Jr., Kohn, K. W., and Kann, H. E., Jr.,** DNA single-strand breaks during repair of UV damage in human fibroblasts and abnormalities of repair in *Xeroderma pigmentosum, Proc. Natl. Acad. Sci. U.S.A.,* 73, 39, 1976.

75. **Kraemer, K. H.,** Progressive degenerative diseases associated with defective DNA repair: *Xeroderma pigmentosum* and ataxia telangiectasia, in *DNA Repair Processes,* Nichols, W. W. and Murphy, D. G., Eds., Symposia Specialists, Miami, 1977, 37.

76. **Regan, J. D. and Setlow, R. B.,** Repair of human DNA: radiation and chemical damage in normal and *Xeroderma pigmentosum* cells, in *Biology of Radiation Carcinogenesis,* Yuhas, J. M., Tennant, R. W., and Regan, J. D., Eds., Raven Press, New York, 1976, 103.

77. **Painter, R. B. and Young, B. R.,** Radiosensitivity in ataxia-telangiectasia: a new explanation, *Proc. Natl. Acad. Sci. U.S.A.,* 77, 7315, 1980.

78. **Paterson, M. C., Smith, B. P., Lohman, P. H. M., Anderson, A. K., and Fishman, L.,** Defective excision repair of γ-ray-damaged DNA in human (ataxia telangiectasia) fibroblasts, *Nature (London),* 260, 444, 1976.

79. **Zwelling, L. A. and Mattern, M. R.,** DNA-repair deficiencies do not affect intercalator-induced cytotoxicity or DNA scission in human cells, *Mutat. Res.,* 104, 295, 1982.

80. **Bradley, M. O. and Erickson, L. C.,** Comparison of the effects of hydrogen peroxide and X-ray irradiation on toxicity, mutation, and DNA damage/repair in mammalian cells (V-79), *Biochim. Biophys. Acta,* 654, 135, 1981.

81. **Cook, P. R. and Brazell, I. A.,** Supercoils in human DNA, *J. Cell Sci.,* 19, 261, 1975.

82. **Cook, P. R. and Brazell, I. A.,** Detection and repair of single-strand breaks in nuclear DNA, *Nature (London),* 263, 679, 1976.

83. **Bowden, G. T., Garcia, D., Peng, Y.-M., and Alberts, D. S.,** Molecular pharmacology of the anthracycline drug 9,10-anthracenedicarboxaldehyde bis[(4,5-dihydro-1-H-imidazole-2-yl)hydrazone] dihydrochloride (CI 216, 942), *Cancer Res.,* 42, 2660, 1982.

84. **Levin, M., Silber, R., Israel, M., Goldfeder, A., Khetarpal, V. K., and Potmesil, M.,** Protein-associated DNA breaks and DNA-protein cross-links caused by DNA nonbinding derivatives of adriamycin in L1210 cells, *Cancer Res.,* 41, 1006, 1981.

85. **Kanter, P. M. and Schwartz, H. S.,** Effects of N-trifluoroacetyladriamycin-14-valerate and related agents on DNA strand damage and thymidine incorporation in CCRF-CEM cells, *Cancer Res.,* 39, 448, 1979.

86. **Waldes, H. and Center, M. S.,** Adriamycin-induced compaction of isolated chromatin, *Biochem. Pharmacol.,* 31, 1057, 1982.

87. **Cozzarelli, N. R.,** DNA gyrase and the supercoiling of DNA, *Science,* 207, 953, 1980.

88. **Gellert, M.,** DNA topoisomerases, *Ann. Rev. Biochem.,* 50, 879, 1981.

89. **Fisher, L. M., Mizuuchi, K., O'Dea, M. H., Ohmori, H., and Gellert, M.,** Site-specific interaction of DNA gyrase with DNA, *Proc. Natl. Acad. Sci. U.S.A.,* 78, 4165, 1981.

90. **Morrison, A. and Cozzarelli, N. R.,** Site-specific cleavage of DNA by E. coli DNA gyrase, *Cell,* 17, 175, 1979.

91. **Morrison, A., Higgins, N. P., and Cozzarelli, N. R.,** Interaction between DNA gyrase and its cleavage site on DNA, *J. Biol. Chem.,* 255, 2211, 1980.

92. **Mattern, M. R., Paone, R. F., and Day, R. S., III,** Eucaryotic DNA repair is blocked at different steps by inhibitors of DNA topoisomerases and of DNA polymerases α and β, *Biochim. Biophys. Acta,* 697, 6, 1982.

93. **Creissen, D. and Shall, S.,** Regulation of DNA ligase activity by poly (ADP-ribose), *Nature (London),* 296, 271, 1982.

94. **Sinden, R. R., Carlson, J. O., and Pettijohn, D. E.,** Torsional tension in the DNA double helix measured with trimethylpsoralen in living E. coli cells: analogous measurements in insect and human cells, *Cell,* 21, 773, 1980.

95. **Wang, A. H.-J., Quigley, G. J., Kokpak, F. J., Crawford, J. L., van Boom, J. H., van der Marel, G., and Rich, A.,** Molecular structure of a left-handed double-helical DNA fragment at atomic resolution, *Nature (London),* 282, 680, 1979.

Chapter 9

GROWTH INHIBITORY EFFECTS OF INTERFERONS AND (2',5')OLIGOADENYLATE AND ITS ANALOGS

Mrunal S. Chapekar and Robert I. Glazer

TABLE OF CONTENTS

I. INTRODUCTION

Interferons (IFNs) are host cell proteins and glycoproteins which were initially recognized and grouped together by their ability to block the replication of viruses.[1] The recent nomenclature[2] classifies IFNs as three general types called α, β, and γ corresponding to virus-induced IFNs produced by leukocytes (α), virus-induced IFNs produced by fibroblasts (β), and IFNs produced by leukocytes in response to lectins or an antigenic stimulus (γ). Recently, gene cloning has revolutionized the interferon field. Pioneered by Weissmann and co-workers,[3] numerous investigators have used the powerful recombinant DNA methodology to clone all three species of IFN. While there is a single cloned species of human IFNβ, there is diversity in the subspecies of IFNα. These singular cloned subspecies have been designated as IFNα_1, IFNα_2, etc. by Brack et al.,[3] whereas Goeddel and co-workers[4] have used the designations IFNαA, IFNαB, etc. to distinguish their cloned IFNs. Nevertheless, it is largely through the current recombinant DNA technology that large quantities of IFNs have been made available for in vitro and clinical studies and, thus far, the future of IFN in cancer therapy appears encouraging.

Though IFN as an antiviral agent was introduced in 1957, it did not gain importance as a growth-inhibitor until 1972. The interesting finding by Paucker et al.[5] that IFN possessed antiproliferative activity remained unattended mainly because IFN was considered not to have any effects on normal physiological functions. Moreover, IFN preparations at that time were impure and several investigators raised the objection of whether the contaminating factors could have contributed to growth inhibition. Years later, the antiproliferative function of IFN was extensively studied by Gresser[6] and his studies were a key factor in establishing IFN as a growth inhibitor.

In this chapter we will present a review of the investigations on the growth inhibitory effects in vitro and the antitumor effects in vivo of IFNs. We will also discuss some of the molecular mechanisms of action, as well as recent pharmacological studies of the (2',5')oligoadenylate metabolites which are thought to mediate, in part, the antiproliferative and antiviral actions of IFN.

II. MOLECULAR MECHANISMS OF INTERFERON ACTION

A. (2',5')Oligo(A) and Protein Kinase Pathways

The early observations that viral RNA and protein synthesis were impaired in IFN-treated cells prompted several investigators to compare cell-free extracts from IFN-treated and untreated cells for their ability to process, translate, and cleave viral and host mRNA. These experiments resulted in the discovery of two double-stranded RNA-dependent enzymes[7] whose levels are enhanced after IFN treatment (Figure 1): a protein kinase which catalyzes phosphorylation of two endogenous polypeptides, one between 65,000 and 75,000 daltons depending on the animal species,[8] and the other a 35,000-dalton polypeptide which is the smallest subunit of one of the initiation factors (eIF$_{2\alpha}$) involved in protein synthesis.[9,10] This protein kinase also phosphorylates histones added as an exogenous substrate.[10,11] The second enzyme pppA(2'p5'A)$_n$ synthetase [(2',5')oligo(A) synthetase] uses ATP as a substrate to produce (2',5')oligo(A)$_n$ (where n = 2 to 5).[12,13] Among the products of the enzyme, di-, tri-, and tetraadenylates are the most abundant. (2',5')oligo(A)$_n$ ($\geq$3) acts as an activator of a latent endoribonuclease (RNase L), a 185,000-dalton protein present in both untreated and IFN-treated cells, and results in degradation of various single-stranded viral RNAs, cellular messenger RNA, and ribosomal RNA,[14,15] but not double-stranded RNA.[16] RNA degradation leads to inhibition of protein synthesis both in cell-free extracts[13,17] and in intact cells.[18-20] (2',5')Oligo(A)synthetase has been found in diverse cell types such as reticulocytes, lymphocytes, chick oviducts, and human lymphoblastoid cells, and the enzyme activity was

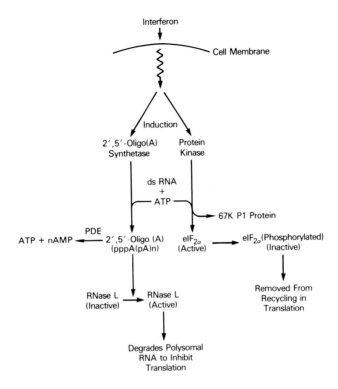

FIGURE 1. Double-stranded RNA-dependent pathways induced by interferon treatment; dsRNA double-stranded RNA.

reported to vary markedly from one tissue to another.[21] Upon IFN treatment, the enzyme activity is induced severalfold and the extent of induction depends on the cell type. An apparently homogeneous enzyme has been obtained from IFN-treated Ehrlich ascites tumor cells and its molecular weight has been reported to be 85,000 daltons as determined by sucrose density gradient centrifugation, and 105,000 daltons by gel electrophoresis.[22] Another important enzyme of the $(2',5')$oligo(A)-RNase L pathway which indirectly influences $(2',5')$oligo(A) levels and hence, RNase L activity, is $(2',5')$ oligo(A)phosphodiesterase $[(2',5')$oligo(A)PDE]. This enzyme has a molecular weight of 40,000 daltons and hydrolyzes $(2',5')$oligo(A)$_n$ to ATP and nAMP.[23,24] The $(2',5')$oligo(A)-RNase L system appears to be a major pathway in IFN-mediated inhibition of translation in mouse L cells, wherein elevated $(2',5')$oligo(A)$_n$ levels have been detected after IFN treatment and encephalomyocarditis virus infection.[25] In HeLa cells, the combination of IFN and polyriboinosinic:polyribocytidylic acid (poly I·C) resulted in an increase in the level of $(2',5')$oligo(A)$_n$ and enhancement of mRNA cleavage and polysome degradation.[26]

The role of the $(2',5')$oligo(A)-RNase L pathway in growth inhibition was even more evident from the studies performed with synthetic $(2',5')$oligo(A)$_n$. Several investigators observed inhibition of protein synthesis by addition of $(2',5')$oligo(A)$_3$ to permeabilized cells with a concomitant increase in RNase L activity.[19,27] Moreover, the dephosphorylated trimer core of $(2',5')$oligo(A)$_n$ (which can presumably pass through the cell membrane) has been shown to inhibit the growth of human lymphoma Daudi cells[28] and of lectin-stimulated lymphocytes[29] and this activity appeared to be analogous to the growth inhibition produced by IFN. Shimizu and Sokawa[30] found high endogenous levels of $(2',5')$oligo(A)synthetase in unstimulated lymphocytes. According to Kimchi et al.,[31] concanavalin A (conA)-stimulated lymphocytes contain higher levels of $(2',5')$oligo(A)PDE; their data support the theory that $(2',5')$oligo(A)$_n$ is normally involved in keeping lymphocytes quiescent and that its level is subsequently reduced after blastogenesis has begun. Similar growth-related changes in

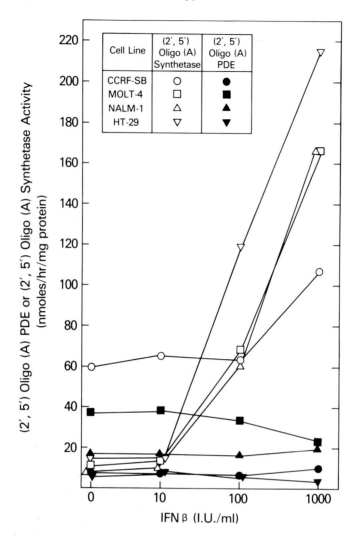

FIGURE 2.   Effect of IFNβ on the activities of (2′,5′)oligo(A)synthetase and (2′,5′)oligo(A)PDE. Tumor cells were treated with 10, 100, and 1000 IU/mℓ IFNβ for 1 day. Extracts from IFNβ-treated and untreated cells were prepared and assayed for (2′,5′)oligo(A)synthetase and (2′,5′)oligo(A)PDE, using the procedures described in Reference 126.

(2′,5′)oligo(A)synthetase and (2′,5′)oligo(A)PDE levels were observed in BSC-1 cells.[31] In the latter study, (2′,5′)oligo(A)synthetase activity was lower in rapidly dividing vs. confluent cells, while the converse was true for (2′,5′)oligo(A)PDE activity. As a result, the (2′,5′)oligo(A)synthetase: (2′,5′)oligo(A)PDE ratio was fivefold greater in rapidly dividing vs. confluent cells. Thus, these data suggest that both enzyme activities may control the degree of involvement of the (2′,5′)oligo(A)-RNase L pathway during cellular proliferation, as well as the IFN-mediated anticellular response.

In recent studies, we have determined the relationship between changes in (2′,5′)oligo(A)synthetase and (2′,5′)oligo(A)PDE activities and the growth inhibitory effects of IFNβ in human tumor cells in culture (Figure 2). The basal (2′,5′)oligo(A)synthetase activities in two B-cell leukemias (CCRF-SB and NALM-1), a T-cell leukemia (MOLT-4) and a colon carcinoma (HT-29), varied from 7 to 22 units/mg except in CCRF-SB cells where the high endogenous enzyme activity was determined to be attributable to a low constitutive production of IFNα (4 IU/mℓ). In this cell line, synthetase activity was inhibited

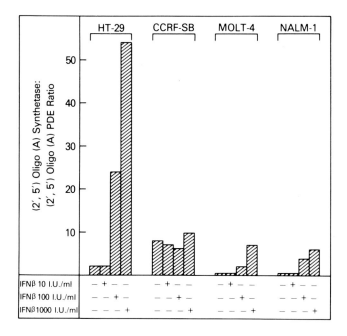

FIGURE 3. Effect of IFNβ on (2',5')oligo(A)synthetase: (2',5')oligo(A)PDE ratios in human tumor cell lines. Cells were treated with 10, 100, and 1000 IU/mℓ of IFNβ for 1 day.

by 50% upon 3-day treatment of the cells with 1000 units/mℓ of anti-IFNα IgG. Conversely, endogenous IFNα secretion was enhanced 162- and 62-fold, respectively, by infection of CCRF-SB cells with Newcastle disease or Sendai viruses, an effect comparable to the response of Namalva cells.[32] Treatment of these cell lines for 1 day with 1000 IU/mℓ of IFNβ induced (2',5')oligo(A)synthetase activity 15-fold in HT-29 cells, but only 2-fold in CCRF-SB cells. Upon similar treatment, (2',5')oligo(A)PDE was not increased in any of the cell lines but instead was reduced by 40% in HT-29 and MOLT-4 cells. The basal activity of (2',5')oligo(A)PDE did vary considerably among the various cell lines, where MOLT-4 cells possessed the highest, and HT-29 cells the lowest, activity. Consequently, the (2',5')oligo(A)synthetase:(2',5')oligo(A)PDE ratio (54) was greatest in HT-29 cells in comparison to the other cell lines where the ratio was 6 to 10. Therefore, it was of no surprise when we discovered that HT-29 cells were sensitive to the cytostatic effect of IFNβ upon 3-day exposure to 1000 IU/mℓ, whereas the other cell lines were refractory; however, no cytocidal activity by IFNβ was noted under these conditions.

In contrast to these studies with IFNβ, as well as recombinant IFNαA, IFNγ appeared to possess significant cytostatic and cytocidal activity against HT-29 cells (Table 1). However, the cytotoxic effects of IFNγ may not be totally reflected in the activity of the (2',5')oligo(A)-RNase L pathway as reflected in the ratios of (2',5')oligo(A)synthetase:(2',5')oligo(A)PDE. At IFNγ concentrations (25 IU/mℓ) which produced a 50% reduction in growth and colony formation in soft agar (a reflection of cell lethality) of HT-29 cells, similar 3-day treatment with 1000 IU/mℓ of IFNβ or recombinant IFNαA produced a 40% decrease in cell growth and a 20% reduction in colony formation, despite the greater synthetase:PDE ratios produced by IFNβ and IFNαA in comparison to IFNγ.

The role of double-stranded RNA-dependent protein kinase in the antiproliferative effects of IFN has been less extensively studied. Carcinoma stem cells which were resistant to IFN did not show elevated kinase activity after IFN treatment in contrast to the induction of kinase levels in sensitive cells.[33] In L1210 cells resistant to the anticellular effects of IFNβ, IFNγ was still capable of inducing (2',5')oligo(A)synthetase and double-stranded RNA-

Table 1
**THE EFFECT OF DIFFERENT TYPES OF IFN ON CELL GROWTH,
VIABILITY, AND (2′5′)Oligo(A) SYNTHETASE AND
PHOSPHODIESTERASE ACTIVITIES IN HUMAN COLON CARCINOMA
CELLS**

IFN	Growth inhibition: IC_{50} (IU/mℓ)	Viability: LC_{50} (IU/mℓ)	(2′,5′)Oligo(A) synthetase (units/mg)	(2′5′)Oligo(A) PDE (units/mg)	Ratio of synthetase: PDE
IFNαA	>2000[a]	>2000[a]	140	5	28
IFNβ	2000	>2000[a]	200	4	50
IFNγ	30	14	80	5	16

Note: Exponentially growing HT-29 cells were treated for 3 days with varying concentrations of IFNs. Enzyme activities were determined after 3-day treatment with 1000 IU/mℓ of IFNαA or IFNβ or 25 IU/mℓ of IFNγ as described in Reference 126.

[a]   Only 30% growth inhibition was observed with 2000 IU/mℓ IFNαA and a 20% reduction in cell viability was found with 2000 IU/mℓ IFNαA or IFNβ.

dependent protein kinase activities, although both IFNs induced these activities to the same extent in sensitive cells.[34] Obviously, a great deal more investigation into the role of the protein kinase pathway, particularly in vivo, is necessary for establishing its definitive role in the antiproliferative activity of IFN.

B. (2′,5′)Oligo(A) Analogs

Although, (2′,5′)oligo(A) appears to mediate growth inhibition in vivo, its direct application as an anticancer drug is limited by its poor cellular uptake and its rapid hydrolysis intracellularly by phosphodiesterases. Hence, several recent studies have been directed toward the synthesis of (2′,5′)oligo(A) analogs which are more resistant to degradation, yet still possess equal or greater antiproliferative activity. Doetsch et al.[35] have reported the enzymatic synthesis of the cordycepin analog of (2′,5′)oligo(A)$_3$, ppp3′dA-(2′p5′-3′dA)$_2$, and demonstrated it to be a far more stable and more potent inhibitor of protein synthesis in vitro in comparison to (2′,5′)oligo(A)$_3$, and as equipotent as (2′,5′)oligo(A)$_4$. Of particular significance was the finding that the 5′-dephosphorylated core of cordycepin trimer prevented the transformation of Epstein-Barr virus-infected human lymphocytes, while showing no cytotoxicity to uninfected lymphocytes.[36]

As an extension of these studies, Eppstein et al.[37] investigated the biological activity in vitro and in vivo of a series of terminally modified cordycepin trimer analogs. As found previously, the cordycepin trimer core was 30-fold more stable to hydrolysis, but was 2-fold *more* active in 3T3 fibroblasts than (2′,5′)oligo(A)$_3$. In contrast, the cordycepin trimer analog introduced by calcium phosphate coprecipitation was actually 10-fold *less* potent than (2′,5′)oligo(A)$_3$ in inhibiting protein synthesis in L929 cells. The cordycepin trimer core with a 2′deoxy terminus instead of a 3′deoxy terminus was 15-fold more stable to degradation, but showed no growth inhibitory activity. The greatest biological activity was achieved by a xylosyladenine trimer core where a 5-fold greater potency and 120-fold greater stability was observed in comparison to (2′5′)oligo(A)$_3$.[37]

In contrast to these results, Sawai et al.[38] found that although the cordycepin trimer and tetramer analogs were hydrolytically stable and capable of binding to RNase L, they were inactive as inhibitors of protein synthesis in L cell extracts.

Baglioni et al.[39] synthesized 3′-O-methylated derivatives of (2′,5′)oligo(A)$_3$ and found that the 5′-triphosphorylated analog with a terminal 3′-O-methyl substitution was tenfold more potent than $(2',5')$oligo(A) in inhibiting protein synthesis in human diploid fibroblasts following calcium phosphate coprecipitation. This increase in activity correlated with the resistance of the $3'$-monomethylated analog to degradation in HeLa cell extracts.

Recently, Imai et al.[40] synthesized a $(2',5')$oligo(A) analog wherein the terminal ribose was derivatized to an N-hexylmorpholinyl (azahexapyranose) substituent. The $5'$-monophosphates of these "tailed" analogs were very resistant to phosphodiesterase, as might be expected from the aforementioned analog studies, and were potent antagonists of the inhibitory effect of $(2',5')$oligo(A) on protein synthesis in vitro. A similarly modified tetramer $5'$-triphosphate was tenfold more active as an inhibitor of protein synthesis, as an activator of RNase L, and as an inhibitor of viral mRNA-dependent translation in vitro in L cell extracts.

It is apparent from these initial studies with $(2',5')$oligo(A) analogs that their biological activity will depend heavily on the cell line and in vitro cell-free system used to assess the drug, as well as the method of introducing the analog into cells. Although, the core analogs should be taken up by the cell more readily than the calcium phosphate coprecipitated triphosphate derivative, it has not been established if the core analog gets rephosphorylated to the $5'$-triphosphate, is degraded to the monomer analog, or acts as the unphosphorylated trimer via some other as yet unidentified mechanism. However, it has been established that the $3'$-deoxy-terminated analogs are far more stable to hydrolysis, although this property in itself does not necessarily confer to the analog biological activity. Further structure-activity studies will undoubtedly yield additional insight into the role of the $(2',5')$oligo(A)-RNase L system and the antiproliferative activity of IFNs.

III. INTERFERON AND THE IMMUNE SYSTEM

Although direct growth inhibition is one of the important factors in the antitumor effect of IFN, several studies have implied a significant role of the immune system of tumor-bearing hosts receiving IFN therapy.[41] The observation that mice inoculated with IFN-resistant tumor cells were protected against neoplastic disease by daily administration of IFN suggested that the antitumor effect of IFN is partly mediated by the host.[42,43] This response is characterized by increased phagocytosis of carbon particles,[44,45] and of Ehrlich ascites and RC19 cells[46] by peritoneal macrophages in IFN-treated tumor-bearing mice.[46] IFN is also capable of modulating the host immune response via the activation of macrophages, and syngenic or allogenic sensitized or nonsensitized (natural killer) lymphocytes, thus producing lysis of tumor cells.[47,48]

The view that immune reactions play an important role in modifying and even controlling malignant neoplasms is gaining wide acceptance. Thus, investigations of the combination of specific and nonspecific immunotherapy with IFN treatment merits serious consideration.

IV. GROWTH INHIBITION IN VITRO BY INTERFERON

Several methods have been used for the quantitation of the antiproliferation activities of IFN and these include direct cell counting,[5,6] colony formation with[49] and without agar,[50] and macromolecular synthesis measured by incorporation of radioactive precursors.[51-54] Gresser and associates[55-57] studied several murine cell lines in suspension cultures and observed that treatment with IFN at relatively high concentrations resulted in a slower growth rate and a lower final cell density. Such cytostatic effects were also observed in monolayer cultures of normal and transformed cells,[51,58,59] where the saturation densities of transformed cells were lowered by IFN, while normal untransformed cells were not affected.[59] Other investigators reported reduced colony formation by murine L1210 leukemia cells after IFN treatment.[49,60] Recently, several reports using diverse tumor systems confirmed that the antiproliferative effects of IFN are caused by the IFN molecule itself rather than by contaminants.[50,59,61-63] Growth inhibition by IFN has been reported in a variety of human tumor cell lines.[53,61,64-74] Human lymphoblastoid cell lines derived from Burkitt's lymphoma were tested by Adams et al.[67] for their susceptibility to the antiproliferative effect of IFN, and were found to vary significantly in their sensitivity to IFNα. Hilfenhaus et al.[53] used the sensitive Daudi lymphoblastoid cell line for studying growth inhibition by [14C]thymidine incorporation and found that 15 IU/mℓ of IFNα reduced [14C]thymidine uptake by 50%. Strander and Einhorn[71] investigated the growth inhibitory effects of human IFNα in vitro in nine cell lines derived from osteosarcoma patients and all were found to be sensitive. Buffet et al.[50] tested four human tumor cell lines for their sensitivity to the growth inhibitory action of purified human IFNβ. Using [3H]thymidine incorporation into acid-insoluble material as an indicator of growth, two cell lines were found to be significantly sensitive, whereas the other two responded poorly.

IFNγ produced by immunocompetent cells and characterized by its lability at pH 2 was found to exert antiviral and anticellular activity in L1210 leukemia cells resistant to IFNα and IFNβ,[34,75] and was shown to be a more potent antiproliferative agent than either IFNβ or IFNα in certain mouse and human cell systems.[76-79] In our recent investigations, human IFNγ was found to be highly cytostatic as well as cytocidal to a human colon adenocarcinoma (HT-29) cell line which showed little sensitivity to the growth inhibitory action of IFNβ and recombinant IFNαA (Table 1).

Experiments performed with asynchronously dividing cells,[80-82] as well as with synchronized cell populations,[83] indicate that IFN does not block the cells in one phase of the cell cycle but rather results in an extension of the G_1 and $S + G_2$ phases with a resultant increased length of the cell cycle. However, the relative extent to which the G_1 and G_2 phases are affected depends on the cell type.[84,85] Leanderson and Lundgren[86] have reported that IFNα treatment results in the entry of cells into the resting G_0 state. Interestingly, (2′,5′)oligo(A) trimer core inhibited the progression of a human lymphoma cell line through S phase rather than allowing an accumulation of cell in G_0 as found with treatment by IFNα.[28] Thus, it seems that IFNs effects on the cell cycle appear to be different depending on the cell line studied, and this fact should be considered in designing clinical trials where IFN might be combined with other cytostatic agents.

V. ANTITUMOR EFFECTS

The antitumor activity of IFN preparations was documented several years before it became accepted that IFN possessed more than just antiviral activity; however, most investigators were unconvinced of the antitumor activity of IFN since it was assumed that the impurities in the IFN preparations were responsible for the antitumor activity. With more extensive documentation in various animal tumor systems, it was eventually confirmed that IFNs were able to exert definite antitumor effects. The following sections will describe some of the antitumor effects of IFNs in various experimental tumor systems.

A. Viral Leukemogenesis

Gresser et al.[87-90] studied the effects of IFN on viral carcinogenesis in Friend and Rauscher murine leukemia systems and demonstrated that continuous suppression of virus growth by IFN was an essential factor for the prevention of leukemogenesis in mice. These investigators also studied the effects of IFN on spontaneous lymphoid leukemia in AKR mice and observed that daily therapy with IFN from birth until 1 year of age reduced the incidence of spontaneous leukemia from 95% in untreated controls to 63% in IFN-treated mice.[91] Similar treatment reduced the development of spontaneous mammary carcinoma in C3H mice.[92] Daily doses of 6×10^6 units of IFN given after the diagnosis of lymphoma in AKR mice also significantly delayed the evolution of the tumor and increased survival by 100%.[93]

B. Transplanted Tumors

The antitumor action of IFN against oncogenic virus-induced tumors has generally been interpreted to be a consequence of inhibition of viral multiplication. However, the antitumor effects of IFN against transplanted tumors suggest that mechanisms other than antiviral activity could also play an important role. Gresser et al.[47,94-96] studied the effect of IFN on the growth of a number of transplanted murine tumors and demonstrated that repeated daily injections of IFN prevented the growth of Ehrlich, RC19, EL4, and L1210 ascites tumors. The most significant effect was observed in the Ehrlich ascites tumor, where the mean survival time of mice inoculated with 10^4 tumor cells was increased 12-fold and 90% of the IFN-treated mice survived more than 6 months.[46] Several principles important to the practical application of IFN therapy emerged from these experiments: (1) the greatest antitumor effects were obtained when contact between IFN and tumor cells was maximum, (2) IFN treatment was ineffective when it was limited to the periods preceding the inoculation of tumor cells, and (3) IFN therapy was less effective in mice bearing solid tumors than in mice inoculated with ascites tumor cells. However, it was later reported[97] that IFN treatment, even beginning 6 days after s.c. implantation of the Lewis lung carcinoma, was effective in preventing the development of the primary tumor and in inhibiting the development of pulmonary metastases.[97] Yokota et al.[98] reported that mouse IFN treatment (2.5×10^4 units twice weekly for 3 weeks administered i.p.) starting after tumor nodules became palpable was significantly inhibitory to the growth of S-180 cells transplanted in normal or nude mice, whereas human IFN treatment was ineffective; however, human tumor cells (HeLa) transplanted into nude mice were sensitive to human IFN, suggesting that IFN acts directly on the tumor cells rather than on the host.

C. Chemical and Radiation Carcinogenesis

IFN treatment was reported to be highly effective in inhibiting the development of 3-methylcholanthrene-induced[99] and 20-methylcholanthrene-induced[100] tumors in mice. Lieberman et al.[101] reported that i.p. injections of low doses of IFN (300 units) immediately after X-irradiation of mice and continued three times a week throughout a 3-month period significantly decreased the incidence of lymphomas.

D. Combination Chemotherapy

Chirigos and Pearson[102] reported that IFN was ineffective against murine leukemia when the host tumor burden was large; however, after the tumor burden was reduced by 1,3-bis(2-chloroethyl)-1-nitrosourea (BCNU), subsequent IFN therapy led to a significant number of cures, and suggested that the combined effect of BCNU + IFN treatment was synergistic. Gresser et al.[103] demonstrated that combined IFN and cyclophosphamide treatment was therapeutically effective, even after the diagnosis of lymphoma in AKR mice. A single injection of cyclophosphamide increased survival from 17 to 29 days, whereas cyclophosphamide treatment followed by daily injections of 3×10^6 units of IFN increased survival to about 53 days.

Thus, it appears that in animals exogenous interferon can reduce the incidence and development of tumors even after they are well advanced, but does not produce cures. These experimental data suggest that IFN should be useful, particularly subsequent to and in combination with anticancer agents which reduce the tumor burden of the host.

E. Combinations of Different Interferons

Potentiation by the combined use of different species of IFN was first observed in mouse L cells where the combination of mouse IFNβ and IFNγ resulted in a synergistic antiviral response.[104] The potentiation of the anticellular activity of IFN was subsequently examined in vitro in mouse B16 melanoma cells where IFNβ and IFNγ resulted in a significant synergistic growth inhibitory effect.[105] Daily injections of IFNγ and IFNβ for 2 weeks into mice bearing P388 lymphocytic leukemia also produced a synergistic antitumor effect as shown by a delay in tumor growth and an increased survival time.[105] A similar effect was observed in a squamous cell carcinoma transplanted into nude mice following i.v. treatment with IFNβ (3000 units/day), IFNγ (10 units/day) or a combination of both IFNs.[106] The combined treatment resulted in a 69% reduction in tumor size, whereas a 38 and 20% reduction was produced by IFNβ and IFNγ, respectively. Synergism by combined administration of IFNβ and IFNγ was also observed on the growth of spontaneous mammary tumors in mice, with a concomitant decrease in the incidence of lung metastases.[107] Thus far, the mechanism of this potentiation is unclear; however, the synergistic effect produced by combinations of different types of IFN should have obvious advantages for clinical therapy in terms of both therapeutic response and drug resistance.

VI. POLY(I·C) AND INTERFERON ACTIVITY

Polynucleotides that induce IFN also manifest cytotoxic effects which increase in parallel with, and are inseparable from, their ability to induce IFN.[108,109] The synthetic double-stranded RNA, poly (I·C), was active against the development of Rauscher[110] and Friend leukemias.[111] Repeated injections of poly(I·C) induced regression of established murine sarcoma virus-induced tumors.[112-114]

Poly(I·C) has been shown to inhibit the growth of a number of transplanted tumors such as murine B16 melanoma[115] and L1210 leukemia,[116] and has induced regression of reticulum cell sarcoma by apparently causing tumor necrosis.[117,118] Most of these effects were due to IFN induction by poly(I·C). Gresser et al.[119] demonstrated that coadministration of antitumor antibodies with poly(I·C) to mice eliminated the antitumor effect.

Poly(I·C) inhibited chemical carcinogenesis in mice treated with dimethylbenzanthracene[120] and methylcholanthrene.[121] Repeated poly(I·C) injections were shown to be effective in inhibiting 3-methylcholanthrene-induced tumors only if given during the early stage of tumor promotion.[122]

Stewart et al.[123] showed that concentrations of poly(I·C) which exerted no detectable toxicity in normal L929 cells were toxic in IFN-treated cells. This enhanced sensitivity to toxicity was specific for double-stranded RNA and was not seen with DNA, single-stranded RNA, and other agents like cycloheximide, actinomycin D, or diphtheria and cholera toxins.[124] Attempts were also made to generate the toxicity-enhancing effect of IFN against Moloney virus-induced tumors in mice.[125] Mice developing autochthonous tumors were given intratumoral injections of IFN and poly(I·C). The sequential local treatment with IFN and poly(I·C) was more effective than treatment with either agent alone. In our experiments with human colon adenocarcinoma (HT-29) cells, a significantly greater growth inhibition was observed with combinations of IFNβ or recombinant IFNα and poly(I·C) in comparison to a marginal effect with either agent alone.[126] The increased growth inhibition by IFNβ or recombinant IFNαA and poly(I·C) was associated with a greater ratio of (2',5')oligo(A)synthetase: (2',5')oligo(A)PDE as a result of inhibition of the latter enzyme activity.

VII. CLINICAL TRIALS

Most of the clinical trials conducted so far have used IFNα which is a mixture of at least eight interferons.[127,128] Purified IFNα from the Namalva lymphoblastoid cell line[129,130] is also now used clinically and contains several subtypes.[131] IFNβ has been produced and purified on a large scale from human foreskin fibroblasts and is being used for clinical trials.[133] The main problem with the clinical use of IFNβ is its instability in vivo and only trace amounts are detected after intramuscular injections.[133,134] In spite of this, a considerable number of patients have been treated with human IFNβ after the observation was made that it can inhibit development of solid tumors if injected intralesionally. The preparation of IFNβ made from tissue culture has only one major molecular species and is similar to the species cloned in bacteria.[135,136] With the advent of recombinant DNA technology some species of human IFNα have been cloned, viz., IFNαA by Genetech and Hoffmann La-Roche[137] and IFNα₂ by Biogene and Schering,[4] and are presently being investigated in clinical trials. The following section will illustrate some of the studies which suggest the usefulness of IFN in cancer treatment.

A. Solid Tumors

One of the earliest evaluations of IFN therapy was in the treatment of patients with osteosarcoma. This trial was initiated at the Karolinska Hospital in Stockholm by Strander[138] and has been continued for 9 years. This is an adjuvant trial where IFNα is given postoperatively for 1.5 years (3×10^6 units/day i.m. three times per week). Two different groups serve as controls: one is a historic group of 35 patients treated at Karolinska hospital from 1952 to 1971, and the second a concurrent group of all other osteosarcoma patients who received no adjuvant therapy in the Swedish hospital. Since the natural history of this disease has changed, the historic control and study group may not be truly comparable. However, even when compared to the current controls (patients in Swedish hospitals), patients receiving IFN therapy showed a greater survival and developed fewer metastases. Promising results were also observed by Christopherson et al.[139] where six osteosarcoma patients were treated i.m. with IFNα at a dose of 4×10^6 IU/day for up to 1 month, and then three times per week for a period ranging from 2 to 28 months. Of these six patients, four did not develop metastases. Ito et al.[140] studied the effect of human leukocyte interferon in three osteosarcoma patients with pulmonary metastases, and in two of the patients the size of the metastasized tumor mass diminished temporarily 6 to 8 months after interferon treatment. Gutterman et al.[141] studied the effect of IFNα therapy in breast cancer patients (3 to 9×10^6 IU/day i.m. for 8 weeks) and observed regression in some patients. Borden et al.[142] undertook a clinical trial with IFNα in patients with disseminated human breast carcinoma and observed partial remission in some of these patients receiving IFNα i.m. (3×10^6 IU/day/28 days). Thus, the results obtained from the clinical trials with IFNα in breast cancer patients appear somewhat promising. This cell type is also significantly sensitive to human IFNα in culture and in the athymic nude mouse.[143,144]

Very few clinical trials have been performed with IFNβ, mainly as a result of an inadequate supply and because of its lability in the circulation. In spite of this, i.v. administration of IFNβ resulted in complete remission in a patient with nasopharyngeal carcinoma that had metastasized to the brain[145] The patient subsequently developed antibodies to IFNβ which apparently did not seem to alter the efficacy of the treatment. This observation suggests that IFNβ, after i.v. administration, though rapidly cleared from the circulation, could still generate long lasting antitumor effects. In a study with IFNβ used intratumorally in a patient with a nasopharyngeal carcinoma, complete disappearance of the tumor resulted.[146] Nakamura et al.[147] observed partial remission in a patient with glioblastoma after intratumoral administration of IFNβ, and objective responses were observed in patients with metastatic breast cancer after i.m. administration of IFNβ.[148]

B. Hematological Malignancies

Myeloma and non-Hodgkin's lymphoma are hematological neoplasms in which IFN therapy has proved to be successful. Of the nine multiple myeloma patients that were given IFNα therapy, five responded favorably and serum Bence Jones protein disappeared in one case.[141] Significant tumor regression was also observed by Mellstedt et al.[149] in a group of multiple myeloma patients treated with IFNα. These investigators reported that IgG-producing myelomas do not respond well to IFNα therapy and IFN trials are now confined to patients with myelomas producing IgA or Bence Jones proteins. Gutterman et al.[141] observed tumor regression with IFNα treatment in a clinical trial with 11 non-Hodgkin's lyphoma patients, and Merigan et al.[150] reported lymphocytic lymphomas to be more sensitive than histiocytic lymphomas to IFNα therapy. The more detailed classification of lymphomas with the use of immunological markers might lead to better selection of lymphoma patients for IFN therapy.

Besides eliciting antitumor activity, IFNα also produces some toxic side effects, most of which are similar to those seen in influenza infections, such as fatigue, chills, fever, etc.[151] These effects have also been observed after treatment with cloned human IFN[152] and suggest that they are not due to contaminants. Although these side effects are commonly seen as a result of systemic administration, very high doses of IFN can be applied intralesionally without any serious side effects.

VIII. CONCLUSION

IFNs appear to be a promising adjunct to the cancer chemotherapy armamentarium as evidenced by their in vitro effects in numerous cell systems, their in vivo activity in animal tumor models, and ultimately by their activity in preliminary clinical trials. Studies showing the great variability in the sensitivity of human tumor cells would suggest a need for a simple screening assay, e.g., the use of the (2′,5′)oligo(A)-RNase L system, for the selection of patients for clinical trials who might show the greatest sensitivity to IFN treatment. The molecular locus of action of IFN appears to involve, at least in part, the (2′,5′)oligo(A) pathway, but this has not been unequivocally established. Nevertheless, this unique oligonucleotide has served as a model for the development of pharmacologically active analogs which possess IFN-like activity yet obviate the need for IFN treatment of the tumor. It is obvious that there is much that is not known about the mode of action of IFNs and there will undoubtedly be many more therapeutic applications derived from the interesting biochemistry associated with this biological response modifier.

REFERENCES

1. **Isaacs, A. and Lindenmann, J.,** Virus interference. 1. The interferon, *Proc. R. Soc. London Ser. B,* 147, 258, 1957.
2. **Stewart, W. E., Falcott, E., Friedman, R. M., Glasso, G. J., Joklik, W. K., Vilcek, J. T., Younger, J. S., and Zoon, K. C.,** Interferon nomenclature, *Nature (London),* 286, 110, 1980.
3. **Brack, C., Nagata, S., Mantei, N., and Weissmann, C.,** Molecular analysis of the human interferon-α gene family, *Gene,* 15, 379, 1981.
4. **Goeddel, D. V., Leung, D. W., Dull, T. J., Gross, M., Lawn, R. M., McCandliss, R., Seeburg, P. H., Ultrich, A., Yelverton, E., and Gray, P. W.,** The structure of eight distinct cloned human leukocyte interferon cDNAs, *Nature (London),* 290, 20, 1981.
5. **Paucker, K., Cantell, K., and Henle, W.,** Quantitative studies on viral interference in suspended L cells. III. Effect of interfering viruses and interferon on the growth rate of cells, *Virology,* 17, 324, 1962.
6. **Gresser, I.,** Antitumor effects of interferons, *Adv. Cancer Res.,* 16, 97, 1972.
7. **Baglioni, C.,** Interferon induced enzymatic activities and their role in the antiviral state, *Cell,* 17, 255, 1979.
8. **Lebleu, B., Sen, G. C., Shaila, S., Cabrer, B., and Lengyel, P.,** Interferon dsRNA, and protein phosphorylation, *Proc. Natl. Acad. Sci. U.S.A.,* 73, 3107, 1976.
9. **Copper, J. A. and Farell, P. J.,** Extracts of interferon treated cells can inhibit reticulocyte lysate protein synthesis, *Biochem. Biophys. Res. Commun.,* 77, 124, 1977.
10. **Hovanessian, A. G. and Kerr I. M.,** The 2′,5′ oligoadenylate synthetase and protein kinase from interferon treated cells, *Eur. J. Biochem.,* 93, 515, 1979.

11. **Roberts, W. K., Hovanessian, A. G., Brown, R. E., Clemens, M. J., and Kerr, I. M.,** Interferon mediated protein synthesis, *Nature (London)*, 264, 477, 1977.

12. **Hovanessian, A. G., Brown, R. E., and Kerr, I. M.,** Synthesis of a low mol. wt. inhibitor of protein synthesis with enzymes from interferon treated cells, *Nature (London)*, 268, 537, 1977.

13. **Kerr, I. M., and Brown, R. E.,** pppA2′p5′A2′p5′A, inhibitor of protein synthesis synthesized with an enzyme fraction from interferon treated cells, *Proc. Natl. Acad. Sci. U.S.A.*, 75, 256, 1978.

14. **Floyd-Smith, G., Slattery, E., and Lengyel, P.,** Interferon Action: RNA cleavage pattern of a (2′,5′)oligoadenylate-dependent endonuclease, *Science*, 212, 1030, 1981.

15. **Chernajovsky, Y., Kimchi, A., Schmidt, A., Zilberstein, A., and Revel, M.,** Differential effects of two interferon-induced translational inhibitors on initiation of protein synthesis, *Eur. J. Biochem.*, 96, 35, 1979.

16. **Ratner, L., Sen, G. C., Brown, G. E., Lebleu, B., Kawakita, M., Cabrer, B., Slattery, E., and Lengyel, P.,** Interferon, double stranded RNA and RNA degradation, *Eur. J. Biochem.*, 79, 565, 1977.

17. **Ball, L. A. and White, C. N.,** Oligonucleotide inhibitor of protein synthesis made in extracts of interferon treated chick embryo cells: comparison with the mouse low molecular weight inhibitor, *Proc. Natl. Acad. Sci. U.S.A.*, 75, 1167, 1978.

18. **William, B. R. G., Golgher, R. R., and Kerr, I. M.,** Activation of a nuclease by pppA2′p5′A2′p5′A in intact cells, *FEBS Lett.*, 105, 47, 1979.

19. **Hovanessian, A. G., Wood, J. N., Meurs, E., and Montagnier, L.,** Increased nuclease activity in cells treated with pppA2′p5′A2′5′A, *Proc. Natl. Acad. Sci. U.S.A.*, 76, 3261, 1979.

20. **Hovanessian, A. G. and Wood, J. N.,** Anticellular and antiviral effects of pppA(2′p5′A)n, *Virology*, 101, 81, 1981.

21. **Stark, G. R., Dower, W. J., Schimke, R. T., Brown, R. E., and Kerr, I. M.,** 2′,5′A synthetase: assay, distribution and variation with growth or hormone status, *Nature (London)*, 278, 471, 1979.

22. **Dougherty, J. P., Samanta, H., Farrel, P. J., and Lengyel, P.,** Interferon, double stranded RNA, and RNA degradation, *J. Biol. Chem.*, 255, 3813, 1980.

23. **Kimchi, A., Shulman, L., Schmidt, A., Chernajovsky, Y., Fradin, A., and Revel, M.,** Kinetics of the induction of three translation-regulatory enzymes by interferon, *Proc. Natl. Acad. Sci. U.S.A.*, 76, 3208, 1979.

24. **Schmidt, A., Chernajovsky, Y., Shulman, L., Federman, P., Berissi, H., and Revel, M.,** Interferon induced phosphodiesterase degrading (2′,5′)oligoadenylate and CCA terminus of tRNA, *Proc. Natl. Acad. Sci. U.S.A.*, 76, 4788, 1979.

25. **Torrence, P. F., Imai, J., and Johnston, M. I.,** 5′-O-monophosphoryladenylyl-(2′ → 5′)adenylyl(2′ → 5′)adenosine is an antagonist of the action of 5′-O-triphosphoryladenylyl-(2′5′)adenylyl(2′5′)adenosine and double-stranded RNA, *Proc. Natl. Acad. Sci. U.S.A.*, 78, 5993, 1981.

26. **Nilsen, T. W., Maroney, P. A., and Baglioni, C.,** Double-stranded RNA causes synthesis of (2′,5′)oligo(A) and degradation of messenger RNA in interferon-treated cells, *J. Biol. Chem.*, 256, 7806, 1981.

27. **William, B. R. G. and Kerr, I. M.,** Inhibition of protein synthesis by 2′,5′-linked adenine oligonucleotides in intact cells, *Nature (London)*, 276, 88, 1978.

28. **Leanderson, T., Nordfelth, R., and Lundgren, E.,** Antiproliferative effect of (2′-5′)oligoadenylate distinct from that of interferon in lymphoid cells, *Biochem. Biophys. Res. Commun.*, 107, 511, 1982.

29. **Kimchi, A., Shure, H., and Revel, M.,** Regulation of lymphocyte mitogenesis by (2′,5′)oligo-isoadenylates, *Nature (London)*, 282, 849, 1979.

30. **Shimizu, N. and Sokawa, Y.,** (2′,5′)oligoadenylate synthetase activity in lymphocytes from normal mouse, *J. Biol. Chem.*, 254, 12034, 1980.

31. **Kimchi, A., Shure, H., and Revel, M.,** Antimitotic function of interferon induced (2′,5′)oligo(adenylate) and growth-related variations in enzymes that synthesize and degrade this oligonucleotide, *Eur. J. Biochem.*, 114, 5, 1981.

32. **Zoon, K. C., Buckler, C. E., Bridgen, R. J., and Gurari-Rotman, D.,** Production of human lymphoblastoid interferon by Namalva cells, *J. Clin. Microbiol.*, 7, 44, 1977.

33. **Wood, J. N. and Hovanessian, A. G.,** Interferon enhances (2′,5′)oligoA synthetase in embryonal carcinoma cells, *Nature (London)*, 282, 74, 1979.

34. **Hovanessian, A. G., LaBonnardiere, C., and Falcoff, E.,** Action of murine γ (immune) interferon on β (fibroblast)-interferon resistant L1210 and embryonal carcinoma cells, *J. Interferon Res.*, 1, 125, 1980.

35. **Doetsch, P. W., Wu, J. M., Sawada, Y., and Suhadolnik, R. J.,** Synthesis and characterization of (2′-5′)ppp3′dA(p3′dA)n, an analogue of (2′-5′)pppA(pA)n, *Nature (London)*, 291, 355, 1981.

36. **Doetsch, P. W., Suhadolnik, R. J., Sawada, Y., Mosca, J. D., Flick, M. B., Reichenbach, N. L., Dang, A. Q., Wu, J. M., Charubala, R., Pfleiderer, W., and Henderson, E. E.,** Core (2′-5′) oligoadenylate and the cordycepin analog: inhibitors of Epstein-Barr virus-induced transformation of human lymphocytes in the absence of interferon, *Proc. Natl. Acad. Sci. U.S.A.*, 78, 6699, 1981.

37. **Eppstein, D. A., Marsh, Y. V., Schryrer, B. B., Larsen, M. A., Barnett, J. W., Verheyden, J. P. H., and Prisbe, E. J.,** Analogs of (A2′p)nA: correlation of structure of analogs of ppp(A2′p)2A and (A2′p)2A with stability and biological activity, *J. Biol. Chem.*, 257, 13390, 1982.

38. **Sawai, H., Imai, J., Lesiak, K., Johnston, M. I., and Torrence, P. F.,** Cordycepin analogs of 2′-5′A and its derivatives: chemical synthesis and biological activity, *J. Biol. Chem.,* 258, 1671, 1983.

39. **Baglioni, C., D'Alessandro, S. B., Nilsen, T. W., den Hartog, J. A. J., Crea, R., and Van Boom, J. H.,** Analogs of (2′-5′)oligo A: endonuclease activation and inhibition of protein synthesis in intact cells, *J. Biol. Chem.,* 256, 3253, 1981.

40. **Imai, J., Johnston, M. I., and Torrence, P. F.,** Chemical modification potentiates the biological activities of 2′-5′A and its congeners, *J. Biol. Chem.,* 257, 12739, 1982.

41. **Gresser, I.,** On the varied biological effects of interferon, *Cell Immunol.,* 34, 406, 1977.

42. **Gresser, I., Bourali, C., and Chouroulin, K. V.,** Treatment of neoplasia in mice with interferon preparations, *Ann. N.Y. Acad. Sci.,* 173, 694, 1970.

43. **Lindahl, P., Leary, P., and Gresser, I.,** Enhancement by interferon of the specific cytotoxicity of sensitized lymphocytes, *Proc. Natl. Acad. Sci. U.S.A.,* 69, 721, 1972.

44. **Huang, K. Y., Donahoe, R. M., Goldon, B. F., and Dressler, H. R.,** Enhancement of phagocytosis by interferon-containing preparations, *Infect. Immunol.,* 4, 581, 1971.

45. **Imanishi, J., Yokota, Y., Kishida, T., Mukainaka, T., and Matsuo, A.,** Phagocytosis enhancing effect of human leukocyte interferon preparation of human peripheral monocytes in vitro, *Acta Virol.,* 19, 52, 1975.

46. **Gresser, I. and Bourali, C.,** Antitumor effects of interferon preparations in mice, *J. Natl. Cancer Inst.,* 45, 365, 1970.

47. **Svet-Moldavsky, G. J. and Chernyakhovskaya, I. J.,** Interferon and the interaction of allogenic normal and immune lymphocytes with L cells, *Nature (London),* 215, 1299, 1967.

48. **Chernyakhovskaya, I. J., Slavina, E. G., and Svet-Moldavsky, G. J.,** Antitumor effect of lymphoid cells activated by interferon, *Nature (London),* 228, 71, 1970.

49. **Gresser, I., Thomas, M. T., Brouty-Boye, D., and Macieira-Coelho, A.,** Interferon and cell division. V. Titration of anticellular action of interferon preparations, *Proc. Soc. Exp. Biol. Med.,* 137, 1258, 1976.

50. **Buffet, R. M., Ito, M., Cairo, A. M., and Carter, W. A.,** Antiproliferative activity of highly purified mouse interferon, *J. Natl. Cancer Inst.,* 60, 243, 1978.

51. **O'Shaughnessy, M. V., Easterbrook, K. B., Lee, S. H. S., Kartz, L. J., and Rozee, K. R.,** Interferon inhibition of autogenously induced virons (C particles) in synchronized L929 cell cultures, *J. Natl. Cancer Inst.,* 53, 1687, 1974.

52. **Tovey, M., Brouty-Boye, D., and Gresser, I.,** Interferon and cell division. X. Early effects of interferon on mouse leukemia cells cultivated in a chemostat, *Proc. Natl. Acad. Sci. U.S.A.,* 72, 2265, 1975.

53. **Hilfenhaus, J., Pamm, H., Karges, H. E., and Manthey, K. R.,** Growth inhibition of human lymphoblastoid Daudi cells *in vitro* by interferon preparations, *Arch. Virol.,* 51, 87, 1976.

54. **Fuse, A. and Kuwata, I.,** Effects of interferon on the human clonal cell line RSa, *J. Gen. Virol.,* 33, 17, 1976.

55. **Gresser, I., Brouty-Boye, D., Thomas, M. T., and Macieira-Coelho, A.,** Interferon and cell division. I. Inhibition of the multiplication of mouse leukemia L1210 cells *in vitro* by interferon preparations, *Proc. Natl. Acad. Sci. U.S.A.,* 66, 1052, 1970.

56. **Gresser, I., Brouty-Boye, D., Thomas, M. T., and Macieira-Coelho, A.,** Interferon and cell division. II. Influence of various experimental conditions on the inhibition of L1210 cell multiplication *in vitro* by interferon preparations, *J. Natl. Cancer Inst.,* 45, 1145, 1970.

57. **Gresser, I., Thomas, M., and Brouty-Boye, D.,** Effect of interferon treatment of L1210 cells *in vitro* on tumor and colony formation, *Nature (London),* 231, 20, 1971.

58. **Lindahl-Magnusson, P., Leary, P., and Gresser, I.,** Interferon and cell division. VI. Inhibitory effect of interferon on the multiplication of mouse embryo and mouse kidney cells in primary cultures, *Proc. Soc. Exp. Biol. Med.,* 138, 1044, 1971.

59. **Knight, E., Jr.,** Interferon: effect on the saturation density to which mouse cells will grow *in vitro, J. Cell Biol.,* 56, 846, 1973.

60. **Gresser, I., Bandu, M., and Brouty-Boye, D.,** Interferon and cell division. IX. Interferon-resistant L1210 cells, characteristics and origin, *J. Natl. Cancer Inst.,* 52, 553, 1974.

61. **Tan, Y. H.,** Chromosome 21 and the cell growth inhibitory effect of human interferon preparations, *Nature (London),* 260, 141, 1976.

62. **Stewart, W. E., II, Gresser, I., Tovey, M. G., Bandu, M., and LeGott, S.,** Identification of the cell multiplication inhibitory factors in interferon preparations as interferons, *Nature (London),* 262, 300, 1976.

63. **Knight, E., Jr.,** Antiviral and cell growth inhibitory activities reside in the same glycoprotein of human fibroblast interferon, *Nature (London),* 262, 302, 1976.

64. **Lee, S. H. S., O'Shaughnessy, M. V., and Rozee, K. R.,** Interferon induced growth depression in diploid and heteroploid human cells, *Proc. Soc. Exp. Biol. Med.,* 139, 1438, 1972.

65. **Gaffney, E. V., Picciano, P. T., and Grant, C. A.,** Inhibition of growth and transformation of human cells by interferon, *J. Natl. Cancer Inst.,* 50, 871, 1973.

66. **Hilfenhaus, J. and Karges, H. E.,** Growth inhibition of human lymphoblastoid cells by interferon preparations obtained from human leukocytes, *Naturforscher,* 29C, 618, 1974.

67. **Adams, A., Strander, H., and Cantell, K.,** Sensitivity of Epstein Barr virus-transformed human lymphoid cell lines to interferon, *J. Gen. Virol.,* 28, 207, 1975.

68. **Dahl, H. and Degre, M.,** Separation of antiviral activity of human interferon from cell growth inhibitory effect, *Nature (London),* 257, 799, 1975.

69. **Kuwata, T., Fuse, A., and Morinaga, N.,** Effects of interferon on cell and virus growth in transformed human cell lines, *J. Gen. Virol.,* 33, 7, 1976.

70. **Dahl, H. and Degre, M.,** Human interferon and cell growth inhibition. I. Inhibitory effect of human interferon on the growth rate of cultured human cells, *Acta Pathol. Microbiol. Scand.,* 84, 285, 1976.

71. **Strander, H. and Einhorn, S.,** Effect of human leukocyte interferon on the growth of human osteosarcoma cells in tissue culture, *Int. J. Cancer,* 19, 468, 1977.

72. **Hilfenhaus, J., Damm, H., and Johannsen, R.,** Sensitivity of various human lymphoblastoid cells to the antiviral and anticellular activity of human leukocyte interferon, *Arch. Virol.,* 54, 271, 1977.

73. **Dahl, M.,** Human interferon and cell growth inhibition. II. Biological and physicochemical properties of the growth inhibitory components, *Acta Pathol. Microbiol. Scand.,* 85, 54, 1977.

74. **Einhorn, S. and Strander, H.,** Is interferon tissue specific? Effect of human leukocyte and fibroblast interferons on the growth of lymphoblastoid and osteosarcoma cell lines, *J. Gen. Virol.,* 35, 573, 1977.

75. **Ankel, H., Krishnamurti, C., Besancon, F., Stefancs, S., and Falcoff, E.,** Mouse fibroblast (type I) and immune (type II) interferons. Pronounced differences in affinity for gangliosides and antiviral and antigrowth effects on mouse leukemia L-1210 cells, *Proc. Natl. Acad. Sci.,* 77, 2528, 1980.

76. **Crane, J. L., Jr., Glasgow, L. A., Kern, E. R., and Youngner, J. S.,** Inhibition of murine osteogenic sarcomas by treatment with type I or type II interferon, *J. Natl. Cancer Inst.,* 61, 871, 1978.

77. **Blalock, J. E., Georgiades, J. A., Langford, M. P., and Johnson, M. M.,** Purified human immune interferon has more potent anticellular activity than fibroblast or leukocyte interferon, *Cell Immunol.,* 49, 390, 1980.

78. **Bourgeade, M. F., Chany, C., and Merigan, T. C.,** Type I and Type II interferons: differential antiviral actions in transformed cells, *J. Gen. Virol.,* 46, 449, 1980.

79. **Rubin, B. Y. and Gupta, S. L.,** Differential efficacies of human type I and type II interferons as antiviral and antiproliferative agents, *Proc. Natl. Acad. Sci. U.S.A.,* 77, 5928, 1980.

80. **Killander, D., Lindahl, P., Lundin, L., Leary, P., and Gresser, I.,** Relationship between the enhanced expression of histocompatibility antigens on interferon-treated L1210 cells and their position in the cell cycle, *Eur. J. Immunol.,* 6, 56, 1976.

81. **Matarese, G. P. and Rossi, G. B.,** Effect of interferon on growth and division cycle of Friend erythroleukemic murine cells *in vitro, J. Cell Biol.,* 75, 344, 1977.

82. **Balkwill, F. R., Watlin, D., and Taylor-Papadimitriou, J.,** Inhibition by lymphoblastoid interferon of growth of cells derived from the human breast, *Int. J. Cancer,* 22, 258, 1978.

83. **Sokawa, Y., Watanabe, Y., and Kawada, Y.,** Interferon suppresses the transition of quiescent 3T3 cells to a growing state, *Nature (London),* 268, 236, 1977.

84. **Coollyn d'Hooghe, M., Brouty-Boye, D., Malause, E. P., and Gresser, I.,** Prolongation by interferon of the intermitotic time of mouse mammary tumor cells *in vitro.* Microcinematographic analysis, *Exp. Cell Res.,* 105, 73, 1977.

85. **Balkwill, F. R. and Taylor-Papadimitriou, J.,** Interferon affects both G_1 and $S + G_2$ in cells stimulated from quiescence to growth, *Nature (London),* 274, 798, 1978.

86. **Leanderson, T. and Lundgren, E.,** Growth inhibition by interferon achieved by collecting cells in G_0, *J. Interferon Res.,* 2, 21, 1982.

87. **Gresser, I., Coppey, J., and Bourali, C.,** Interferon and murine leukemia. III. Efficacy of interferon preparations administered after inoculation of Friend virus, *Nature (London),* 215, 174, 1967.

88. **Gresser, I., Coppey, J., Falcoff, E., and Fontaine, D.,** Interferon and murine leukemia. I. Inhibitory effect of interferon preparations on development of Friend leukemia in mice, *Proc. Soc. Exp. Biol. Med.,* 124, 84, 1967.

89. **Gresser, I., Falcoff, R., Brouty-Boye, D., Zaydela, F., Coppey, Y., and Falcoff, E.,** Interferon and murine leukemia. IV. Further studies on the efficacy of interferon preparations administered after inoculation of Friend virus, *Proc. Soc. Exp. Biol. Med.,* 126, 791, 1967.

90. **Gresser, I., Berman, L., deThe, G., Brouty-Boye, D., Coppey, Y., and Falcoff, E.,** Interferon and murine leukemia. V. Effect of interferon preparations on the evolution of Rauscher disease in mice, *J. Natl. Cancer Inst.,* 41, 505, 1968.

91. **Gresser, I., Coppey, J., and Bourali, C.,** Interferon and murine leukemia. VI. Effect of interferon preparations on the lymphoid leukemia of AKR mice, *J. Natl. Cancer Inst.,* 48, 1151, 1972.

92. **Came, P. E. and Moore, D. M.,** Effect of exogenous interferon treatment on mouse mammary tumors, *J. Natl. Cancer Inst.,* 48, 1151, 1972.

93. **Gresser, I., Maury, G., and Tovey, M.,** Interferon and murine leukemia. VII. Therapeutic effect of interferon preparations after diagnosis of lymphoma in AKR mice, *Int. J. Cancer,* 17, 647, 1976.

94. **Gresser, I., Bourali, C., and Levy, J. P.,** Increased survival in mice inoculated with tumor cells and treated with interferon preparations, *Proc. Natl. Acad. Sci.,* 63, 51, 1969.

95. **Gresser, I. and Bourali, C.,** Exogenous interferon and inducers of interferon in the treatment of Balb/c mice inoculated with RC19 tumor cells, *Nature (London),* 223, 844, 1969.

96. **Gresser, I., Bourali, C., Chouroulinkow, I., Fontaine-Brouty-Boye, D., and Thomas, M. T.,** Treatment of neoplasia in mice with interferon preparation, *Ann. N.Y. Acad. Sci.,* 173, 694, 1970.

97. **Gresser, I. and Bourali-Maury, C.,** Inhibition by interferon preparations of a solid malignant tumor and pulmonary metastasis in mice, *Nature New Biol.,* 236, 78, 1972.

98. **Yokota, Y., Kishida, T., Esaki, K., and Kawamata, J.,** Antitumor effects of interferon on transplanted tumors in congenitally athymic nude mice, *Biken J.,* 19, 125, 1976.

99. **Salerno, R. A., Whitmire, C. E., Garcia, I. M., and Heubner, R. J.,** Chemical carcinogens in mice inhibited by interferon, *Nature New Biol.,* 239, 31, 1972.

100. **Kishida, T., Tada, S., Toida, T., and Hattori, T.,** Effect of interferon on malignant mouse cells, *C. R. Soc. Biol. (Paris),* 165, 1489, 1971.

101. **Lieberman, M., Merigan, T. C., and Kaplan, H. S.,** Inhibition of radiogenic lymphoma development in mice by interferon, *Proc. Soc. Exp. Biol. Med.,* 138, 575, 1976.

102. **Chirigos, M. A. and Pearson, J. W.,** Cure of murine leukemia with drug and interferon treatment, *J. Natl. Cancer Inst.,* 51, 1367, 1973.

103. **Gresser, I., Maury, C., and Tovey, M. G.,** Efficacy of combined interferon cyclophosphamide therapy after diagnosis of lymphoma in AKR mice, *Eur. J. Cancer,* 14, 97, 1978.

104. **Fleischmann, W. R., Jr., Georgiades, J. A., Osborne, L. C., and Johnson, H. M.,** Potentiation of interferon activity by mixed preparations of fibroblast and immune interferon, *Infect. Immun.,* 26, 248, 1979.

105. **Fleischmann, W. R., Jr.,** Potentiation and inhibition of interferon action — antiviral and antitumor studies, *Med. Pediatr. Oncol.,* 9, 89, 1981.

106. **Brysk, M. M., Tschen, E. H., Hudson, R. D., Smith, E. B., Fleischmann, W. R., Jr., and Black, H. R.,** The activity of interferon on UV light-induced squamous carcinoma in mice, *J. Am. Acad. Dermatol.,* 5, 61, 1981.

107. **DeClercq, E., Zhang, Z.-X., Huygen, K., and Leyten, R.,** Inhibitory effect of interferon on the growth of spontaneous mammary tumors in mice, *J. Natl. Cancer Inst.,* 69, 653, 1982.

108. **Niblack, J. F. and McCreary, M. B.,** Relationship of biological activities of poly I.C. to homopolymer molecular weights, *Nature New Biol.,* 233, 52, 1971.

109. **Declercq, E. and Stewart, W. E., II,** Interferon production linked to toxicity of polyriboinosinic·polyribocytidylic acid, *Infect. Immun.,* 6, 344, 1972.

110. **Youn, J. K., Barski, G., and Huppert, J.,** Inhibition of viral leukemogenesis in mice by treatment with synthetic polynucleotides, *C. R. Acad. Sci., (Paris) D,* 267, 816, 1968.

111. **Larson, V. M., Clark, W. R., Dagle, G. E., and Hilleman, M. R.,** Influence of synthetic double-stranded ribonucleic acid (poly I·C) on Friend leukemia in mice, *Proc. Soc. Exp. Biol. Med.,* 132, 602, 1969.

112. **Sarma, P. S., Neubauer, R. H., and Rabstein, L.,** Inhibitory effect of interferon on murine sarcoma virus infection *in vitro, Proc. Soc. Exp. Biol. Med.,* 137, 469, 1971.

113. **Sarma, P. S., Shiu, G., Baron, S., and Huebner, R. J.,** Inhibitory effect of interferon in murine sarcoma virus infection *in vitro, Nature (London),* 223, 845, 1969.

114. **Rhim, J. S. and Huebner, R. J.,** Comparison of the antitumor effect of interferon and interferon inducers, *Proc. Soc. Exp. Biol. Med.,* 136, 524, 1971.

115. **Bart, R. S. and Kopf, A. W.,** Inhibition of the growth of murine malignant melanoma with synthetic double-stranded ribonucleic acid, *Nature (London),* 224, 372, 1969.

116. **Zeleznick, L. D. and Bhuyan, B. K.,** Treatment of leukemic (L1210) mice with double-stranded polyribonucleotides, *Proc. Soc. Exp. Biol. Med.,* 130, 126, 1969.

117. **Levy, H. G., Law, L., and Wand-Robson, A. S.,** Inhibition of tumor growth by polyinosinic-polycytidylic acid, *Proc. Natl. Acad. Sci. U.S.A.,* 62, 357, 1969.

118. **Levy, H. B., Asofsky, R., Riley, F., Garapin, A., Cantor, H., and Adamson, R.,** The mechanism of the antitumor action of poly IC, *Ann. N.Y. Acad. Sci.,* 173, 640, 1970.

119. **Gresser, I., Maury, C., Bandu, M. T., Tovey, M., and Maunory, M. T.,** Role of endogenous interferon in the antitumor effect of poly I·C and statolon as demonstrated by the use of antimouse interferon serum, *J. Natl. Cancer Inst.,* 21, 71, 1978.

120. **Gelboin, H. V. and Levy, H. B.,** Polyinosinic-polycytidylic acid inhibits chemically induced tumorigenesis in mouse skin, *Science,* 167, 205, 1970.

121. **Kreibich, G., Suss, R., Kinzel, V., and Hecker, E.,** On the biochemical mechanism of tumorogenesis in mouse skin. III. Decrease in tumor yields by poly I·C administered during initiation of skin by an intragastric dose of 7,12 dimethylbenz[a]anthracene, *Z. Krebsforsch.,* 74, 383, 1970.

122. **Elgjo, K. and Degre, M.,** Polyinosinic-polycytidylic acid in two stage skin carcinogenesis effect on epidermal growth parameters and interferon induction in treated mice, *J. Natl. Cancer Inst.,* 51, 171, 1973.

123. **Stewart, W. E., II, Declercq, E., Billiau, A., Desmyter, J., and Desomer, P.,** Increased susceptibility of cells treated with interferon to the toxicity of polyriboinosinic-polyribocytidylic acid, *Proc. Natl. Acad. Sci. U.S.A.,* 69, 1851, 1972.

124. **Stewart, W. E., II, Declercq, E., and Desomer, P.,** Specificity of interferon induced enhancement of toxicity for double-stranded ribonucleic acids, *J. Gen. Virol.,* 18, 237, 1973.

125. **Stewart, W. E., II,** *Interferon Systems,* Springer-Verlag, New York, 1979, 248.

126. **Chapekar, M. S. and Glazer, R. I.,** The effects of fibroblast and recombinant leukocyte interferons and double-stranded RNA on (2′,5′)oligo(A) synthesis and cell proliferation on human colon carcinoma cells *in vitro, Cancer Res.,* 43, 2683, 1983.

127. **Rubinstein, M., Levy, W. P., Moschera, J., Lai, C.-Y., Rubenstein, S., Familletti, P. C., Hershberg, R. D., Bartlett, R. T., and Pestka, S.,** Human leukocyte interferon: isolation and characterization of several molecular forms, *Arch. Biochem. Biophys.,* 210, 307, 1981.

128. **Berg, K. and Heron, I.,** The complete purification of human leukocyte interferon, *Scand. J. Immunol.,* 11, 489, 1980.

129. **Strander, H., Mogensen, K. E., and Cantell, K.,** Production of human lymphoblastoid interferon, *J. Clin. Microbiol.,* 1, 116, 1975.

130. **Finter, N. B., Fantes, K. H., and Johnston, M. D.,** Human lymphoblastoid cells as a source of interferon, *Dev. Biol. Stand.,* 38, 343, 1978.

131. **Allen, G. and Fantes, K. H.,** A family of structural genes for human lymphoblastoid (leukocyte type) interferon, *Nature (London),* 287, 408, 1980.

132. **Leong, S. S. and Horoszewicz, J. S.,** Production and preparation of human fibroblast interferon for clinical trials, *Meth. Enzymol.,* 78, 87, 1981.

133. **Edy, V. G., Biliau, A., and Desomer, P.,** Nonappearance of injected fibroblast interferon in circulation, *Lancet,* 21, 451, 1978.

134. **Lucero, M. A., Magdelenat, H., Fridman, W. H., Poulliart, P., Billardon, C., Biliau, A., Cantell, K., and Falcoff, E.,** Comparison of effects of leukocyte and fibroblast interferon on immunological parameters in cancer patients, *Eur. J. Cancer,* 18, 243, 1982.

135. **Derynck, R., Content, J., Declercq, E., Volckaert, G., Tavernier, J., Devos, R., and Fiers, W.,** Isolation and structure of a human fibroblast gene, *Nature (London),* 285, 542, 1980.

136. **Taniguchi, T., Mantei, N., Schwarzstein, M., Nagata, S., Muramatsu, M., and Weissmann, C.,** Human leukocyte and fibroblast interferons are structurally related, *Nature (London),* 285, 547, 1980.

137. **Streuli, M., Nagata, S., and Weissmann, C.,** At least three human type α interferons: structure of α2, *Science,* 209, 1343, 1980.

138. **Strander, H.,** Interferons: antineoplastic drugs, *Blut.,* 35, 277, 1977.

139. **Christopherson, I. S., Jordal, R., Osther, K., Lindenberg, J., Pedersen, P. H., and Berg, K.,** Interferon therapy in neoplastic disease, *Acta Med. Scand.,* 204, 471, 1978.

140. **Ito, H., Murakami, K., Yanagawa, T., Ban, S., Sawamura, H., Sakakida, K., Matsuo, A., Imanishi, J., and Kishida, T.,** Effect of human leukocyte interferon on the metastatic lung tumor of osteosarcoma, *Cancer,* 46, 1562, 1980.

141. **Gutterman, J. U., Blumenschein, G. R., Alexanian, R., Yap, H. Y., Buzdar, A. U., Cabanillas, F., Hortobagyi, G. M, Hersh, E. M., Rasmussen, S. L., Harmon, M., Kramer, M., and Pestka, S.,** Leukocyte interferon-induced tumor regression in human metastatic breast cancer multiple myeloma and malignant lymphoma, *Ann. Intern. Med.,* 93, 399, 1980.

142. **Borden, E. C., Holand, J. F., Dao, T. L., Gutterman, J. U., Wiener, L., Chang, Y., and Patel, J.,** Leukocyte-derived interferon (Alpha) in human breast carcinoma, *Ann. Intern. Med.,* 97, 1, 1982.

143. **Shibata, H. and Taylor-Papadimitriou, J.,** Effects of human lymphoblastoid interferon on cultured breast cancer cells, *Int. J. Cancer,* 28, 447, 1981.

144. **Balkwill, F., Taylor-Papadimitriou, J., Fantes, K. H., and Sebesteny, A.,** Human lymphoblastoid interferon can inhibit the growth of human breast cancer xenografts in athymic (nude) mice, *Eur. J. Cancer,* 16, 569, 1980.

145. **Vallbracht, A., Treuner, J., Flehmig, B., Joester, K. E., and Niethammer, D.,** Interferon-neutralizing antibodies in a patient treated with human fibroblast interferon, *Nature (London),* 289, 496, 1981.

146. **Treuner, J., Niethammer, D., Dannecker, G., Hagmann, R., Neff, V., and Hofschneider, P. H.,** Successful treatment of nasopharyngeal carcinoma with interferon, *Lancet,* 1, 817, 1980.

147. **Nakamura, O., Takakura, K., and Kobayashi, S.,** Effect of human interferon-β in the treatment of malignant brain tumors, in *Interferons,* Merigan, T. C. and Friedman, R. C., Eds., Academic Press, New York, 1982, 465.

148. **Quesada, J. R., Gutterman, J. U., and Heysh, E. M.,** Clinical and immunological study of beta interferon by intramuscular route in patients with metastatic breast cancer, *J. Interferon Res.,* 2, 593, 1982.
149. **Mellstedt, H., Ahre, A., Bjorkholm, M., Holm, G., Johansson, B., and Strander, H.,** Interferon therapy in myelomatosis, *Lancet,* 1, 245, 1979.
150. **Merigan, T. C., Sikora, K., Breeden, J. H., Levy, R., and Rosenberg, S. A.,** Preliminary observations on the effect of human leukocyte interferon in non-Hodgkin's lymphoma. IV, *N. Engl. J. Med.,* 299, 1449, 1978.
151. **Priestman, T. J.,** Initial evaluation of human lymphoblastoid interferon in patients with advanced malignant disease, *Lancet,* 2, 113, 1980.
152. **Gutterman, J. U., Fine, S., Quesada, J., Horning, S. J., Levine, J. L., Alexanian, R., Bernhardt, L., Kramer, M., Spiegel, H., Colburn, W., Trown, P., Merigan, R., and Dziewanowska, Z.,** Recombinant leukocyte A interferon: pharmacokinetics, single-dose tolerance, and biologic effects in cancer patients, *Ann. Intern. Med.,* 96, 549, 1981.

Chapter 10

THE 2',5'-OLIGOADENYLATES AND THEIR ANALOGS: BIOCHEMICAL PROBES IN THE TREATMENT OF CANCER AND VIRUS-RELATED DISEASES

Robert J. Suhadolnik

TABLE OF CONTENTS

I. INTRODUCTION

Nature offers a wide variety of compounds that inhibit bacteria, inactivate viruses, and are cytotoxic to tumors. There naturally occurring metabolites have attracted much attention in terms of their mechanism of action. These compounds act in mammalian cells by inhibiting various phases of the cell cycle. With tumor and cancer cells, which are continuously growing and dividing, DNA becomes a critical macromolecule in the use of many antitumor agents that have found successful use in tumor biology. Some naturally occurring drugs act at the level of nucleotide metabolism, some inhibit DNA replication, some interact with the double helix of the DNA to destabilize the DNA by either intercalation or formation of covalent bonds with the purine and pyrimidine bases, some act by cleaving DNA or cleaving the ribosyl moiety, and some act by removal of the purines and/or pyrimidines.

One of the more recently investigated groups of inhibitors of cellular function is the family of proteins, the interferons. Interferons are not only antiviral agents, but also modify cell functions.[1,2] For example, interferon inhibits cell growth and tumor cell proliferation,[3-7] activates natural killer cells,[8,9] modulates immune responses,[8,10-12] increases binuclear cell formation,[5,13] and delays entry of the cell into the S phase of the cell cycle.[14-17] The antiviral function of interferon has been shown to involve the induction of two enzymes: a dsRNA dependent protein kinase and a dsRNA dependent $2',5'$-A_n synthetase.[18] The protein kinase phosphorylates eIF-2 and inhibits protein synthesis. The $2',5'$-A_n synthetase polymerizes ATP into oligonucleotides called $2',5'$-$pppA(pA)_n$. These oligonucleotides are unique in that they have a $2',5'$-phosphodiester bond. One function of these $2',5'$-oligonucleotides involves the activation of a latent endoribonuclease (RNase L). RNase L hydrolyzes mRNA which eventually inhibits protein synthesis. Because interferon is known to have antiviral activity, interest has developed in its use in cancer chemotherapy.[19,20] However, the use of interferon is limited due to delivery to target cells, antibody formation, scarcity, and other adverse effects.[21,22] Because of these limitations, the ideal circumstance would be to bypass interferon by designing antiviral nucleotides with a $2',5'$-phosphodiester bond that would be active in virus-infected cells. With the above as background information, this chapter will be concerned with the role of the $2',5'$-oligoadenylate molecule and the $5'$-dephosphorylated ''core'' molecule, and their analogs in cancer and diseases of viral origin. The relationship between the structure, activity, metabolic stability, and toxicity of the $2',5'$-oligoadenylate molecule will also be described.

Our experience in the biosynthesis of the naturally occurring nucleoside antibiotics and their use in prokaryotic and eukaryotic systems attracted us to the study of structurally modified $2',5'$-oligoadenylates as biological probes of the development of the antiviral/antitumor state of mammalian cells. This chapter will present studies concerning:

1. The enzymatic synthesis of the structurally modified $2',5'$-p_3A_n molecules, $2',5'$-$p_33'dA_3$ and $2',5'$-$p_33'dA_4$, that are metabolically more stable than the naturally occurring $2',5'$-p_3A_n
2. The inhibition of protein synthesis by $2',5'$-$p_33'dA_3$ and $2',5'$-$p_33'dA_4$ in lysates from rabbit reticulocytes, L cells, and fibroblasts
3. The inhibition of transformation of Epstein-Barr virus (EBV)-infected human lymphocytes by the $2',5'$-A_n core and its analogs
4. The binding and metabolism of $2',5'$-A_3 and $2',5'$-$3'dA_3$ cores in lymphocytes and lymphoblasts
5. The augmentation of natural killer cell activity by the $2',5'$-A_n core and its analogs
6. The intracellular accumulation of the cordycepin analog in HeLa cells treated with human fibroblast interferon and dsRNA
7. The activity of the $2',5'$-A_n synthetase in cutaneous T-cell lymphoma cell extracts
8. The inhibition of tumor growth in animals by $2',5'$-$3'dA_3$ core

II. ENZYMATIC SYNTHESIS OF THE CORDYCEPIN ANALOGS OF $2',5'$-p_3A_n, $2',5'$-$p_3 3'dA_3$, AND $2',5'$-$p_3 3'dA_4$, AND INHIBITION OF PROTEIN SYNTHESIS

In view of the reports on the rapid hydrolysis of $2',5'$-p_3A_n by $2',5'$-phosphodiesterase, we reasoned that a minimal structural modification of the ribosyl moiety would be of utmost interest in the design of a functional $2',5'$-oligoadenylate analog that would be metabolically more stable to hydrolysis by $2',5'$-phosphodiesterase, but still retain biological activity. Such a metabolically stable $2',5'$-oligoadenylate molecule could be used as a probe to study the antiviral/antitumor state of the cell, either as the $5'$-triphosphate or as the $5'$-dephosphorylated core nucleotide. There are many ATP analogs that might replace ATP as a substrate for the $2',5'$-A_n synthetase. However, we selected cordycepin $5'$-triphosphate ($3'dATP$). Cordycepin ($3'$-deoxyadenosine) was the first naturally occurring nucleoside antibiotic isolated.[23] It is a cytostatic analog of adenosine.[24,25] The lack of a $3'$-hydroxyl group on $3'$-dATP makes it less likely to be degraded by the $2',5'$-phosphodiesterase present in mammalian cells. In 1965, Suhadolnik and co-workers reported on the isolation of the $2',5'$-phosphodiester bond of cordycepin from H. Ep. #1 cells.[26] Furthermore, they have also reported that replacement of the AMP moiety of NAD^+ by cordycepin monophosphate produced a $3'dNAD^+$ that markedly inhibited DNA repair.[27,28]

When $3'dATP$ was incubated with $2',5'$-A_n synthetase from lysed rabbit reticulocytes bound to poly(rI)·poly(rC)-agarose, $2',5'$-$p_3 3'dA_3$ was isolated following incubation at 30°C for either 5 or 17 hr.[29,30] When incubations were for 5 hr at 37°C, the only product isolated was the tetramer, $2',5'$-$p_3 3'dA_4$[31,32] (Figure 1). The proof of structure of the putative $2',5'$-$p_3 3'dA_3$ and $2',5'$-$p_3 3'dA_4$ was based on comparison with enzymatic and chemical degradations of authentic, chemically synthesized $2',5'$-$p_3 3'dA_3$ and $2',5'$-$p_3 3'dA_4$. When $2',5'$-$p_3 3'dA_4$ (enzymatically or chemically synthesized) was treated with alkali, there was no change in the inhibition of protein synthesis, indicating that there were no adenylate residues present in the molecule.[30,32]

Since our first report on the enzymatic synthesis of $2',5'$-$p_3 3'dA_3$ and its inhibition of protein synthesis,[29,30] other laboratories have expanded studies on the structural modification of the $2',5'$-p_3A_n molecule at the $3'$-terminus or other parts of the molecule.[33-39] Similarly, the synthesis and use of structurally modified $2',5'$-A_n cores has expanded to several other laboratories.[36,39-43]

In previous studies on protein synthesis in lysates from rabbit reticulocytes, polypeptide synthesis was measured by the incorporation of radioactive amino acids into polypeptides, with no concern needed for changes in mRNA concentration and the subsequent effects on the translational machinery. However, in the case of the $2',5'$-oligoadenylate molecule, protein synthesis is inhibited due to the continued hydrolysis of mRNA by the activated $2',5'$-A_n-dependent endoribonuclease. Therefore, it was necessary to establish the optimum concentration of radioactive amino acids added to lysates from rabbit reticulocytes containing $2',5'$-p_3A_n or analogs in order to observe inhibition of translation caused by a limiting amount of mRNA (due to the activated endoribonuclease). A comparison of the inhibition of protein synthesis by $2',5'$-p_3A_4 and $2',5'$-$p_3 3'dA_4$ in lysates from rabbit reticulocytes with differing concentrations of [14C]leucine or valine showed marked differences in inhibition of protein synthesis (Table 1).[32] In lysates I and III, when the concentration of [U-14C]leucine or [U-14C]-valine was 10 and 16 μM, respectively, there was little inhibition of polypeptide synthesis by $2',5'$-p_3A_4 and $2',5'$-$p_3 3'dA_4$ (experiments 1 and 4); however, when the [14C]leucine and [14C]valine concentrations were increased to 90 and 50 μM, respectively, there was a 50% inhibition of protein synthesis at $6.7 \times 10^{-9} M$. With lysate II, experiment 3, there was a 61% inhibition of protein synthesis at $6.7 \times 10^{-10} M$ with $2',5'$-$p_3 3'dA_4$. Under the assay conditions containing 90 μM [U-14C]leucine, $2',5'$-$p_3 3'dA_4$, either enzy-

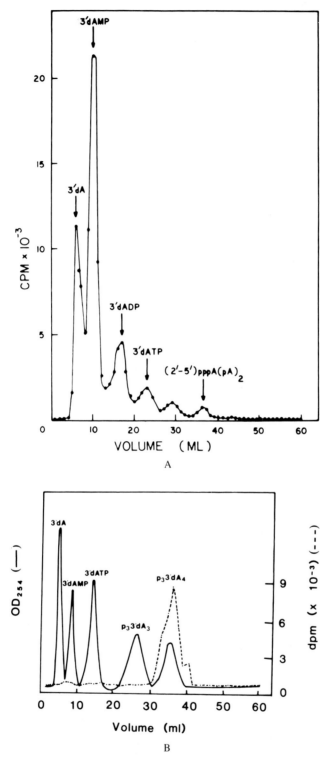

FIGURE 1. DEAE-cellulose chromatographic profile of (A) [³H]2′,5′-p₃3′dA₃ and (B) [³H]2′,5′-p₃3′dA₄ from incubations with [G-³H]3′dATP. The second 1-mℓ fraction displaced from DEAE-cellulose columns with 350 mM KCl was dialyzed, adjusted to 50 mM NaCl, and fractionated on a DEAE-cellulose column as described.[30,32] UV markers are indicated by arrows.

Table 1
INHIBITION OF PROTEIN SYNTHESIS BY
$2',5'$-p_3A_4 AND $2',5'$-$p_3 3'dA_4$ IN LYSATES FROM
RABBIT RETICULOCYTES[32]

Lysate[a] experiment amino acid	I[b]		II[c]	III[d]	
	1	2	3	4	5
	[U-^{14}C]leucine			[U-^{14}C]valine	
Final concentration (μM)	10	90	90	16	50
Specific activity (dpm/pmole)	760	83	83	550	178
pmoles ^{14}C added	300	300	300	1,820	1,820
pmoles Unlabeled amino acid added	0	2,400	2,400	0	3,750
Total pmoles added	300	2,700	2,700	1,820	5,570

pmoles Incorporated Into Polypeptide

Control[e] (no addition)	270	2,090	970	1,460	2,050
$2',5'$-p_3A_4					
$6.7 \times 10^{-9}\ M$	250	850	270	1,280	1,060
$6.7 \times 10^{-10}\ M$	270	1,640	410	1,460	2,010
$6.7 \times 10^{-11}\ M$	270	1,910	980	1,400	2,180
$2',5'$-$p_3 3'dA_4$					
$6.7 \times 10^{-9}\ M$	250	1,040	300	1,390	1,160
$6.7 \times 10^{-10}\ M$	260	1,790	380	1,530	1,880
$6.7 \times 10^{-11}\ M$	260	2,020	860	1,550	2,140

[a] Lysates preincubated with $2',5'$-p_3A_4 or $2',5'$-$p_3 3'dA_4$ at 30°C for 10 min followed by addition of master mix and an additional 60 min incubation. Experiments 1 to 3 according to Doetsch et al.[30]: 30 $\mu \ell$ assay; [U-^{14}C]leucine added: 220,000 dpm. Experiments 4 and 5 according to Safer et al.[87]: 110 $\mu \ell$ assay; [U-^{14}C]valine added: 1×10^6 dpm.

[b] Lysate from Clinical Convenience.

[c] Lysate from phenylhydrazine injection of rabbits.

[d] Lysate, master mix, [U-^{14}C]valine, and $2',5'$-$p_3 3'dA_4$ from Dr. P. Torrence, NIH.

[e] dpm Incorporated into polypeptide per 5 $\mu \ell$ aliquot, experiments 1 to 5: 34,300, 27,870, 12,930, 36,500, and 16,770, respectively.

matically or chemically synthesized, is the most potent inhibitor of protein synthesis in lysates from rabbit reticulocytes. In addition, the enzymatically or chemically synthesized $2',5'$-$p_3 3'dA_4$ binds to and activates the $2',5'$-A_n-dependent endonuclease and degrades VSV mRNA (Figure 2).[32] These data show that the 3'-hydroxyl groups of $2',5'$-p_3A_n are not required for the activation of the $2',5'$-A_n-dependent endonuclease.[32] Several other laboratories have supported the conclusion that the 2'- and 3'-hydroxyl groups of the 2'-terminus of the molecule can be modified without affecting its biological activity.[33-39] $2',5'$-p_3A_n and $2',5'$-$p_3 3'dA_n$ (at $1 \times 10^{-8}\ M$) inhibit protein synthesis in L929 cells and normal human fibroblasts as determined by the calcium phosphate coprecipitation technique (Figure 3).[44]

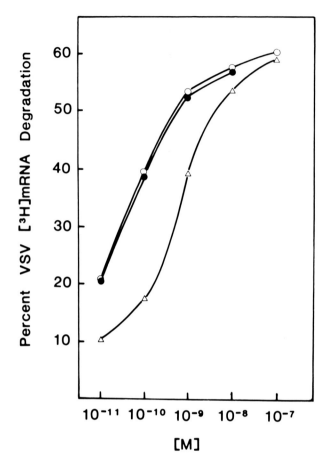

FIGURE 2.   VSV [³H]mRNA hydrolysis by 2′,5′-p₃A₄ and 2′,5′-p₃3′dA₄.
Assays were done as described.³² Chemically synthesized 2′,5′-p₃3′dA₄.
○—○; enzymatically synthesized 2′,5′-p₃3′dA₄, ●—●; 2′,5′-p₃A₄,
△—△. In control assays (nuclease with no addition), 80% of the VSV
[³H]mRNA was recovered.

When $2',5'\text{-}p_3 3'dA_4$ was added to protein synthesizing cell-free extracts of L929 cells there was also an inhibition of protein synthesis, demonstrating that the inhibition of protein synthesis by the cordycepin analog is not limited to lysates from rabbit reticulocytes. At 16 μM [U-¹⁴C]valine, the inhibition of protein synthesis is marginal at best, in agreement with the recent report of Torrence and co-workers.⁴⁵ At low concentrations of amino acids, the results are a reflection of the rate of protein synthesis and are not detectable by mRNA availability. However, at higher concentrations of amino acids (i.e., 63 μM) where there is an increase in translational efficiency, we observe an increased inhibition of protein synthesis by $2',5'\text{-}p_3A_4$ and $2',5'\text{-}p_3 3'dA_4$ (Figure 4).⁸⁹ The increased inhibition indicates that at 63 μM [U-¹⁴C]leucine the rate of protein synthesis is governed by the availability of mRNA.

We now know that the rate of protein synthesis or the efficiency of translation is regulated by the rate of initiation (Table 1, Figure 5). The rate of initiation can be regulated by the rate of formation of either the ternary complex or by binding of mRNA to the 43S initiation complex. Therefore, whenever mRNA is regulated by the activation of the 2′,5′-A dependent endoribonuclease due to the presence of $2',5'\text{-}p_3A_4$ or $2',5'\text{-}p_3 3'dA_4$, protein synthesis may be determined by the binding of the mRNA to the 43S complex. These results will require more detailed studies to clarify the importance of the concentration of the limiting amino acid in the inhibition of protein synthesis by $2',5'\text{-}p_3A_n$ and its analogs.

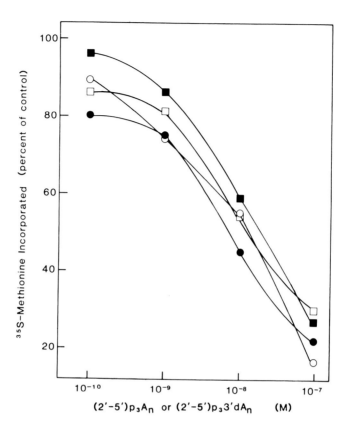

FIGURE 3.   Inhibition of protein synthesis by $2',5'$-p_3A_n and $2',5'$-$p_33'dA_n$ in mouse L929 cells. Inhibition of protein synthesis by $2',5'$-p_3A_3, ●—●; $2',5'$-p_3A_4, ○—○; $2',5'$-$p_33'dA_3$, ■—■; and $2',5'$-$p_33'dA_4$, □—□, was determined in intact L929 cells[44] using the calcium phosphate coprecipitation technique as described by Hovanessian and Wood.[88] Control cultures were treated with calcium phosphate without oligonucleotides and the incorporation of [^{34}S]methionine (2 μCi/assay) into control cultures was taken as 100%.

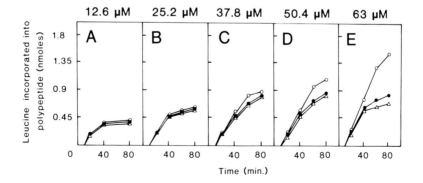

FIGURE 4.   Inhibition of protein synthesis by $2',5'$-p_3A_4 and $2',5'$-$p_33'dA_4$ with increasing concentrations of amino acid in lysates from rabbit reticulocytes.[89] Protein synthesis assays were as described,[30] with varying concentrations of [U-^{14}C]leucine as indicated above each panel; $2',5'$-p_3A_4 or $2',5'$-$p_33'dA_4$ were present at 3×10^{-8} M (concentration expressed as AMP or 3'dAMP equivalents); $2',5'$-p_3A_4, ●—●; $2',5'$-$p_33'dA_4$, △—△; control, ○—○.

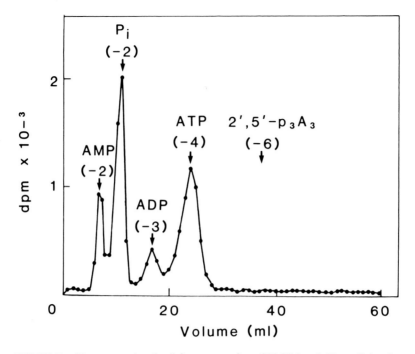

FIGURE 5.   Chromatography of cell-free extracts from C85-5C lymphoblasts 12 hr after treatment with [^{32}P]2′,5′-A$_3$ core. The cytoplasmic trichloroacetic acid-soluble extract from 2′,5′-[^{32}P]A$_3$ core-treated C85-5C lymphoblasts was applied to a DEAE cellulose column and the nucleotides displaced as described.[30] Arrows indicate displacement of charge markers.

III. INHIBITION OF TRANSFORMATION OF EPSTEIN-BARR VIRUS-INFECTED LYMPHOCYTES BY 2′,5′-A$_3$ CORE AND 2′,5′-3′dA$_3$ CORE

Because of the report by Revel and co-workers[46] that mitogenesis of lymphocytes was inhibited by 2′,5′-A$_n$ core following concanavalin A treatment, we reasoned that the 2′,5′-A$_n$ core and its analogs might be excellent probes for the study of the inhibition of transformation of virus-infected cells and the inhibition of virus replication. For these studies, we selected the Epstein-Barr virus (EBV)-infected lymphocyte. Epstein-Barr virus is a lymphotropic dsDNA virus of the herpes group.[47] EBV infection is the cause of infectious mononucleosis and has been implicated as the cause of three human cancers.[47] When lymphocytes are infected with EBV, they are morphologically transformed into immortalized lymphoblasts. One advantage to the use of EBV-infected lymphocytes is that we observed that the lymphocytes do not require any pretreatment (i.e., calcium phosphate coprecipitation or permeabilization) to measure the effect of the 2′,5′-A$_n$ cores and 2′,5′-A$_n$ core analogs. When the 5′-dephosphorylated 2′,5′-A$_n$ cores were added to EBV-infected lymphocytes, there was a dose-dependent inhibition of EBV-induced DNA synthesis by 2′,5′-A$_3$, 2′,5′-A$_4$, and 2′,5′-3′dA$_3$ cores (Table 2).[48] The transformed centers assay was also used to determine the effect of the 2′,5′-A$_3$ core and 2′,5′-3′dA$_3$ core on EBV-induced transformation. The 2′,5′-A$_n$ and 2′,5′-3′dA$_3$ cores inhibited the appearance of transformed colonies.[48] Of interest was the observation that whereas the naturally occurring 2′,5′-A$_3$ and 2′,5′-A$_4$ cores were toxic to Raji and BJA-B lymphoblasts, the 2′,5′-3′dA$_3$ core was not cytotoxic. More recently, Sharma and Goswami,[39] have extended the 2′,5′-A$_n$ core studies. They reported that vaccinia virus replication is inhibited by 2′,5′-A$_n$ and 2′,5′-3′dA$_3$ cores. Furthermore, Imbach et al.,[40] Eppstein et al.,[36] and Jurovčik and Smrt[49] have also shown that 2′,5′-A$_n$ and 2′,5′-A$_n$ core analogs inhibit DNA and protein synthesis in mammalian cells without any pretreatment (i.e., calcium phosphate coprecipitation or permeabilization).

Table 2
EFFECT OF IFN-β AND CORE 2′,5′-OLIGONUCLEOTIDES ON SPONTANEOUS AND EBV-INDUCED DNA SYNTHESIS IN LYMPHOCYTES[51]

| | [³H]Thymidine incorporation | | | |
| | Infected | | Uninfected | |
Treatment	cpm	ratio[a]	cpm	ratio
None (control)	17,450	1.00	7,390	1.00
IFN-β				
10 units/mℓ	15,000	0.86	9,090	1.22
100 units/mℓ	11,990	0.60	10,460	1.41
250 units/mℓ	10,420	0.60	16,550	2.23
2′,5′-A₃ core				
25 μM	7,950	0.45	5,050	0.68
50 μM	4,013	0.23	4,411	0.59
200 μM	1,770	0.10	1,870	0.25
2′,5′-A₄ core				
5 μM	10,580	0.60	6,190	0.84
25 μM	6,460	0.37	3,560	0.48
100 μM	740	0.04	1,560	0.21
2′,5′-3′dA₃ core				
5 μM	17,790	1.02	7,420	1.00
100 μM	13,380	0.77	7,760	1.03
200 μM	8,150	0.47	11,580	1.56

[a] Ratio of treated to untreated cells.

In contrast, Ts'o and co-workers[34] reported that the $2',5'$-A₃ core did not inhibit human HF926 fibroblast cells treated with calcium phosphate. However, Williams and Kerr,[50] using permeabilized BHK cells with ATP, GTP, and creatine phosphate, reported an inhibition of protein synthesis. They suggested that these cells convert the $2',5'$-A₃ core to the triphosphate by rephosphorylation. Furthermore, some researchers,[43,49,50] using either permeabilized or untreated cells in culture, suggested that the antimitogenic effect of $2',5'$-Aₙ core and analogs was inhibiting DNA and protein sythesis by rephosphorylation at the $5'$-hydroxyl group.

A most significant finding is that the $2',5'$-A₃ core and the $2',5'$-3′dA₃ core also inhibit tobacco mosaic virus replication in tobacco plants.[41,42] These reports are unique in that the $2',5'$-Aₙ core nucleotides are active in both animal and plant systems. However, this need not mean that the antiviral mechanisms are the same in both systems.

To determine the mechanism by which the $2',5'$-A₃ and $2',5'$-3′dA₃ cores inhibited EBV-induced transformation, we designed experiments to determine if the $2',5'$-A₃ and $2',5'$-3′dA₃ cores inhibit the expression of Epstein-Barr virus-associated nuclear antigen (EBNA) in EBV-infected human peripheral blood leukocytes.[51] Human leukocyte interferon (IFN-α) also inhibited EBNA expression. We observed that the $2',5'$-A₃ core and $2',5'$-3′dA₃ core inhibited EBNA formation.[51]

In a preliminary study, we have shown that the addition of $2',5'$-[³²P]A₃ core, if taken up by lymphocytes, is not rephosphorylated at the $5'$-position (Figure 5).[52] Whereas only inorganic ³²P-phosphate was observed in the TCA-soluble cytoplasmic extracts of lymphocytes treated with $2',5'$-[³²P]A₃ core, about 1.3% of the $2',5'$-[³²P]3′dA₃ core was isolated from the TCA-soluble cytoplasmic extracts of lymphoblasts as the unmodified $2',5'$-3′dA₃ core.[52] It is not known if the ³²P isolated represents true uptake or binding to membrane receptors. These findings do suggest, however, that the $2',5'$-Aₙ cores are functioning by a mechanism different from interferon.

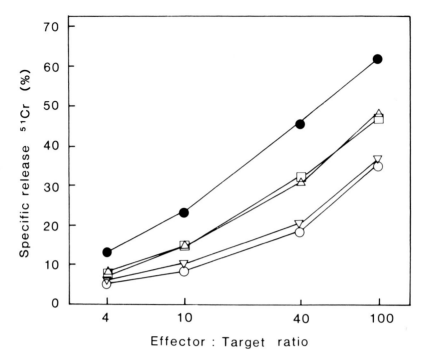

FIGURE 6. Increased tumoricidal activity of 2',5'-A₃ core, □—□; 2',5'-3'dA₃ core, △—△; 3',5'-A₃ core, ▽—▽; and IFN-α, ●—● (control, ○—○) on natural killer cell activity.[62] Peripheral blood lymphocytes were treated for 1 hr with the 2',5'-oligo nucleotides (50 μ*M*) or IFN-α (500 units/m*ℓ*), washed and assayed for cytolytic activity against K562 cells in a 4-hr ⁵¹Cr release assay.

IV. EFFECT OF 2',5'-A₃ CORE AND 2',5'-3'dA₃ CORE ON AUGMENTATION OF NATURAL KILLER CELL ACTIVITY

One of the effects of interferon is to augment natural killer (NK) cell activity directed towards tumor and virus-infected target cells.[53] Human NK cells are Fc receptor-bearing lymphocytes with a low affinity for binding sheep erythrocytes. They show spontaneous tumoridical activity against a variety of tumor cell lines in the absence of any apparent immunization.[54] There is considerable evidence to suggest that NK cells are important in the mechanism of the immune surveillance against cancer.[54-58] Furthermore, NK cells can kill EBV-infected target cells.[59] Sullivan et al.[60] have reported that patients with X-linked lymphoproliferative syndrome who suffer from chronic EBV infection have defective NK cell activity. Therefore, because of our studies on the inhibition of transformation of EBV-infected lymphocytes by the 2',5'-Aₙ cores, we determined the effect of the 2',5'-Aₙ cores on the lytic activity of NK cells. We have been able to show that the 2',5'-A₃ core and 2',5'-3'dA₃ core, but not the 3',5'-A₃ core, cause a consistent augmentation of the lytic activity of human NK cells as measured in a 4-hr⁵¹ Cr release microtoxicity assay.[61,62] K562 cells derived from a patient with acute myelogenous leukemia served as target cells because of their susceptibility to lysis by NK cells[63] (Figure 6).

V. INTRACELLULAR ACCUMULATION OF THE CORDYCEPIN ANALOG, 2',5'-p₃3'dAₙ, IN HeLa CELLS TREATED WITH HUMAN FIBROBLAST INTERFERON AND dsRNA

Because of the increased metabolic stability of the 2',5'-p₃3'dA₃ analog, we reasoned that it might be possible to observe an intracellular accumulation of 2',5'-p₃3'dAₙ in mam-

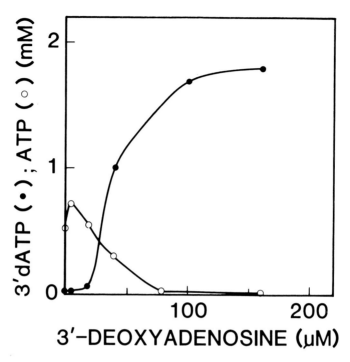

FIGURE 7.   Changes in intracellular concentrations of ATP, ○—○, and 3'dATP, ●—●, in HeLa cells treated with deoxycoformycin (2 μM) and cordycepin (80 μM).[64]

malian cells. The accumulation of such a metabolically stable analog of $2',5'$-p_3A_n could be useful in the study of viral infection of cells, with the eventual goal of designing a drug that could be a chemotherapeutic agent that would inhibit virus infections and cancer. When 2 μM deoxycoformycin and 80 μM cordycepin were added to HeLa cells, there was an increase in the intracellular concentration of 3'dATP to 1.7 mM, while the ATP concentration decreased to a level too low to detect by HPLC (Figure 7).[64] Deoxycoformycin was added to inhibit the deamination of cordycepin. The decrease in intracellular concentration of ATP might be explained by the report of Bagnara and Hershfield.[65] They reported that increased concentrations of 2'dAMP in human lymphoblastoid cells decreased intacellular ATP due to the inhibition of *de novo* synthesis of ATP and the subsequent hydrolysis of AMP to hypoxanthine. The hypoxanthine is then excreted into the medium. When [8-³H]3'-deoxyadenosine (80μM) was added to HeLa cells treated with human fibroblast interferon (200 units/mℓ for 17 hr) followed by 200 μg/mℓ of poly(rI)·poly(rC) for 3 hr and deoxycoformycin (2 μM), $2',5'$-$p_3$3'dA_n was isolated by displacement with 350 mM KCl buffer from DEAE-cellulose columns, as described.[30] Synthesis of $2',5'$-$p_3$3'dA_n was further verified by dialysis of the 350 mM KCl eluant and enzyme hydrolysis (SVPD, BAP, T2 RNase) as previously described.[30] When $2',5'$-$p_3$3'dA_n of known concentration was added to lysates from rabbit reticulocytes, protein synthesis was inhibited. The antiviral state, based on plaque forming units per milliliter, decreased 600-fold when compared to untreated HeLa cells. Furthermore, the treated cells showed an induced $2',5'$-A_n synthetase. Most important was the observation that the treated HeLa cells were viable as determined by Trypan blue exclusion. Although the intracellular accumulation of $2',5'$-$p_3$3'dA_n may not represent the ideal analog of the $2',5'$-p_3A_n molecule to accumulate in mammalian cells, this is a new approach to the intracellular accumulation of a metabolically stable, structurally modified and biological active $2',5'$-p_3A_n analog to be used in the study of the regulation of virus protein synthesis, virus replication, and prevention of virus diseases and cancer.

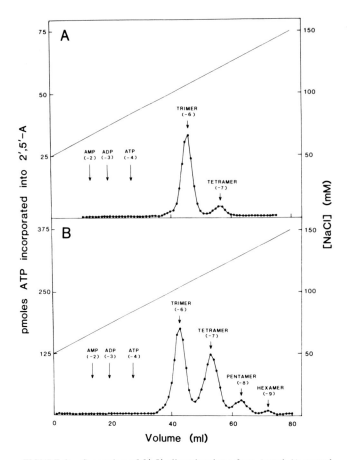

FIGURE 8. Separation of 2′,5′-oligoadenylates from (panel A) normal and (panel B) cutaneous T-cell lymphoma PBMC extracts.[67] Oligonucleotides displaced from DEAE cellulose columns by 350 mM KCl were separated as described.[30] Charge markers added to the samples are indicated with arrows.

VI. 2′,5′-A$_n$ SYNTHETASE FROM CUTANEOUS T-CELL LYMPHOMA: BIOSYNTHESIS, CHARACTERIZATION, AND INHIBITION OF PROTEIN SYNTHESIS

Retroviruses have been implicated as the agents that cause leukemias, lymphomas, and sarcomas in animals.[66] Although the presence of retrovirus particles has recently been demonstrated in T-cell lymphomas, and there is good evidence that these leukemias and lymphomas are viral in origin, in a majority of cutaneous T-cell lymphomas there is no detectable retrovirus particle. Therefore, we have completed a detailed biochemical analysis of cell-free extracts from peripheral blood mononuclear cells (PBMC) from cutaneous T-cell lymphoma blood samples by studying the activity of the 2′,5′-A$_n$ synthetase, quantity of 2′,5′-p$_3$A$_n$ synthesized, and the molecular size of the 2′,5′-p$_3$A$_n$ synthesized in cell-free extracts of mammalian cells compared to normal PBMC. The purpose of this study was to establish if there was a biochemical relationship between the cancerous state of the cutaneous T-cell lymphoma patient and the antiviral state as determined by 2′,5′-A$_n$ synthetase activity. We have shown that there is a tenfold increase in the synthesis of 2′,5′-p$_3$A$_n$ in PBMC cell-free extracts from cutaneous T-cell lymphoma samples compared to cell-free extracts from normal samples.[67] To determine the molecular size and percent composition of the 2′,5′-oligoadenylates synthesized, gradient DEAE-cellulose chromatography was performed (Figure 8).[67]

With PBMC cell-free extracts from normals, only the trimer and tetramer were isolated, whereas in the PBMC cell-free extracts from T-cell lymphomas the trimer, tetramer, pentamer, and hexamer $2',5'-p_3A_n$ were isolated. Again, there was a tenfold increase in the total $2',5'$-oligoadenylates isolated from cutaneous T-cell lymphoma samples compared with normals. The proof of structure of the $2',5'$-oligoadenylates following biosynthesis from ATP was determined by classical digestion with BAP, SVPD, and T2 RNase, followed by chromatography.[30] To determine if this increased synthesis of $2',5'-p_3A_n$ in PBMC cell-free extracts from cutaneous T-cell lymphomas represented a true biological effect, the binding to and activation of the latent $2',5'-A_n$-dependent endoribonuclease, hydrolysis of mRNA, and inhibition of protein synthesis in lysates from rabbit reticulocytes was studied. When a 2500-fold dilution of the $2',5'-p_3A_n$ displaced by 350 mM KCl from PBMC of cutaneous T-cell lymphoma samples was added to lysates from rabbit reticulocyte protein synthesis assays there was an inhibition of protein synthesis, whereas there was no inhibition of protein synthesis by a 2500-fold dilution of the $2',5'-p_3A_n$ from PBMC cell-free extracts from normal samples.[67] Cell-free extracts from lymphocytes of patients with psoriasis showed no elevation of the $2',5'-p_3A_n$ synthetase activity. While these studies were in progress, proviral DNA was found in adult T-cell leukemia patients.[68] Cloning and sequence analysis of the adult T-cell leukemia provirus DNA suggests that adult T-cell leukemia is unlike all known avian, murine, or primate retroviruses except bovine leukemia virus.[69,70]

Our results show that whereas the proviral DNA was not isolated from the PBMC samples obtained from patients with cutaneous T-cell lymphoma, we were able to determine dramatic differences in the biochemistry of cells from cutaneous T-cell lymphoma PBMC as measured by the concentration of the $2',5'$-oligoadenylates synthesized and the type and size of the $2',5'$-oligoadenylate molecule. Therefore, measuring increased synthetase activity by examining the $2',5'$-oligoadenylate profile may be a reliable method to substantiate viral etiology in this human T-cell lymphoma virus that cannot be detected by immunological methods. Finally, when PBMC cell-free extracts from a patient with stage IV cutaneous T-cell lymphoma were examined after treatment with interferon, the tenfold elevation of $2',5'-A_n$ synthetase decreased to normal levels.[67]

VII. INHIBITION OF CELL PROLIFERATION FOLLOWING TREATMENT OF HeLa CELLS WITH HUMAN FIBROBLAST INTERFERON

Interferons are not only known for their antiviral action, but also for their ability to inhibit cell growth and tumor cell proliferation.[1,2] In order to more clearly understand how interferon inhibits cell proliferation, we have examined thymidine nucleoside/nucleotide metabolism, DNA synthesis, DNA processing, and changes in the chromatin structure of HeLa cells treated with human fibroblast interferon. When interferon was added at the S/G_2 boundary of the synchronized HeLa cells maintained on 7% serum, interferon had a mitogenic effect (Figure 9).[71] The mitogenic effect of interferon has also been observed in interferon-treated normal uninfected lymphocytes.[48] The addition of interferon at the S/G_2 boundary of the cell cycle resulted in a marked increased in the incorporation of tracer amounts of [^{3}H]thymidine into the trichloroacetic acid precipitate of HeLa cells. When the interferon was added at the G_1/S boundary (Figure 9, solid arrow), there was no increased incorporation of [^{3}H]thymidine into the DNA at the time of the second round of cell division. To establish that HeLa cells maintained on 7% serum were not altered from cells maintained on 10% serum, the antiviral state was examined by determining the antiviral activity and the induction of $2',5'-A_n$ synthetase. The antiviral activity of the interferon-treated HeLa cells maintained on 7% serum was the same as for cells maintained on 10% serum. Furthermore, the induction of $2',5'-A_n$ synthetase in the synchronized HeLa cells maintained on 7% serum was similar to that of cells maintained on 10% serum.

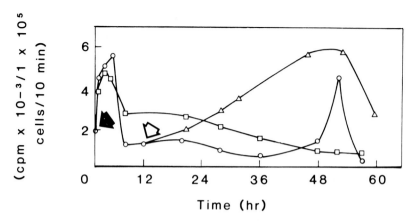

FIGURE 9.   Effect of IFN-β on the incorporation of [³H]thymidine into TCA-precipitates of synchronously grown HeLa cells.[71] HeLa cells maintained on 7% serum were synchronized by a double block with 1 m*M* hydroxyurea and resuspended in fresh medium (2 × 10⁵ cells/ m*ℓ*). IFN-β (100 units/m*ℓ*) was added at either the early S phase (solid arrow) or at the S/ G₂ boundary (open arrow) 12 hr after release from the second hydroxyurea block; ○—○, untreated; □—□, IFN-β added at early S phase; △—△, IFN-β added at S/G₂ boundary.

At first appearance, the increased incorporation of [³H]thymidine into the DNA of intact HeLa cells and the increased incorporation of [³H]dTTP into the DNA of nuclei isolated from interferon-treated cells appeared to be due to a stimulation of DNA synthesis. However, when the intracellular pool was flooded with excess thymidine, there was no difference in DNA synthesis between the untreated and interferon-treated cells.[71] To reconcile the differences in the thymidine nucleoside/nucleotide metabolism and increased DNA synthesis in the interferon treated cells, we examined the processing of the newly synthesized DNA strands in the HeLa cells. The DNA synthesized in interferon-treated cells was replicative, as measured by cesium chloride buoyant density centrifugation. However, size analysis of the newly synthesized DNA of the interferon-treated HeLa cells showed an accumulation of low-molecular-weight DNA (Figure 10).[71] Apparently, the synchronously grown HeLa cells to which interferon was added at the S/G₂ boundary can synthesize DNA; however, either the processing of the Okazaki fragments (lagging strand), or the repair process of the leading strand, is inhibited in such a way that following excision of a modified base, i.e., dUMP, reinsertion of dTTP to synthesize longer DNA strands does not occur. These findings are supported by the following three studies with interferon-treated cells. Lewis et al.[72] showed that there is a requirement for thymidine kinase for interferon action. Miyoshi et al.,[73] using 5-fluorouracil in combination with interferon, suggested that nucleotide pools in HeLa cells might be altered by interferon. Furthermore, the studies of Goulian et al.[74] suggest that the misincorporation of dUMP into DNA in place of dTMP may be occurring in interferon-treated cells because of decreased dTTP. Once the dUMP is removed from the DNA, the ligation process cannot occur due to a lack of dTTP. Evidence that the decreased *de novo* synthesis of dTMP from dUMP could be attributed to a decreased tetrahydrofolate one-carbon pool is based on the report of deFerra and Baglioni.[75] They demonstrated that VSV-infected HeLa cells treated with interferon produced VSV mRNA lacking the 7-methyl group in the 5′-terminal guanosine. They showed that there was an intracellular accumulation of *S*-adenosyl homocysteine in these cells. *S*-adenosyl homocysteine accumulates when 5-methyltetrahydrofolate cannot transfer its methyl group to B₁₂ coenzyme to form methyl-B₁₂. When this occurs, homocysteine cannot be methylated to form methionine. The accumulation of 5-methyltetrahydrofolate would prevent thymidylate synthetase from catalzing the *de novo* methylation of dUMP to dTMP because of an insufficient supply of N^5,N^{10}-methylenetetrahydrofolate. Clemens and co-workers[76,77] have also reported on the accu-

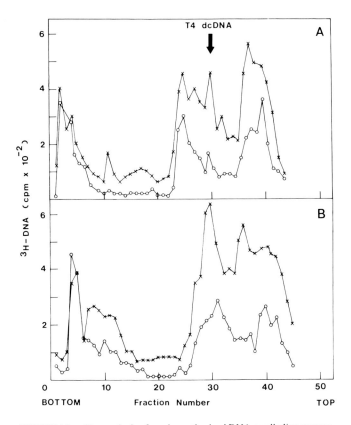

FIGURE 10.   Size analysis of newly synthesized DNA on alkaline sucrose gradients.[71] Synchronously grown HeLa cells were treated with [^{14}C]thymidine for 11 hr during the S phase (O—O). The [^{14}C]thymidine in the medium was removed by centrifugation and the cells were resuspended with fresh medium to 2×10^5 cells/mℓ and divided in half. Panel A: one half of the cells was not treated with IFN-β; Panel B: one half of the cells was treated with IFN-β (100 units/mℓ);13 hr later, 3×10^6 cells (treated and untreated) were centrifuged, resuspended in fresh medium, pulsed with [^{3}H]thymidine, and chased (x—x). Lysed cells were treated with protease K and size analysis of the newly synthesized DNA was performed on alkaline sucrose gradients. The arrow shows the position of a [^{3}H]T4 dcDNA, single stranded, 56×10^6 daltons.

mulation of small "Okazaki fragments" of newly synthesized DNA in interferon-treated Daudi cells. In conjunction with the effect of interferon on DNA synthesis, we have also observed changes in the chromatin structure as measured by circular dichroism and by a 70% decrease in the postsynthetic modification of nuclear proteins as measured by poly(ADP-ribosylation).[71] Using 3T3 cells and mouse interferon, Butt and Sreevalsan[78] also showed an inhibition of the automodification of the poly(ADP-ribose) synthetase. The decrease in the molar ellipticity of the circular dichroism spectra of the chromatin observed following interferon treatment of HeLa cells represents a more condensed chromatin structure than is observed in untreated cells. Our findings are in agreement with previous circular dichroism studies by Fasman and co-workers,[79] who reported that a more negative molar ellipticity in circular dichroism spectra indicates a more condensed chromatin structure. Ishimi et al.[80] reported that a more relaxed chromatin structure is associated with an increased molar ellipticity. The decreased ADP-ribosylation, decreased molar ellipticity indicating a more condensed chromatin conformation, and an increase in the newly synthesized low-molecular-weight DNA may all be related to the antiproliferative properties of interferon.

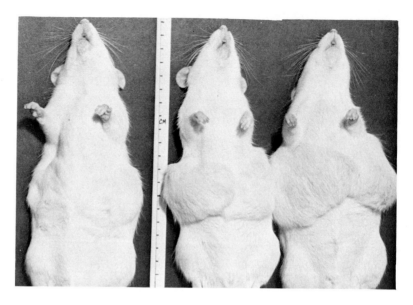

FIGURE 11.   Photographs of rats bearing Swarm chondrosarcoma: effect of treatment with
$2',5'-3'dA_3$ core. Rats treated with (left to right): 5 μmol/100 g body weight per tumor of
$2',5'-3'dA_3$ core, 0.5 μmol/100 g body weight per tumor of $2',5'-3'dA_3$ core, and untreated.
Photograph taken of anesthetized rats 22 days after treatment with oligonucleotide.

VIII. INHIBITION OF SWARM CHONDROSARCOMA TUMOR GROWTH IN RATS BY 2′,5′-3′-DEOXYADENYLATE TRIMER CORE

In view of the inhibition of transformation of EBV-infected lymphocytes and the antimitogenic effects in tissue culture by the $2',5'-A_n$ and $2',5'-3'dA_3$ core, it was critical to
determine the effects of the $2',5'-A_3$ core and analogs on rapidly proliferating tumor tissues
in the intact animal.

Because we were able to show that the $2',5'-A_3$ and $2',5'-3'dA_3$ core inhibit transformation
of EBV-infected lymphocytes, and because the intratumoral injection of cyclic $3',5'$-nu-
cleotide analogs is known to inhibit tumor growth,[81-83] we reasoned that the direct injection
of the $2',5'-3'dA_3$ core might be effective in inhibiting growth of an animal tumor. We
selected Swarm chondrosarcoma for these studies. Swarm chondrosarcoma is a solid cartilage
tumor derived from a naturally occurring osteochondrosarcoma.[84] It is a well-differentiated,
stable, transplantable, naturally occurring tumor well suited for in vivo or in vitro studies
with tumor pieces.

When $2',5'-3'dA_3$ core was injected intratumorally into rats bearing Swarm chondrosarcoma at a concentration of 0.5 or 5 μmol/100 g body weight per tumor, there was a marked
inhibition of tumor growth in the tumor-bearing animals (Figure 11).[85,86] A study of the
tumor growth vs. time indicated that there was a regression of tumor growth for 14 days
following the injection of $2',5'-3'dA_3$ core. After 14 days, the inhibitory effect of $2',5'-
3'dA_3$ core was no longer observed (Figure 12). In control experiments with $2',5'-A_3$ and
$3',5'-A_3$ core, there was no inhibition of tumor growth. When cordycepin or 3′dAMP (5
μmol/100 g body weight per tumor) was injected intratumorally, there was an inhibition of
tumor growth, but not as pronounced an effect as observed with the $2',5'-3'dA_3$ core. The
inhibition of tumor growth of the animals treated with cordycepin and 3′dAMP suggests
that the inhibition observed with $2',5'-3'dA_3$ core may be due to its metabolic products,
cordycepin and 3′dAMP. However, whereas $2',5'-3'dA_3$ core inhibits DNA and protein
synthesis, cordycepin and 3′dAMP do not act by the same mechanism.[86,87] To determine
whether the $2',5'-3'dA_3$ core following intratumoral injection was distributed intact through-

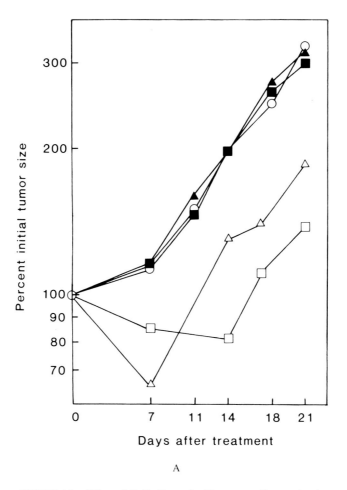

A

FIGURE 12. Effect of 2′,5′-oligonucleotide cores on Swarm chondro-sarcoma growth. Rats bearing bilateral subcutaneous chondrosarcoma tumors were treated by intratumoral injection. The doses (expressed as μmoles per 100 g body weight per tumor) were administered 6 days after tumor implantation. Equal volumes of saline were injected into control tumors. Tumor size was measured along the longitudinal axis of the tumor. Results are expressed as percent of the initial tumor size at the time of treatment (control = 2.5 cm). (A) Effect of 2′,5′-oligonucleotide cores injected bilaterally. Control, ○—○; 2′,5′-3′dA$_3$ core (0.5 μmol), △—△; 2′,5′-3′-dA$_3$ core (5 μmol), □—□; 2′,5′-A$_3$ core (5 μmol), ▲—▲; 3′,5′-A$_3$ core (5 μmol), ■—■. (B) Effect of 2′,5′-3′dA$_3$ core injected at a single tumor site. Control, ○—○; 2′,5′-3′dA$_3$ core (5 μmol), △—△.

out the animal, the following experiments were done. Seven days after implantation of 2 g of tumor tissue bilaterally, 5 μmol/100 g body weight per tumor of 2′,5′-3′dA$_3$ core was injected into one tumor. The inhibition of tumor growth was limited to the site of injection; the second tumor grew as in the untreated animals. These data strongly suggest that the 2′,5′-3′dA$_3$ core, once injected into the tumor site, is not distributed to peripheral tissues. When a second dose of 2′,5′-3′dA$_3$ core was injected into tumors 22 days after implantation, there was no inhibition of growth. This also indicates that there is a time dependence in that once the tumor is established and growing, its growth cannot be controlled. The extended effect of the 2′,5′-3′dA$_3$ core on tumor growth indicates that the effect of the 2′,5′-3′dA$_3$ core is immediate and irreversible for at least 14 days. The data also indicate that if the inhibition of tumor growth is due to the intracellular or extracellular metabolism of the 2′,5′-3′dA$_3$ core to cordycepin, 3′dAMP, or 3′dATP, these metabolic products are not distributed

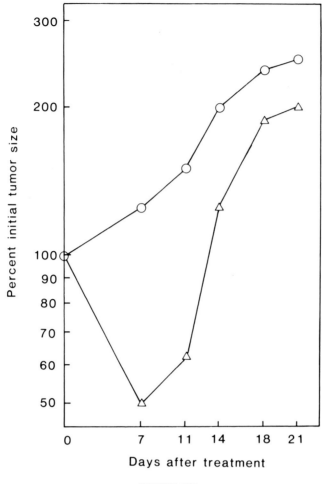

FIGURE 12B.

throughout the animal in sufficient concentrations to affect the growth of the noninjected tumor. Because of the dramatic effects of the $2',5'$-$3'dA_3$ core on the inhibition of a naturally occurring animal tumor, studies are currently underway with tumors caused by chemicals or ionizing radiation.

The results presented here clearly demonstrate that the structurally modified $2',5'$-oligoadenylate core molecule (i.e., $2',5'$-$3'dA_3$ core) is a potent inhibitor of tumor growth in tumor-bearing animals. Moreover, as we found in tissue culture studies, the $2',5'$-$3'dA_3$ core is not toxic to the animal, nor is it distributed throughout the animal. These results emphasize the potential value of the $2',5'$-oligoadenylate molecule in the treatment of cancer or diseases of viral origin. The major impact of these findings may be in determining whether $2',5'$-$3'dA_3$ core acts in the intact cell, acts by binding to cell membrane receptors, or acts by alternate mechanisms.

IX. CONCLUSION

Although the treatment of cancer is often successful following chemotherapy, it must be kept in mind that a single tumor might be a mixture of subpopulations of cells that differ in their susceptibility of drug therapy as well as their ability to metastasize to other organs in the body. Therefore, because cancer actually may be a combination of diseases, the ultimate goal is to design molecules to effectively treat all of these disease states. One such molecule could be the $2',5'$-oligoadenylate molecule, synthesized in the mammalian cell in response to interferon. This molecule could prevent virus DNA from being incorporated into the human genome. This chapter has described the exciting progress in the use of the $2',5'$-oligoadenylate molecule and its analogs. These structurally modified $2',5'$-oligoadenylates have contributed greatly to our understanding of the regulation of virus infections. It is interesting that, once more, the naturally occurring nucleoside antibiotics have proven useful biological probes in these complex cellular processes.

ACKNOWLEDGMENTS

The author expresses appreciation to research colleagues who have played vital roles in the studies reported here: P. Black, A. Q. Dang, Y. Devash, P. W. Doetsch, M. B. Flick, J. Gabriel, E. E. Henderson, C. Lee, J. D. Mosca, W. Pfleiderer, N. L. Reichenbach, Y. Sawada, I. Sela, D. H. Willis, Jr., and J. M. Wu. The additional assistance of N. L. Reichenbach in the preparation of this manuscript is gratefully acknowledged. Research in this laboratory has been supported in part by research grants GM-26134 from the National Institutes of Health and PCM-8111752 from the National Science Foundation, training grant AM-07162 from the U.S. Public Health Service, Biomedical Research Support Grant 507-RR05417 from the Division of Research Resources, National Institutes of Health, and federal work study awards.

REFERENCES

1. **Pestka, S., Ed.,** Interferons, part A, *Meth. Enzymol.*, 78, 1981.
2. **Pestka, S., Ed.,** Interferons, part B, *Meth. Enzymol.*, 79, 1981.
3. **Gewert, D. R., Shah, S., and Clemens, M. J.,** Inhibition of cell division by interferon: changes in the transport and intracellular metabolism of thymidine in human lymphoblastoid (Daudi) cells, *Eur. J. Biochem.*, 116, 487, 1981.
4. **Gresser, I.,** On the varied biologic effects of interferon, *Cell. Immunol.*, 34, 406, 1977.
5. **Panniers, L. R. V. and Clemens, M. J.,** Inhibition of cell division by interferon: changes in cell cycle characteristics and in morphology of Ehrlich ascites tumour cells in culture, *J. Cell Sci.*, 48, 259, 1981.
6. **Paucker, K., Cantell, K., and Henle, W.,** Quantitative studies on viral interference in suspended L cells. III. Effect of interfering viruses and interferon on the growth rate of cells, *Virology*, 17, 324, 1962.
7. **Pfeffer, L. M., Murpy, J. S., and Tamm, I.,** Interferon effects on the growth and division of human fibroblasts, *Exp. Cell Res.*, 121, 111, 1979.
8. **Gresser, I., Brouty-Boye, D., Thomas, M.-T., and Macieira-Coelho, A.,** Interferon and cell division. I. Inhibition of the multiplication of mouse leukemia L 1210 cells *in vitro* by interferon preparations, *Proc. Natl. Acad. Sci. U.S.A.*, 66, 1052, 1970.
9. **Herberman, R. B., Ortaldo, J. R., Mantovani, A., Hobbs, D. S., Kung, H., and Pestka, S.,** Effect of human recombinant interferon on cytotoxic activity of natural killer (NK) cells and monocytes, *Cell. Immunol.*, 67, 160, 1982.
10. **Gresser, I. and Tovey, M. G.,** Antitumor effects of interferon, *Biochim. Biophys. Acta*, 516, 231, 1978.
11. **Harfast, B., Huddlestone, J. R., Casali, P., Merigan, T. C., and Oldstone, M. B. A.,** Interferon acts directly on human B lymphocytes to modulate immunoglobulin synthesis, *J. Immunol.*, 127, 2146, 1981.
12. **Sehgal, P. B., Pfeffer, L. M., and Tamm, I.,** Interferon and its inducers, in *Chemotherapy of Viral Infections*, Came, P. E. and Caliguiri, L. A., Eds., 1982, 205.
13. **Wang, E., Pfeffer, L. M., and Tamm, I.,** Interferon increases the abundance of submembranous microfilaments in HeLa-S_3 cells in suspension culture, *Proc. Natl. Acad. Sci. U.S.A.*, 78, 6281, 1981.
14. **Creasey, A. A., Bartholomew, J. C., and Merigan, T. C.,** Role of G_0-G_1-arrest in the inhibition of tumor cell growth by interferon, *Proc. Natl. Acad. Sci. U.S.A.*, 77, 1471, 1980.
15. **Creasey, A. A., Bartholomew, J. C., and Merigan, T. C.,** The importance of G_0 in the site of action of interferon in the cell cycle, *Exp. Cell Res.*, 134, 155, 1981.
16. **Leandersson, T. and Lundgren, E.,** Antiproliferative effects of interferon on a Burkitt's lymphoma cell line, *Exp. Cell Res.*, 130, 421, 1980.

17. **Sawada, Y., Suhadolnik, R. J., Todd, P., and Kunze, M. R.,** The effect of human fibroblast interferon on the cell cycle of HeLa cells as determined by laser flow cytometry, manuscript in preparation.

18. **Baglioni, C.,** Interferon-induced enzymatic activities and their role in the antiviral state, *Cell,* 17, 255, 1979.

19. **Strander, H.,** Interferons: antineoplastic drugs, *Blut,* 35, 277, 1977.

20. **Marx, J. L.,** Interferon. I. On the threshold of clinical application, *Science,* 204, 1183, 1979.

21. **Vallbracht, A., Treuner, J., Flehming, B., Joester, K.-E., and Neithammer, D.,** Interferon-neutralizing antibodies in a patient treated with human fibroblast interferon, *Nature (London),* 289, 496, 1981.

22. **Cantell, K.,** Towards the clinical use of interferon, *Endeavour,* 2, 27, 1978.

23. **Cunningham, K. G., Hutchinson, S. A., Manson, W., and Spring, F. S.,** Cordycepin, a metabolic product isolated from cultures of *Cordyceps militaris, J. Chem. Soc.,* p. 2299, 1951.

24. **Suhadolnik, R. J.,** *Nucleoside Antibiotics,* John Wiley & Sons, New York, 1970.

25. **Suhadolnik, R. J.,** *Nucleosides as Biological Probes,* John Wiley & Sons, New York, 1979.

26. **Cory, J. G., Suhadolnik, R. J., Resnick, B., and Rich, M. A.,** Incorporation of cordycepin (3'-deoxyadenosine) into ribonucleic acid and deoxyribonucleic acid of human tumor cells, *Biochim. Biophys. Acta,* 103, 646, 1965.

27. **Suhadolnik, R. J., Lennon, M. B., Uematsu, T., Monahan, J. E., and Baur, R.,** Role of adenine ring and adenine ribose of nicotinamide adenine dinucleotide in binding and catalysis with alcohol, lactate, and glyceraldehyde-3-phosphate dehydrogenase, *J. Biol. Chem.,* 252, 4125, 1977.

28. **Suhadolnik, R. J., Baur, R., Lichtenwalner, D. M., Uematsu, T., Roberts, J. H., Sudhakar, S., and Smulson, M.,** ADP-ribosylation of isolated nuclei from HeLa cells, rat liver, fetal rat liver and Novikoff hepatoma: effect of nicotinamide adenine dinucleotide analogs on template activity for DNA synthesis, incorporation into nuclear proteins, and a new $1' \rightarrow 3''$ osidic linkage, *J. Biol. Chem.,* 252, 4134, 1977.

29. **Doetsch, P., Wu, J., Shockman, G. D., and Suhadolnik, R. J.,** 2',5'-Oligo(cordycepin), an analog of 2',5'-oligo(A): enzymatic synthesis, purification and characterization in lysed rabbit reticulocytes and HeLa cell extracts, *Fed. Proc.,* 39, 1778, 1980.

30. **Doetsch, P., Wu, J. M., Sawada, Y., and Suhadolnik, R. J.,** Synthesis and characterization of $(2',5')ppp3'dA(p3'dA)_n$, an analogue of $(2',5')pppA(pA)_n$, *Nature (London),* 291, 355, 1981.

31. **Suhadolnik, R. J., Devash, Y., Reichenbach, N. L., Lee, C., Wu, J. M., and Flick, M. B.,** The enzymatic synthesis of $2',5'$-$ppp3'dA(p3'dA)_3$, an analog of $2',5'$-$pppA(pA)_3$, from cordycepin 5'-tri-phosphate (3'dATP) by rabbit reticulocyte lysates (LRR): effect of hydrolysis of globin mRNA and inhibition of protein synthesis in LRR and mammalian cells, *Fed. Proc.,* 42, 1918 (abstr. 943), 1983.

32. **Suhadolnik, R. J., Devash, Y., Reichenbach, N. L., Flick, M. B., and Wu, J. M.,** Enzymatic synthesis of the $2',5'$-A_4 tetramer analog, $2',5'$-$ppp3'dA(p3'dA)_3$, by rabbit reticulocyte lysates: binding and activation of the $2',5'$-A_n-dependent nuclease, hydrolysis of mRNA, and inhibition of protein synthesis, *Biochem. Biophys. Res. Commun.,* 111, 205, 1983.

33. **Imai, J., Johnston, M. I., and Torrence, P. F.,** Chemical modification potentiates the biological activities of 2-5A and its congeners, *J. Biol. Chem.,* 257, 12739, 1982.

34. **Drocourt, J.-L., Dieffenbach, C. W., Ts'o, P. O. P., Justesen, J., and Thang, M. N.,** Structural requirements of (2'-5')-oligoadenylate for protein synthesis inhibition in human fibroblasts, *Nucl. Acids Res.,* 10, 2163, 1982.

35. **Baglioni, C., D'Alessandro, S. B., Nilsen, T. W., den Hartog, J. A. J., Crea, R., and van Boom, H. J.,** Analogs of (2'-5')oligo(A): endonuclease activation and inhibition of protein synthesis in intact cells, *J. Biol. Chem.,* 256, 3253, 1981.

36. **Eppstein, D. A., Marsh, Y. V., Schryber, B. B., Larsen, M. A., Barnett, J. W., Verheyden, J. P. H., and Prisbe, E. J.,** Analogs of $(A2'p)_nA$: correlation of structure of analogs of $ppp(A2'p)_2A$ and $(A2'p)_2A$ with stability and biological activity, *J. Biol. Chem.,* 257, 13390, 1982.

37. **Hughes, B. G., Srivastava, P. C., Muse, D. D., and Robins, R. K.,** I. Enzymatic synthesis of 2',5'-oligoadenylates and related 2',5'-oligonucleotide analogues. Substrate specificity of the interferon-induced murine 2',5'-oligoadenylate synthetase, *Biochemistry,* 22, 2116, 1983.

38. **Hughes, B. G. and Robins, R. K.,** II. Effect of 2',5'-oligoadenylates and related 2',5'-oligonucleotide analogues on cellular proliferation, protein synthesis, and endoribonuclease activity, *Biochemistry,* 22, 2127, 1983.

39. **Sharma, O. K. and Goswami, B.,** O-methylated nucleoside and nucleotide analogs as inhibitors of virus replication, 185th ACS Meet. Symp. Antiviral Agents: Chem. Biochem., March 23, Seattle, 1983.

40. **Gosselin, G., Haikal, A., Chavis, C., and Imbach, J. L.,** Unusual nucleoside synthons and oligonucleotide synthesis, 5th Int. Round Table: Nucleosides, Nucleotides, and Their Biological Applications, Burroughs Wellcome Co., October 20, Research Triangle Park, N.C., 1982.

41. **Devash, Y., Biggs, S., and Sela, I.,** Multiplication of tobacco mosaic virus in tobacco leaf discs is inhibited by (2'-5')-oligoadenylate, *Science,* 216, 1415, 1982.

42. **Reichman, M., Devash, Y., Suhadolnik, R. J., and Sela, I.,** Human leukocyte interferon and the antiviral factor from virus-infected plants stimulate plant tissues to produce nucleoties with antiviral activity, *Virology,* 128, 240, 1983.

43. **Kimchi, A., Shure, H., Lapidot, Y., Rapoport, S., Panet, A., and Revel, M.,** Antimitogenic effects of interferon and (2′-5′)oligoadenylate in synchronized 3T3 fibroblasts, *FEBS Lett.,* 134, 212, 1981.

44. **Lee, C. and Suhadolnik, R. J.,** Inhibition of protein synthesis by the cordycepin analog of $(2'-5')p_3A_n$, $(2'-5')p_33'dA_n$, in intact mammalian cells, *FEBS Lett.,* 157, 205, 1983.

45. **Sawai, H., Imai, J., Lesiak, K., Johnston, M. I., and Torrence, P. F.,** Cordycepin analogues of 2-5A and its derivatives: chemical synthesis and biological activity, *J. Biol. Chem.,* 258, 1671, 1983.

46. **Kimchi, A., Shure, H., and Revel, M.,** Regulation of lymphocyte mitogenesis by (2′-5′)oligo-isoadenylate, *Nature (London),* 282, 849, 1979.

47. **Epstein, M. A. and Achong, B. G., Eds.,** *The Epstein-Barr Virus,* Springer-Verlag, New York, 1979.

48. **Doetsch, P. W., Suhadolnik, R. J., Sawada, Y., Mosca, J. D., Flick, M. B., Reichenbach, N. L., Dang, A. Q., Wu, J. M., Charubala, R., Pfleiderer, W., and Henderson, E. E.,** Core (2′-5′)oligoadenylate and the cordycepin analog: inhibitors of Epstein-Barr virus-induced transformation of human lymphocytes in the absence of interferon, *Proc. Natl. Acad. Sci. U.S.A.,* 78, 6699, 1981.

49. **Jurovčik, M. and Smrt, J.,** Inhibition of protein synthesis by exogenous A2′p5′A2′p5′A (2-5 A core) and its bis-phosphoramidate analog in intact mouse lymphocytes, hepatocytes and bone marrow cells, *FEBS Lett.,* 133, 178, 1981.

50. **Williams, B. R. G. and Kerr, I. M.,** Inhibition of protein synthesis by 2′,5′-linked adenine oligonucleotides in intact cells, *Nature (London),* 276, 88, 1978.

51. **Henderson, E. E., Doetsch, P. W., Charubala, R., Pfleiderer, W., and Suhadolnik, R. J.,** Inhibition of Epstein-Barr virus-associated nuclear antigen (EBNA) induction by (2′,5′)-oligoadenylate and the cordycepin analog: mechanism of action for inhibition of EBV-induced transformation, *Virology,* 122, 198, 1982.

52. **Suhadolnik, R. J., Doetsch, P. W., Henderson, E. E., Charubala, R., and Pfleiderer, W.,** [^{32}P]2′,5′-Adenylate and [^{32}P]2′,5′-3′-deoxyadenylate trimer cores: inhibition of cell growth and uptake and/or binding to lymphocytes and lymphoblasts, *Nucleosides and Nucleotides,* 2, 351, 1983.

53. **Djeu, J. Y., Huang, K.-Y., and Herberman, R. B.,** Augmentation of mouse natural killer activity and induction of interferon by tumor cell *in vivo, J. Exp. Med.,* 151, 781, 1980.

54. **Herberman, R. B. and Ortaldo, J. R.,** Natural killer cells: their role in defenses against disease, *Science,* 214, 23, 1981.

55. **Herberman, R. B., Ortaldo, J. R., Mantovani, A., Hobbs, D. S., Kung, H.-F., and Pestka, S.,** Effect of human recombinant interferon on cytotoxic activity of natural killer (NK) cells and monocytes, *Cell. Immunol.,* 67, 160, 1982.

56. **Haliotis, T., Roder, J., Klein, M., Ortaldo, J., Fauci, A. S., and Herberman, R. B.,** Chédiak-Higashi gene in humans. 1. Impairment of natural-killer function, *J. Exp. Med.,* 151, 1039, 1980.

57. **Hanna, N. and Burton, R. J.,** Definite evidence that natural killer (NK) cells inhibit experimental tumor metastasis *in vivo, J. Immunol.,* 127, 1754, 1981.

58. **Warner, J. F. and Dennert, G.,** Effects of a cloned cell line with NK activity on bone marrow transplant, tumour development and metastasis *in vivo, Nature (London),* 300, 31, 1982.

59. **Tanaka, Y., Sugamur, K., Hinuma, Y., Sato, H., and Okochik, K.,** Memory of Epstein-Barr virus-specific cytotoxic T cells in normal seropositive adults as revealed by an *in vitro* restimulation method, *J. Immunol.,* 125, 1426, 1980.

60. **Sullivan, H. L., Byron, K. S., Brewster, F. E., and Purtillo, D. T.,** Deficient natural killer cell activity in X-linked lymphoproliferative syndrome, *Science,* 210, 543, 1980.

61. **Black, P. L., Suhadolnik, R. J., and Henderson, E. E.,** Augmentation of natural killer by interferon-inducible oligonucleotides, *Fed. Proc.,* 42, 678 (Abstr. 2258), 1983.

62. **Black, P. L., Henderson, E. E., Suhadolnik, R. J., Pfleiderer, W., and Charubala, R.,** Effect of interferon-inducible oligonucleotides on natural killer cells, manuscript in preparation, 1983.

63. **Lozzio, C. B. and Lozzio, B. B.,** Human chronic myelogenous leukemia cell-line with positive Philadelphia chromosome, *Blood,* 45, 321, 1975.

64. **Suhadolnik, R. J., Doetsch, P. W., Flick, M. B., Sawada, Y., and Dang, A. Q.,** Intracellular accumulation of 2′,5′-oligo-3′-deoxyadenylate in interferon and double-stranded RNA treated HeLa cells, manuscript in preparation, 1983.

65. **Bagnara, A. S. and Hershfield, M. S.,** Mechanism of deoxyadenosine-induced catabolism of adenine ribonucleotides in adenosine deaminase-inhibited human T lymphoblastoid cells, *Proc. Natl. Acad. Sci. U.S.A.,* 79, 2673, 1982.

66. **Klein, G.,** *Viral Oncology,* Raven Press, New York, 1980.

67. **Suhadolnik, R. J., Flick, M. B., Mosca, J. D., Sawada, Y., Doetsch, P. W., and Vonderheid, E. C.,** 2′,5′-Oligoadenylate synthetase from cutaneous T-cell lymphoma: biosynthesis, identification, quantification, molecular size of the 2′,5′-oligoadenylates, and inhibition of protein synthesis, *Biochemistry,* 22, 4153, 1983.

68. **Yoshida, M., Miyoshi, I., and Hinuma, Y.,** Isolation and characterization of retrovirus from cell lines of human adult T-cell leukemia and its implication in the disease, *Proc. Natl. Acad. Sci. U.S.A.,* 79, 2031, 1982.

69. **Seiki, M., Hattori, S., and Yoshida, M.,** Human adult T-cell leukemia virus: molecular cloning of the provirus DNA and the unique terminal structure, *Proc. Natl. Acad. Sci. U.S.A.,* 79, 6899, 1982.

70. **Popovic, M., Reitz, M. S., Sarngadharan, M. G., Robert-Guroff, M., Kalyanaraman, V. S., Nakao, Y., Miyoshi, I., Minowada, J., Yoshida, M., Ito, Y., and Gallo, R. C.,** The virus of Japanese adult T-cell leukaemia is a member of the human T-cell leukaemia virus group, *Nature (London),* 300, 63, 1982.

71. **Suhadolnik, R. J., Sawada, Y., Gabriel, J., Henderson, E. E., and Reichenbach, N. L.,** Effect of human fibroblast interferon on thymidine metabolism, DNA processing, and chromatin structure in HeLa cells, *J. Biol. Chem.,* in press, 1984.

72. **Lewis, J. A., Mengheri, E., and Esteban, M.,** Induction of an antiviral response by interferon requires thymidine kinase, *Proc. Natl. Acad. Sci. U.S.A.,* 80, 26, 1983.

73. **Miyoshi, T., Ogawa, S., Kanamori, T., Nobuhara, M., and Namba, M.,** Interferon potentiates cytotoxic effects of 5-fluorouracil on cell proliferation of established human cell lines originating from neoplastic tissues, *Cancer Lett.,* 17, 239, 1980.

74. **Goulian, M., Bleile, B., and Tseng, B. Y.,** The effect of methotrexate on levels of dUTP in animal cells, *J. Biol. Chem.,* 255, 10630, 1980.

75. **deFerra, F. and Baglioni, C.,** Increase in S-adenosylhomocysteine concentration in interferon-treated HeLa cells and inhibition of methylation of vesicular stomatitis virus mRNA, *J. Biol. Chem.,* 258, 2118, 1983.

76. **Moore, G., Gewert, D. R., and Clemens, M. J.,** Changes in deoxynucleoside metabolism and DNA synthesis in interferon-treated human lymphoblastoid cells, 597th Meet. Biochem. Soc., 1982.

77. **Moore, G. and Clemens, M. J.,** Inhibition of cell proliferation by human interferon associated with rapid turnover of newly replicated DNA, 598th Meet. Biochem. Soc., 1983.

78. **Butt, R. T. and Sreevalsan, T.,** Interferon and sodium butyrate inhibit the stimulation of poly(ADP-ribose) synthetase in mouse cells stimulated to divide, in press, 1983.

79. **Reczek, P. R., Weissman, D., Hüvös, P. E., and Fasman, G. D.,** Sodium butyrate induced structural changes in HeLa cell chromatin, *Biochemistry,* 21, 993, 1982.

80. **Ishimi, Y., Ohba, Y., Yoshuda, H., and Yamada, M.,** The interaction of H1 histone with nucleosome core, *J. Biochem.,* 89, 1881, 1981.

81. **LePage, G. A. and Hersh, E. M.,** Cyclic nucleotide analogs as carcinostatic agents, *Biochem. Biophys. Res. Commun.,* 46, 1918, 1972.

82. **Cho-Chung, Y. S.,** In vivo inhibition of tumor growth by cyclic adenosine 3′,5′-monophosphate derivatives, *Cancer Res.,* 34, 3492, 1974.

83. **Hughes, R. G., Jr. and Kimball, A. P.,** Metabolic effects of cyclic 9-β-D-arabinofuranosyladenine 3′,5′-monophosphate in L1210 cells, *Cancer Res.,* 32, 1791, 1972.

84. **Smith, B. C., Martin, G. R., Miller, E. J., Dorfman, A., and Swarm, R.,** Nature of the collagen synthesized by a transplanted chondrosarcoma, *Arch. Biochem. Biophys.,* 166, 181, 1975.

85. **Willis, D. H., Pfleiderer, W., Charubala, R., and Suhadolnik, R. J.,** (2′-5′)3′-Deoxyadenylate trimer core inhibits Swarm chondrosarcoma tumor growth *in vivo* and DNA and protein synthesis in isolated tumor pieces, *Fed. Proc.,* 43, 1833(Abstr. 443), 1983.

86. **Willis, D. H., Pfleiderer, W., Charubala, R., and Suhadolnik, R. J.,** (2′-5′)3′-Deoxyadenylate trimer core: inhibition of tumor growth in rats, *Cancer Res.,* in press, 1984.

87. **Safer, B., Jagus, R., and Kemper, W. M.,** Analysis of initiation factor function in highly fractionated and unfractionated reticulocyte lysate system, *Methods Enzymol.,* 60, 61, 1979.

88. **Hovanessian, A. G. and Wood, J. N.,** Anticellular and antiviral effects of pppA(2′p5′A)$_n$, *Virology,* 101, 91, 1980.

89. **Devash, Y., Flick, M. B., Reichenbach, N. L., Wu, J. M., Pfleiderer, W., Charubala, R., and Suhadolnik, R. J.,** Inhibition of protein synthesis, affinity for binding protein, and activation of 2′,5′-A$_n$ dependent endonuclease by the cordycepin analog of 2′,5′-p$_3$A$_n$, manuscript in preparation.

Chapter 11

INDUCTION OF DIFFERENTIATION OF THE HUMAN PROMYELOCYTIC CELL LINE HL-60 AND PRIMARY CULTURES OF HUMAN LEUKEMIA CELLS: A MODEL FOR CLINICAL TREATMENT

Hiromichi Hemmi and Theodore R. Breitman

TABLE OF CONTENTS

I. INTRODUCTION

In recent years the development of human myelomoncytic cell lines has provided useful models for studying regulation of both cell proliferation and differentiation. This can be very important for studies on the treatment of leukemia, because the finding that some of these cell lines can be induced to terminally differentiate by a wide variety of compounds has suggested an alternative approach to the therapy of certain types of leukemias.

The growth advantage that myeloid leukemia cells have *in vivo* over normal cells is not because of a more rapid growth rate, but rather because of an apparent inability to mature to functional, terminally differentiated end cells. It is possible that some leukemia cells do not mature either because they have a decreased ability to respond to exogenous differentiative factors or because the production of specific gene products obligatory for differentiation is altered. The availability of tissue-culture cell lines has made it possible to study the regulation of proliferation and differentiation of specific hematopoietic cell types and the effect on these cells of known mediators and modulators. These studies have had an impact on the approach to the treatment of some leukemias. Cancer treatment has traditionally consisted of a two-pronged attack consisting of surgical removal where applicable and treatment with cytotoxic agents including chemotherapy, ionizing radiation, and immunotherapy. The employment of cytotoxic agents has been the prime treatment for leukemia, but it is associated with many toxic side effects.

In this report, we review our previous work and present new data on the finding that some leukemic cell lines, as well as fresh cells from patients with acute promyelocytic leukemia, are induced to differentiate with physiological concentrations of retinoic acid (RA). This induction is modulated by agents increasing the intracellular level of cyclic AMP and/or by a T-cell lymphokine we call Differentiation Inducing Activity (DIA). Thus, it is feasible that treatment of some leukemias may be approached, not with the aim of killing the leukemic population, but rather to induce them to mature to a more normal and functional nongrowing cell type. With this approach, the hope is that treatment will be more selective, with diminished toxic side effects.

II. HUMAN MYELOMONOCYTIC CELL LINES

Some properties of human myeloid leukemia cell lines are summarized in Table 1.

A. K-562

The first clearly human nonlymphoid leukemia cell line, K562, was established from the

Table 1
SOME PROPERTIES OF HUMAN MYELOID LEUKEMIA CELL LINES

Characteristics	HL-60	U-937	THP-1	KG-1	K-562
Source	APL	Histocytic lymphoma	AMol	AML	CML in blast crisis
Predominant cell	Promyelocyte	Monoblastoid	Monocyte	Myeloblast	Blast cell
Mean doubling-time (hr)	36	50	48	40—50	12
Karyotype	Aneuploid	Aneuploid	Diploid	Hypodiploid	Ph[1]
Lymphocyte makers	None	None	None	None	None
Colony formation in agar					
Spontaneous	Yes	No	No	No	Yes
Induced by CSA	Yes	No	Yes	Yes	No
Differentiation in culture					
Spontaneous	Yes	No	Yes	No	Yes
Induced by DMSO	Yes	No	No	No	No
Induced by hemin	No			No	Yes
Induced by RA	Yes	Yes	Yes	No	No
Induced by DIA	Yes	Yes	Yes	Yes	
Induced cell	G or M	M	M	M	Erythroid, G, or M

Note: Abbreviations: APL, acute promyelocytic leukemia; AMol, acute monocytic leukemia; AML, acute mye-logenous leukemia; CML, chronic myelogenous leukemia; Ph[1], Philadelphia chromosome; G, granulocyte; M, monocyte/macrophage; CSA, colony stimulating activity; DMSO, dimethyl sulfoxide; RA, all-*trans*-β-retinoic acid; DIA, T-lymphocyte-derived differentiation inducing activity.

pleural effusion of a patient with chronic myelogenous leukemia (CML) in blast crisis.[1] These cells are induced to differentiate along the erythroid pathway with the production of hemoglobin when treated with butyric acid or hemin.[2-4] More recently, K562 has been reported to be a multipotential cell line differentiating in long-term culture without added inducers into recognizable progenitors of the granulocytic, monocytic, and erythrocytic series.[5]

B. KG-1

The KG-1 cell line, isolated from a patient with acute myelogenous leukemia (AML),[6] is composed primarily of myeloblasts and promyelocytes and differentiates into nondividing macrophage-like cells by exposure to phorbol diesters.[7] These cells develop many of the characteristics of macrophages including adhesion, phagocytosis, lysozyme secretion, nitroblue tetrazolium (NBT) reduction, Fc receptors, and nonspecific esterase activity.[8]

C. U-937

U-937 is a human histiocytic lymphoma cell line with monoblast-like characteristics.[9] These cells differentiate into morphologically mature macrophage-like cells with increased activity in antibody-dependent cytotoxicity assays after treatment with phorbol diesters[10] or the conditioned medium from mixed-lymphocyte cultures.[11] More recently, U-937 was shown to differentiate into monocyte-like cells by incubation with RA.[12] These induced cells are phagocytic, reduce nitroblue tetrazolium (NBT), and show an increased hexose monophosphate shunt (HMPS) activity, consistent with monocyte-like cells.

D. THP-1

THP-1 is a human acute monocytic leukemia cell line established by Tsuchiya et al.[13] The monocytic nature of this cell line was based on morphology, nonspecific esterase activity, lysozyme production, and phagocytosis of latex beads and sensitized sheep erythrocytes.

When these cells are treated with phorbol diester they become adherent, and there are increases in phagocytosis, nonspecific esterase activity, and HMPS activity.[14] These results have been interpreted to indicate that THP-1 cells can be converted into mature cells with functions of macrophages.

E. HL-60

HL-60 is the *prima donna* of the human myeloid leukemia cell lines. It was the first human cell line with distinct myeloid features to be developed.[15] This cell line, isolated from the blood of a patient with acute promyelocytic leukemia, proliferates continuously in suspension culture and consists predominantly of promyelocytes. HL-60 is induced to terminally differentiate to cells having many of the morphological features of mature granulocyes by exposure to a wide variety of compounds (Table 2), including dimethyl sulfoxide, dimethyl formamide, hypoxanthine, butyric acid, actinomycin D, and RA.[16-18, 30, 31] Moreover, these induced HL-60 cells have many of the functional characteristics of normal human peripheral blood granulocytes including phagocytosis, lysosomal enzyme release, complement receptors, chemotaxis, HMPS activity, superoxide anion generation, and the ability to reduce NBT.[16,17,35] HL-60 lacks leukocyte alkaline phosphatase,[36] and although differentiating HL-60 cells do not develop secondary (specific) granules and the specific protein markers for these granules, lactoferrin, and B_2-binding protein,[35,37,38] They still provide a unique system for studying growth and differentiation of human myeloid cells in vitro.

III. GROWTH OF HL-60 IN DEFINED MEDIUM

A. Growth in Suspension

For the studies on HL-60 reported here, we have used a serum-free nutrient medium supplemented only with 5 μg insulin and 5 μg transferrin per milliliter. The nutrient medium can be either a 1:1 mixture of Dulbecco's modified Eagle medium and Ham's F 12 medium containing 14.3 mM NaHCO$_3$ and 15 mM HEPES at pH 7.2[40] or RPMI 1640. In this insulin- and transferrin-supplemented medium, referred to as defined medium, long-term growth of HL-60 continues at a rate approximately 80% of that occurring in medium supplemented with serum.[39] The saturation density is lower in defined medium (1.5 × 10^6 cells/mℓ) than in serum-supplemented medium (3 × 10^6 cells/mℓ). Growth of HL-60 cells has continued in defined medium for over 30 passages, including at least 60 population-doublings. This translates into a 10^{18}-fold increase in cell number in the absence of serum, making it unlikely that residual serum components are contibuting to the growth of the cells.

There is an absolute requirement for both insulin and transferrin to maintain continuous proliferation of HL-60 cells.[39] These requirements are more pronounced at low cell concentrations where a lag before the onset of growth is also observed. In nutrient medium supplemented with 10% fetal bovine serum (FBS) there is essentially no lag in the growth of HL-60 after cultures are seeded with initial cell concentrations as low as 3000 cells/mℓ[34] However, in defined medium this lag is seen even at initial cell concentrations of 2.5 × 10^5/mℓ and can be decreased but not eliminated by the addition of low concentrations of bovine serum albumin (BSA). The cause of the lag in growth in defined medium appears to involve not only a delay before the onset of growth but a decrease in the number of cells in suspension because of the attachment of cells to the tissue culture vessel surface.[34] The finding that, in the presence of insulin and transferrin, the addition of BSA decreases the lag before the onset of growth indicates that a major function of FBS is to provide a protein-rich environment. Indirect support for this view is that the addition of 1% FBS to defined medium supports growth of HL-60 such that after 4 days it is approximately 90% of the growth obtained in medium with 10% FBS.[34] Medium with 1% FBS has a total protein concentration of approximately 400 μg/mℓ, of which 240 μg/mℓ is serum albumin. Therefore, comparable increases in growth of HL-60 in defined medium occur at similar protein concentrations of either BSA or FBS. The extreme sensitivity of the growth of HL-60 to microgram quantities of various proteins should be taken into consideration if the growth of these cells in defined medium is used for analysis of possible growth factors.

B. Growth in Semisolid Medium

Although growth of HL-60 in suspension culture is supported by defined medium, colony growth of HL-60 in semisolid medium appears to be absolutely dependent on serum.[39] HL-60 cells form colonies in semisolid medium (methylcellulose) supplemented with FBS and their cloning efficiency increases with the addition of colony stimulating activity (CSA).[41,42] However, when HL-60 cells are suspended in a serum-free semisolid medium supplemented with insulin and transferrin, no colonies form even at high cell densities or in the presence of CSA.[39] The addition of BSA to the defined medium has no effect on the number of colonies formed. Thus, it appears clear that factor(s) in serum are required to support colony formation of HL-60. The identification of this activity would be a fruitful area of future investigation. The ability of a defined medium to support the growth of single cells may be considered the penultimate test for the efficacy of a growth medium. By this criterion, serum-free medium supplemented only with insulin and transferrin does not support the growth of individual cells of HL-60 into colonies. This may be a manifestation of what was observed in suspension culture where defined medium did not support maximal growth of HL-60 without an initial lag; the extent of the lag being inversely related to the initial cell concentration.

In spite of these deficiencies, defined medium has been very useful in investigating differentiation of HL-60, as discussed below, where studies have been carried out in the absence of undefined serum inhibitors or enhancers of differentiation, providing a useful means of assessing HL-60 response to physiologic differentiation-inducing compounds having relevance to the control mechanisms of normal granulopoiesis.

IV. DIFFERENTIATION OF HL-60 IN DEFINED MEDIUM

A. RA

Until recently, terminal differentiation of HL-60 could be induced either by nonphysiological compounds, e.g., dimethyl sulfoxide, or by physiological chemicals at markedly greater than physiological concentrations, e.g., hypoxanthine. Recently, all-*trans*-β-RA was found to be the most potent inducer of granulocytic differentiation of HL-60.[30,31] This compound induces differentiation at 10^{-6} to 10^{-3} the concentration of other inducers (Figure 1), induces relatively more extensive morphological differentiaton than other inducers,[30] and probably more important, induces at concentrations that are physiological.[43]

1. Effect of Serum or Albumin

The extent of RA-induced differentiation of HL-60, as was the case with dimethyl sulfoxide-induced differentiation,[30] is the same in defined medium as in serum-supplemented medium (Figure 2). These results are in contrast to those observed with murine F9 embryonal carcinoma cells where the RA requirements for induction of differentiation are markedly decreased in the absence of serum.[44] Because of the high capacity that serum albumin has for binding RA[45], the latter findings are not surprising. However, serum albumin at concentrations as high as 4.5 mg/mℓ has essentially no effect on RA-induced differentiation of HL-60 in defined medium (Figure 3). At the highest concentration of albumin used in this experiment the molar ratio of albumin to RA was 220 (67 μM/0.3 μM). Thus, even though a value for the equilibrium constant for the binding of RA to albumin has not been reported, it would be expected that under these conditions the concentration of free RA would be

Table 2
DIFFERENTIATION INDUCERS OF HL-60

Inducer[a]	Concentration	Percentage differentiation for parameter	Time in culture (days)	Ref.
Nonphysiological Inducers				
Chemicals				
Dimethyl sulfoxide	155—180 mM	94% morphol; 85% phago; 72% NBT-red	6	16, 17
Acetamide	150 mM	71% morphol	6	16
N-Methylacetamide	20 mM	68% morphol	6	16
N,N-Dimethylacetamide	10 mM	73% morphol	6	16
N-Methylformamide	150 mM	81% morphol	6	16
N,N-Dimethylformamide	60 mM	84% morphol	6	16
Piperidone	37.5 mM	78% morphol	6	16
1-Methyl-2-piperidone	4 mM	65% morphol	6	16
Triethylene glycol	100 mM	60% morphol	6	16
Butyric acid	0.6 mM	58% morphol	6	16
Hexamethylene bisacetamide	2 mM	95% morphol; 97% NBT-red	6	18
Methotrexate	14 nM	31% morphol; 31% NBT-red	6	18
2-Ethionine	2—3.2 mM	27—45% NBT-red; 53% C3	4—5	20, 21
Nucleoside analogs				
6-Thioguanine	3 μM	49% morphol; 45% NBT-red	6	18
3-Deazauridine	12 μM	90% morphol; 84% NBT-red	6	19
Pyrazofurin	0.5 μM	60% morphol; 64% NBT-red	6	19
TCN	2 μM	50% morphol; 48% NBT-red	6	19
5-Bromodeoxyuridine	16.2 nM	53% morphol; 33.3% C3	5	22
Antibiotics				
Actinomycin D	0.8 nM	74% morphol; 37.3% C3	5	18
Daunomycin	4 nM	89% morphol; 93% NBT-red	6	23
	19 nM	35% morphol	6	18
Anthracyclines				
Marcellomycin	30 nM	77% NBT-red	5	24
Musettamycin	60 nM	67% NBT-red	5	24
Aclacinomycin A	80 nM	72% NBT-red	5	24

10-Decarbomethoxymarcellomycin	340 nM	46% NBT-red	5	24
Tunicamycin	6 μM	55.2% morphol; 55% phago	6	25
Tumor promoters				
12-*O*-Tetradecanoyl-phorbol-13-acetate(TPA)	0.8 nM	90% morphol; 40% phago	2	26
	160 nM	65% phago; adhesion	4	27
	0.81 nM	88% morphol; 56.8% C3	6	23
Dihydroteleocidin B	0.3 ng/mℓ	51.5% adhesion	2	28
	5 ng/mℓ	55—60% phago	2	29
Lyngbyatoxin A	5 ng/mℓ	45—50% phago	2	29
Tetrahydrolyngbyatoxin A	5 ng/mℓ	55—60% phago	2	29
Teleocidin	5 ng/mℓ	35—40% phago	2	29
Physiological Inducers				
Retinoids				
All-*trans*-β-retinoic acid	1 μM	94% morphol; 95% NBT-red	5	30, 31
13-*cis*-retinoic acid	1 μM	85% NBT-red	5	30
4-Keto-retinoic acid	1 μM	93% NBT-red	5	32
4-Hydroxy-retinoic acid	1 μM	87% NBT-red	5	32
α-Retinoic acid	1 μM	67% NBT-red	5	32
Vitamin D				
1α,25-Dihydroxycholecalciferol	12 nM	44% morphol	3	33
Hypoxanthine	5 mM	86% morphol; 90% NBT-red	6	18
Prostaglandin E_2	1 μM	28% NBT-red	4	34
Dibutyryl cAMP	0.1 mM	33% NBT-red	4	32

Note: Abbreviations — morphol = morphologically mature cells including myelocytes, metamyelocytes, banded and segmented neutrophils, monocytes, and macrophages; phago, phagocytosis; C3, C3 receptors; NBT-red, nitroblue tetrazolium reduction; TCN, 3-amino-1,5-dihydro-5-methyl-1-β-D-ribofuranosyl-1,4,5,6,8-pentaazaacenaphthylene; cAMP, cyclic adenosine 3′:5′-monophosphate.

[a] Inducers producing approximately a 30% increase in one or more of the maturation parameters: nitroblue tetrazolium reduction, phagocytosis, Fc and C3 receptors, and cell adhesion within 6 days of culture.

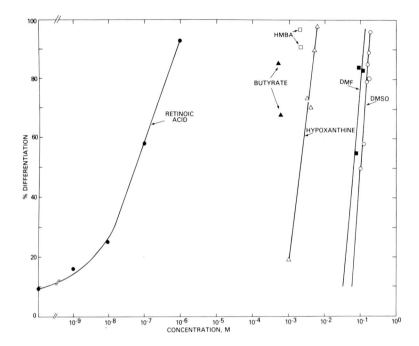

FIGURE 1.   Terminal differentiation of HL-60 cells induced by various compounds. Differentiation was measured at day 5 of incubation and is expressed as the percentage of cells capable of reducing nitroblue tetrazolium (NBT).

decreased. The absence of any major effect by FBS or BSA on RA-induced differentiation raises the possibility that bound RA is as active as the free form and suggests that the "triggering" for differentiation occurs at the plasma membrane.

B. Mechanisms of RA-Induction

1. RA-Binding Protein

Notwithstanding the above speculation, the exact mechanism by which RA enhances differentiation of HL-60 cells or affects other cells is unknown. A proposed mechanism is that RA exerts an effect in the nucleus after binding to a highly specific cytoplasmic receptor (cellular RA-binding protein).[45] However, we have been unable to demonstrate such a binding protein in HL-60 cells, either with the sucrose-density gradient sedimentation assay[46] or with a much more sensitive polyacrylamide gel electrophoresis technique.[47] These results are in conflict with the conclusion of Takenaga et al.[48] who report that HL-60 has RA-binding protein, but are in agreement with Douer and Koeffler[49] who also could not detect this protein.

2. RA Metabolites

The possibility that RA acts on HL-60 after its conversion to 4-hydroxy- and 4-keto-RA[50] was investigated indirectly by testing the ability of these two metabolites to induce differentiation.[32] Both compounds were approximately 1/10 as effective as RA. In the same study, other retinoids were tested and the results indicated that the most effective retinoid inducers of HL-60 differentiation possess a carboxylic acid function at the C-15 terminal carbon (RA and 13-*cis*-RA). This activity was retained, although somewhat diminished, in spite of alterations in the ring as in the 4-hydroxy- and 4-keto-substituted derivatives and α-RA. Substitutions at the C-15 position resulted in essentially a complete loss of activity (retinal, retinol, retinyl acetate). These activity-structure relationships emphasize the specificity of the RA effect on HL-60 and makes more likely the possibility that this phenomenon, observed in vitro, is an expression of a true physiological process.

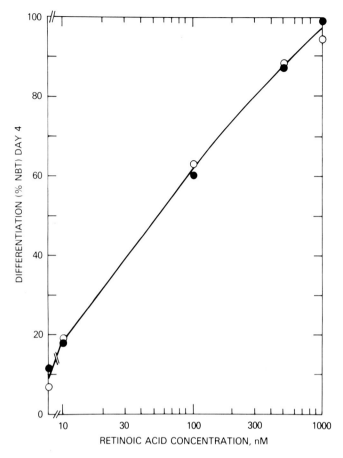

FIGURE 2. RA-induced differentiation of HL-60 in defined medium (○) and in serum-supplemented medium (●).

3. Retinoylation

A very speculative hypothesis for the mechanism of action of RA in some cell types, presently under investigation in this laboratory, is that RA is metabolized in a series of reactions analogous to the activation and transport of fatty acids in mitochondria (Figure 4). Thus, an acyl-CoA synthetase would catalyze the formation of a thioester bond between the carboxyl group of RA and the thiol group of coenzyme A: RA + ATP + CoA-SH ↔ Retinoyl-CoA + AMP + PPi. In the next reaction, similar to the formation of fatty acyl-carnitine, an oxygen ester is formed between the high energy retinoyl-CoA and an hydroxyl group of an acceptor: Retinoyl-CoA + R-OH → Retinoyl-OR + CoA-SH. In the metabolism of fatty acids a high-energy fatty acyl-carnitine ester is formed, but it is possible that with RA the acceptor is an hydroxyl group of a macromolecule, e.g., the threonine, serine, or tyrosine moieties of a protein. This ester would be of low energy, resulting in essentially a one-way reaction for its formation and the formation of a stable covalent bond.

An extension of this hypothesis is that retinoylation and another modification (phosphorylation, methylation, acetylation, etc.) occurs at the same site. When this other modification dominates, the cell continues to proliferate and does not differentiate. In a transformed or neoplastic cell the balance is shifted even further in the direction of the other modification. This could be because of an increase in the capacity of the cell to carry out the other modification or because the information for this modification, carried by an oncogene or an infective virus, is activated or amplified. Under these conditions a higher than normal dose of RA may shift the balance back towards an increase in retinoylation, effectively blocking

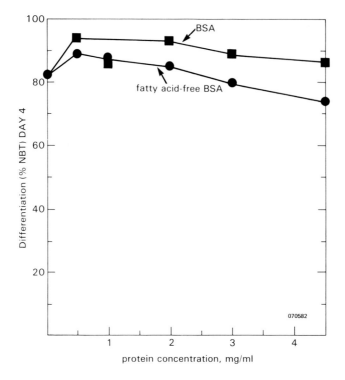

FIGURE 3.   Inability of bovine serum albumin (BSA) to inhibit induction of differentiation of HL-60 by 0.3 μ*M* RA in defined medium.

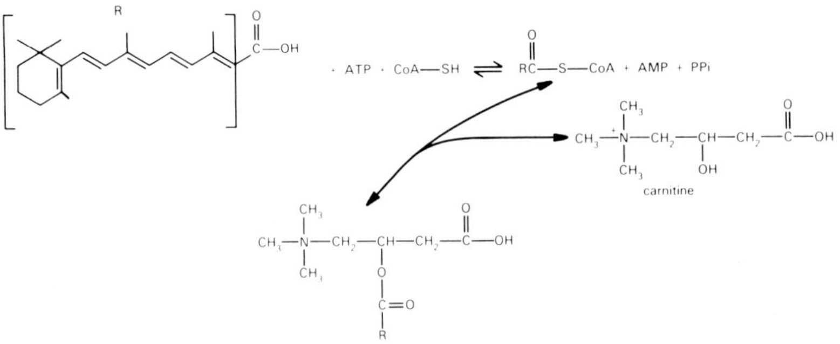

FIGURE 4.   Possible metabolism of RA based on fatty acid activation fatty acyl-S-CoA. With RA, the receptor of the retinoyl moiety may be a a macromolecule. R = decarboxylated portion of RA.

the competing modification, and allowing the cell to differentiate. With some cells, the higher than normal dose of RA may result in a retinoylation that competes with an essential modification, thus, leading to cell death. This model, or one similar to it, can explain why treatment of cells with RA have chemoprevention, differentiation-inducing, and cytotoxic activties.

V. INDUCER-DEPENDENT MORPHOLOGICAL, BIOCHEMICAL, AND FUNCTIONAL CHANGES IN HL-60

A. Chemotactic Peptide Receptor
There is now increasing evidence that there are differences in the properties of HL-60

cells maturing in response to different inducers. Thus, Skubitz et al.[51] report that there is an increase in the activity of HL-60 surface receptors for the f-met-leu-phe chemotactic peptide during induction of differentiation by dimethyl formamide and dimethyl sulfoxide. RA-induced cells exhibit a decrease in this parameter which is a direct function of the concentration of RA. Dexamethasone increases the number of chemotactic peptide receptors in dimethyl sulfoxide- or dimethyl formamide-induced HL-60 cells.[51,52] and this effect is markedly suppressed by RA.[51]

B. Production of Metabolites of Arachidonic Acid

Levine and Breitman[53] have shown that the calcium ionophore A_{23187}- activated production of leukotrienes and thomboxane B_2 is much greater in dimethyl sulfoxide-induced HL-60 than in RA-induced cells. In contrast, prostaglandin $E_2(PGE_2)$ production is much greater in RA-induced cells than in dimethyl sulfoxide-induced cells.

C. Morphological and Biochemical Changes

Comparative morphological and biochemical changes of HL-60 during differentiation induced by RA and dimethyl sulfoxide have been studied by Hemmi et al.[54] Morphological differentiation occurs at a much faster rate in the presence of RA (Figure 5) than with dimethyl sulfoxide (Figure 6). However, increases in biochemical parameters of the phagocytosis-associated "respiratory burst" of mature granulocytes (the generation of superoxide anion as measured either by the reduction of NBT or of ferricytochrome c and an enhanced HMPS) are relatively higher in the more immature dimethyl sulfoxide-treated culture than in the RA-treated culture. This is made clearer when these three biochemical parameters are compared relative to the maturation of the culture (Figure 7). In the normal developing granulocyte, the ability to reduce NBT appears with minimal activity at the metamyelocyte stage and increases in more mature forms.[55] In this respect, RA-induced HL-60 cells more closely follow the normal pattern (Figure 7), while with dimethyl sulfoxide-induced cells it appears that there is a dissociation of these biochemical maturation functions from morphological maturation.

VI. INVOLVEMENT OF INTRACELLULAR CYCLIC ADENOSINE 3′,5′-MONOPHOSPHATE (cAMP) IN DIFFERENTIATION OF HL-60

Agents, such as prostaglandin E (PGE), cholera toxin, and dibutyryl cAMP that increase the intracellular cAMP level, markedly potentiate RA-induced differentiation of HL-60.[32,34,56] PGs E_1, E_2, A_1, and A_2 promote differentiation of HL-60 in a concentration-dependent manner (Figures 8 and 9). Compared with RA, at least 60-fold greater concentrations of PGE are required to promote differentiation to the same extent. The most striking finding is that PGE_1 and PGE_2 are very effective inducers in combination with RA. That this combination is synergistic and not additive is demonstrated clearly by isobolograms (Figure 10). PGE_2 inhibits proliferation of HL-60 without having any effect on viability (Figure 11). RA is present in normal human peripheral blood at 10 nM[43] and PGE_2 is routinely found in human peripheral blood at 1 nM,[57] and can increase to 400 nM in localized areas of trauma, inflammation, or infection.[58] Thus, it is possible that the effects on differentiation with 10 nM RA and various concentrations of PGE (Figures 8 and 10) reflect in vitro what can occur in vivo where concentrations of RA can be expected to be fairly steady and concentrations of PGE vary widely.

The other PGs, either alone or in combination with RA, are much less active than PGE in inducing differentiation of HL-60 (Table 3), indicating a great degree of biological specificity by HL-60 in distinguishing between these structurally similar compounds. This specificity is related to substitutions in the cyclopentane ring, as there are no significant differences in biological activity between the PG-1s and PG-2s in each class.

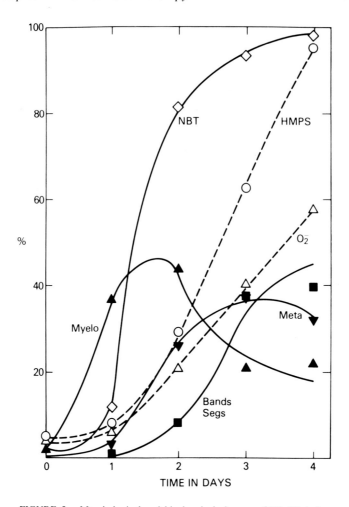

FIGURE 5. Morphological and biochemical changes of HL-60 during differentiation induced by 0.3 μ*M* RA. Morphological changes: ▲, myelocytes; ▼, metamyelocytes; ■, banded and segmented neutrophils. Biochemical changes: ◇, nitroblue tetrazolium (NBT) reduction; ○, hexose monophosphate shunt (HMPS) activity; △, superoxide anion (O_2^-) production. Morphological assessments were performed on Wright-Giemsa stained Cytospin slide preparations. NBT reduction was measured on cells activated with 12-*O*-tetradecanoylphorbol-13-acetate (TPA). The percentage of cells containing blue-black formazan deposits was assessed on Cytospin slide preparations stained with Wright-Giemsa. HMPS activity was measured as the release of $^{14}CO_2$ from glucose-1-^{14}C by intact cells. This activity is expressed as a ratio of the CO_2 released by cells treated with TPA to the CO_2 released by cells not treated with TPA. This ratio was 25:1 for cells incubated with 180 m*M* dimethyl sulfoxide for 4 days and set to 100% for comparisons. Superoxide anion (O_2^-) production was determined with intact cells activated with TPA by measuring the reduction of exogenous ferricytochrome c to ferrocytochrome c. Cells incubated with 180 m*M* dimethyl sulfoxide for 4 days produced 170 nmol (O_2^-) $\times 10^{-6}$ cell/hr and this value was set to 100% for comparisons.

PGE acts on many cell types by activating membrane adenylate cyclase, and increasing intracellular levels of cyclic AMP.[59-61] A similar mechanism is probably operative in HL-60 cells, as PGE_2 promotes a marked increase in cAMP.[34] $PGF_{2\alpha}$ is much less potent than PGE_2 in increasing the cAMP level of HL-60,[62] indicating that for the PGs there is a positive correlation between the extent of the increase in cAMP and the potentiation of RA-induced

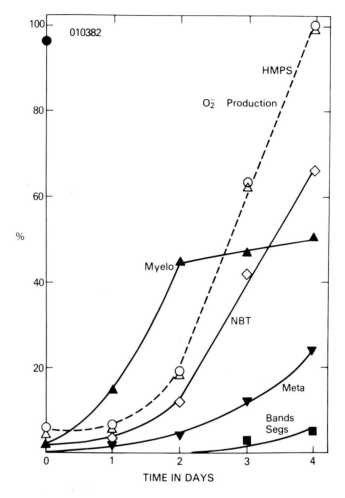

FIGURE 6. Morphological and biochemical changes of HL-60 during differentiation induced by 180 mM dimethyl sulfoxide. Symbols and methods as described in Figure 4; ●, promyelocytes at zero time.

differentiation. RA has no effect on the intracellular cAMP level, either alone or in combination with PGE$_2$. The combination of cholera toxin (which also increases HL-60 intracellular cAMP[62]), or dibutryl cAMP with RA give increases in differentiation of HL-60 that are synergistic (Table 4).[32] These results, and the report of Levine and Ohuchi[63] that in MDCK cells RA enhances the deacylation of cellular lipids with a consequent increase in PG production, suggested the possibility that RA induction of HL-60 is mediated by endogenous synthesis of PG. However, indomethacin and aspirin, inhibitors of the PG synthetic enzyme cyclooxygenase, has no inhibitory effect on RA-induced differentiation of HL-60 (Table 5). The concentration of aspirin and the lowest concentration of indomethacin used here are at least fivefold greater than concentrations reported to completely suppress PG synthesis in a wide variety of cell types and cell lines including rat neutrophils, murine macrophages and human monocytes, MDCK cells, HeLa cells, and human fibroblasts. In addition, Bonser et al.[64] have shown that indomethacin does not block the increases in chemotactic formyl peptide receptor binding and hexose monophosphate shunt activity in HL-60 induced to differentiate by exposure to dimethyl sulfoxide. Thus, it appears unlikely that endogenously synthesized PGs play a role in the induction of differentiation of HL-60. It is more likely that the results we have obtained on HL-60 cells in vitro reflect events occuring during normal granulocytic differentiation in vivo. It is well known that PGE and

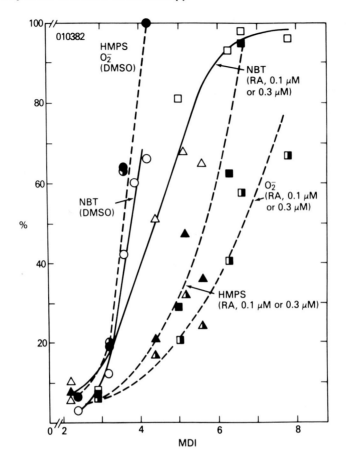

FIGURE 7.   Biochemical parameters as a function of morphology of HL-60 induced to differentiate by 180 mM dimethyl sulfoxide (DMSO) or 0.1 μM and 0.3 μM RA. For cells treated with DMSO: ○, NBT reduction; ●, HMPS, ◖, O_2^-, production. For cells treated with 0.1 μM RA: △, NBT reduction; ▲, HMPS; ◭, O_2^- production. For cells treated with 0.3 μM RA: □, NBT reduction; ■, HMPS; ◩, O_2^- production. MDI is a morphological differentiation index calculated according to the formula: MDI = [(% myelobasts × 0) + (% promyelocytes × 2) + (% myelocytes × 4) + (% metamyelocytes × 6) + (% banded neutrophils × 8) + (% segmented neutrophils × 10)] × 10^{-2}

cAMP are potent inhibitors of both normal bone marrow granulocyte/macrophage colony forming units and of myeloid leukemia cell lines in semisolid medium.[7,65-67] However, these studies have not adequately provided a clear distinction between decreased colony numbers resulting from terminal differentiation and those resulting from cytotoxicity. In the microenvironment of the bone marrow, the interplay between RA derived from the diet, and PGE and colony-stimulating activity derived from monocytes, may be one of the important controls of granulocytic maturation.

VII. DIFFERENTIATION EFFECTS OF AGENTS THAT INCREASE INTRACELLULAR cAMP on HL-60 PRIMED WITH RA

The finding that differentiation of HL-60 by RA is potentiated by agents known to increase intracellular cAMP prompted a study on the effects of sequential treatment with these agents.[56] It was found that HL-60 could be primed for differentiation by treatment for

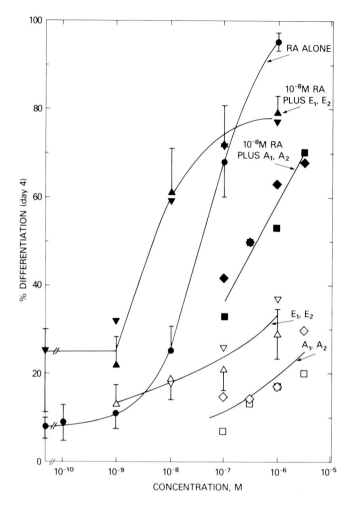

FIGURE 8.   Differentiation of HL-60 induced by various concentrations
of PGE and PGA in the presence and absence of 10 nM RA. Differentiation
is expressed as the percentage of cells reducing NBT.

approximately 1 day with 10 nM RA followed by exposure to a cAMP-inducing agent
(cholera toxin or PGE_2). The reverse sequence was ineffective at the same concentrations.
Thus, HL-60 could be primed by incubation for less than 20 hr with 10 nM RA to respond
by differentiation to the addition of 10 nM PGE_2 or 1 nM cholera toxin, whereas 10 nM
RA alone was inactive. Priming of HL-60 did not depend on the normal rate of protein
synthesis, as it occurred even better in the presence of 1 μg/mℓ cycloheximide, a concentration that inhibited growth completely and protein synthesis by 86%. However, the resulting
maturation was inhibited by cycloheximide. These results suggest that a decrease in synthesis
of some protein(s) favors RA-induced differentiation. The nature of these proteins is unknown, as is the direct consequences of inhibition of their synthesis. One possibility is that
differentiation in HL-60 is inhibited by a polypeptide. Inhibition of protein synthesis by
cycloheximide could diminish the production of this inhibitor and facilitate the modulating
activities on differentiation by cAMP-inducing agents. Another untested hypothesis is that
RA induces the production of a mRNA whose translation initiates the phenotypic changes
characteristic of differentiated cells; cycloheximide could increase the production and the
half-life of this mRNA as has been reported for human fibroblast interferon mRNA.[68]

It is possible that the effects of RA and cAMP-inducing agents on HL-60 may be explained
on the basis of a cAMP-dependent protein kinase activity. The phosphorylation of specific

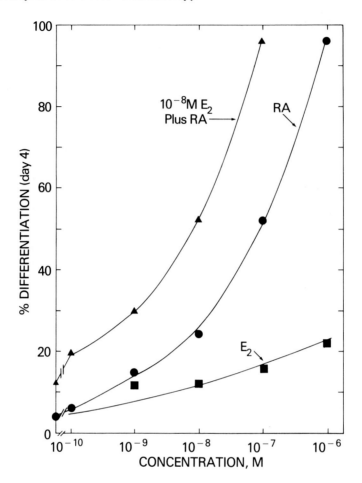

FIGURE 9.   Differentiation of HL-60 induced by various concentrations
of RA or PGE$_2$ and by RA in the presence of 10 nM PGE$_2$. Differentiation
is expressed as the percentage of cells reducing NBT.

proteins has been implicated as playing a central role in a large number of biological
processes, and most, if not all, effects of cAMP are thought to be mediated by cAMP-
dependent protein kinases.[69] In murine melanoma cells, RA increases cAMP-dependent
protein kinase activity[70] with no change in intracellular cAMP levels.[70, 71] In HL-60, RA
may also induce or increase the synthesis of a specific protein kinase. The activity of this
enzyme would be dependent on the intracellular level of cAMP, which in vitro is increased
by adding PGE, cholera toxin, or dibutyryl cAMP to HL-60 cultures. Alternatively, RA
may induce the production of a product which is phosphorylated in the process of differentiation. Recent findings[56] have shown that exogenous ATP or dATP have differentiation-
inducing effect on HL-60, either in the presence of a low concentration of RA or on cells
primed with RA. Because nucleotides are not transported into the intracellular space, and
because cAMP-dependent protein kinases are present on the outer surface of the plasma
membrane of some cells,[72, 73] these results give indirect support for the involvement of
phosphorylation reactions on the plasma membrane in the differentiation of HL-60.

VIII. MONOCYTIC DIFFERENTIATION OF HL-60 BY T-LYMPHOCYTE DERIVED DIFFERENTIATION INDUCING ACTIVITY (DIA)

HL-60 is also induced to differentiate into cells having many of the functional and mor-

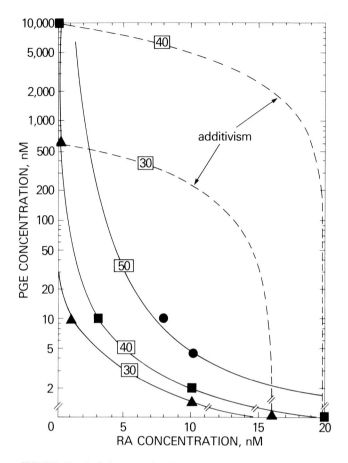

FIGURE 10. Isobolograms showing synergy for induction of differentiation of HL-60 cells by combinations of PGE and PGA. The experimental points were obtained from the data shown in Figures 7 and 8 and other experiments, and are the concentrations of PGE and RA in combination inducing 30% (▲), 40% (■), and 50% (●) differentiation as indicated by the boxed values on each curve. The dashed lines connecting the values of PGE and RA alone would have been obtained if the two compounds in combination were additive.

phological characteristics of mature monocyte-like cells by conditioned media of activated mononuclear cells (Table 6).[23, 74-77] The morphological changes include diminished cytoplasmic basophilia, less prominent granules, and decreased nuclear-cytoplasmic ratios.[74] Functional changes include increase in the proportion of cells: positive for nonspecific esterase;[74, 75] with Fc and C3 receptors and capable of immunophagocytosis,[23] reducing NBT,[77] and expressing surface antigens of monocytes or macrophages.[76,78]

We have named the activity of these conditiond media Differentiation Inducing Activity or DIA. This activity is associated with a protein(s) and is distinct from colony stimulating activity (CSA) as these two activities are separated by gel-permeation chromatography.[77]

The human T-lymphocytic leukemia cell line, HUT-102, established from a patient with cutaneous T-cell lymphoma,[79] is a constitutive producer of DIA.[56] DIA, partially purified from serum-free conditioned medium of HUT-102, has been used for the experiments described below.

While DIA alone induces differentiation of HL-60, its most marked effect is in combination with RA[80] (Figure 12). The synergy of this combination is similiar to the synergy observed with combinations of RA and cAMP-inducing agents (see above), and the apparent synergy

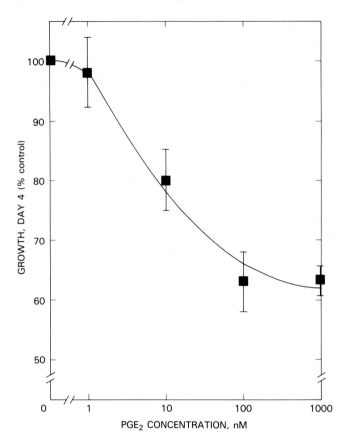

FIGURE 11. Inhibition by PGE_2 of growth of HL-60 cells. Cells (2.5 × 10^5/mℓ) were grown for 4 days in defined medium containing the indicated concentration of PGE_2. At day 4, control cells had grown to a concentration of 8 × 10^5 cells/mℓ (mean of five experiments). Bars: SE of five experiments. Viability, measured by trypan blue exclusion, was >90% under all conditions.

Table 3
DIFFERENTIATION OF HL-60 CELLS BY COMBINATIONS OF RA, PGF, PGB, AND PGA

		Differentiation, day 4 (% NBT) PG concentration, μM			
PG	RA, 10 nM	0	1	3	10
$F_{1\alpha}$	−	8	4	7	11
	+	25	24	25	53
$F_{2\alpha}$	−		12	16	25
	+		26	27	47
B_1	−		12	20	33
	+		26	37	82
B_2	−		9	11	23
	+		34	52	76
A_1	−		19	25	
	+		62	68	
A_2	−		18	25	
	+		53	70	

Table 4
MODULATION OF RA-INDUCED DIFFERENTIATION OF HL-60 BY DIBUTYRYL cAMP (dbcAMP)

Condition	Differentiation, day 4 (% NBT)
Control	8 ± 3
RA, 10 nM	25 ± 6
dbcAMP	
10 μM	12
100 μM	33 ± 5
dbcAMP, 100 μM	
plus 10 nM RA	92 ± 7

Table 5
EFFECTS OF ASPIRIN AND INDOMETHACIN ON RA-INDUCED DIFFERENTIATION OF HL-60 CELLS

Condition	Differentiation, day 4 (% NBT)
Control	8 ± 3
RA, 0.1 μM	68 ± 8
1 μM	95 ± 2
Aspirin, 0.56 mM	7
plus RA, 1 μM	95
Indomethacin, 2.8 μM	10 ± 3
plus RA, 0.1 μM	76
plus RA, 1 μM	90
Indomethacin, 14 μM	9
plus RA, 0.1 μM	88
Indomethacin, 28 μM	10
plus RA, 0.1 μM	94

observed with combinations of RA and α- or β-interferon.[81] DIA also promotes differentiation of RA-primed HL-60.[56] However, DIA has no effect on the intracellular level of cAMP.[82] Therefore, its mechanism of action is probably different from that of PGE, cholera toxin, and dibutyryl cAMP.

From experiments similiar to the one described in Figure 12, a unit of DIA is defined as an amount increasing differentiation of HL-60 (measured as the percentage of NBT-positive cells) by 1% when cells are incubated in serum-free defined medium containing 10 nM RA for 4 days. Based on this definition, the DIA preparation used in the experiment shown in Figure 12 contains approximately 10 units of DIA per microliter.

We studied the effects of DIA alone and in combination with 10 nM RA on three markers of differentiation (Figure 13). HL-60 cultures treated with 1 μM RA show time-dependent increases in the percentage of cells: reducing NBT, exhibiting Fc receptors, and capable of immunophagocytosis (Figure 13A). Under this condition there was no increase in the activities of two markers of monocytes/macrophages: 5'-nucleotidase[83] and nonspecific esterase (data not shown). DIA alone (60 units/mℓ of culture) increases the proportion of cells with Fc receptors, and to a lesser extent increases immunophagocytosis and NBT reduction (Figure

Table 6
DIFFERENTIATION INDUCING ACTIVITY(DIA) FOR HL-60 CELLS

Name	Source[a]	Stimulated with	Concentration	Differentiation parameter	Time in culture (days)	Ref.
MGI(LCM)	Lymphocytes	PHA	50%	80% morphol, 52.9% Fc, 45.4% C3, increased lysozyme activity	6	23
LCM	Mononuclear cells	2-ME	20 or 40%	40—50% morphol, increased lysozyme activity	6	74
LCM	Lymphocytes or T-lymphocytes	PHA or MLC	30%	40—47% morphol, 37—48% C3	4, 5	75
LCM	Leukocytes	PHA	10%	macrophage surface antigens	5	76
LCM	Mononuclear cells	PWM	10%	morphol, increased granule protein	4—6, 3—10	38
DIFs	LCM of mononuclear cells	Con A, PWM or protein A	10%	35—40% morphol, 35—45% NBT-red	5	77
DIFs	LCM of HUT 102	None	50 µg/mℓ	40% NBT-red	4	56
DIFs(LCM)	Mononuclear cell	PHA	50%	monocyte/macrophage surface antigens, 83—93% NBT-red	3—5, 5	78

Note: Abbreviations — MGI, normal protein inducer of differentiation to macrophages or granulocytes; LCM, leukocyte or lymphocyte conditioned medium; PHA, phytohemagglutinin; 2-ME, 2-mercaptoethanol; MLC, mixed lymphocyte culture; PWM, pokeweed mitogen; Con A, concanavalin A; NBT-red, nitroblue tetrazolium reduction; DIFs, T-lymphocyte-derived differentiation inducing factors; morphol, morphologically mature cells including: myelocytes, metamyelocytes, banded and segmented neutrophilis, monocytes, and macrophages; C3, C3 receptors; Fc, Fc receptors.

[a]   Cells were isolated from human peripheral blood except for the cell line HUT 102.

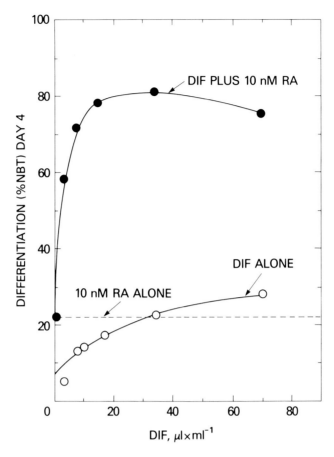

FIGURE 12.   Differentiation of HL-60 induced by various concentrations
of DIA (DIF) with (●) and without (○) 10 n*M* RA. This DIA preparation
had approximately 10 units/μℓ.

13C). The combination of 10 n*M* RA [which alone elicits only slight increases in these
parameters (Figure 13B)] and DIA markedly increases the rate of appearance and the extent
of both phagocytosis and NBT reduction (Figure 13D) compared to the effect of each of
these agents alone. HL-60 cells treated with RA alone exhibit low levels of positivity for
5′-nucleotidase and nonspecific esterase. HL-60 treated with DIA alone exhibits moderate
levels of activity for these two markers, but the combination of DIA and 10 n*M* RA promotes
large increases in both markers that essentially parallel the increases in phagocytosis and
NBT reduction shown in Figure 13D.

The finding that DIA alone and in combination with RA induces differentiation of HL-
60 to cells with many properties of monocytes/macrophages raises the possibility that DIA
may be a normal physiological agent acting via the phorbol diester receptor. HL-60 cells,
like virtually all mammalian cells except erythrocytes, have phorbol diester receptors.[84-86]
Phorbol diesters induce HL-60 to differentiate into cells with a macrophage morphology and
with macrophage characteristics, such as adherence, and increases in cellular activities for
nonspecific esterase, lysozyme, 5′-nucleotidase, and acid phosphatase.[23, 27, 87] These cells
are, however, deficient in some important macrophage biochemical and functional characteristics such as immunophagocytosis, reduction of NBT, HMPS activity, superoxide generation, and Fc receptors.[27, 87] These latter markers are the very markers appearing (in addition
to adherence, 5′-nucleotidase, nonspecific esterase, and monocyte/macrophage morphology)
when HL-60 cells are induced to differentiate with a combination of DIA and RA (Figure

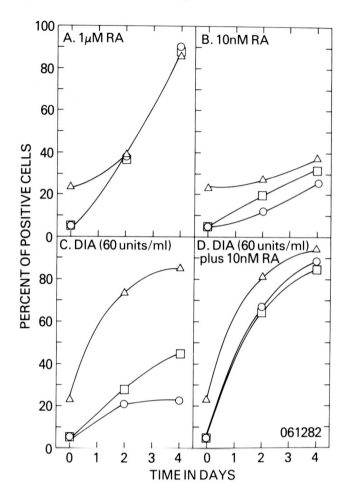

FIGURE 13. Increases in biochemical and functional parameters of HL-60 treated with DIA and RA alone and in combination. Fc receptors, ($\triangle$); immunophagocytosis, ($\square$); NBT reduction, ($\bigcirc$).

13D). Thus, the combination of RA (at a physiological concentration) and DIA (a lymphokine with an unknown physiological concentration) promotes differentiation of HL-60 to cells having a more complete catalog of monocyte/macrophage properties than the HL-60 cells produced by the tumor-promoting phorbol diesters. Because the phorbol diesters appear to act by binding to specific high-affinity cellular receptors, we speculate that the mechanism of action of both phorbol diester and DIA may involve the same receptor.

IX. RA-INDUCED DIFFERENTIATION OF FRESH HUMAN ACUTE PROMYELOCYTIC LEUKEMIA CELLS IN PRIMARY CULTURE

The finding that RA is a potent inducer of HL-60 terminal differentiation prompted an investigation to determine whether fresh human leukemic cells shared this response. In a recent report,[46] we incubated fresh human myeloid leukemia cells in short-term suspension cultures in the presence of RA: 21 leukemic patients were studied. The diagnosis was acute myelocytic leukemia in 13 patients, acute myelomonocytic leukemia in 2 patients, acute promyelocytic leukemia (APL) in 2 patients, chronic myelocytic leukemia in blastic phase in 3 patients, and chronic myelomonocytic leukemia in accelerated phase in 1 patient. Differentiation of the leukemic cells from 2 of the 21 patients was induced by RA. The only

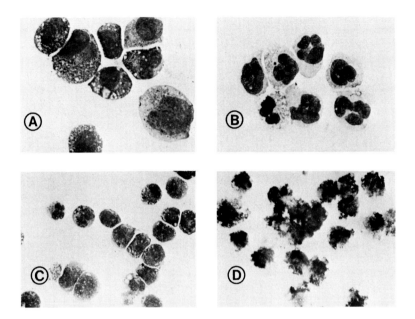

FIGURE 14. Morphological and functional maturation of leukemic cells obtained from a patient with acute promyelocytic leukemia. Cells were incubated in serum-containing medium for 5 days. Cytospin slide preparations were stained with Wright-Geimsa (A) Cells cultured without RA consisting of promyelocytes with characteristic granules. (B) Cells cultured with 1 μM RA showing maturation to banded and segmented neutrophils. (C) Absence of NBT reduction by cells cultured without RA. (D) NBT reduction by cells incubated with 1 μM RA. The magnification in (A) and (B) is approximately 2.8-fold greater than in (C) and (D).

inducible specimens were from the two patients with APL, both of whose cells incubated in the absence of RA did not morphologically differentiate and did not reduce NBT (Figure 14).

None of the other patients cells showed any significant granulocytic differentiation induced by RA. In no specimen did RA significantly affect viability or the total cell counts. In several of the cultures, especially those diagnosed as myelomonocytic leukemia, cells morphologically resembling monocytes and macrophages developed after a few days in suspension culture. These cells were NBT positive, also a biochemical marker of monocytes and macrophages.[55] Similiar spontaneous differentiation of fresh human leukemic cells in short-term culture has been described.[88] However, RA had essentially no effect on this spontaneous differentiation.

Since this initial report we have studied ten peripheral blood and/or marrow samples from six patients with APL. The cells from all of these patients differentiated in vitro in response to RA (Table 7 and data not shown). Cells from some of these patients were also tested for effects of PGE$_2$ and DIA (Table 7). The cells in all of these samples responded with differentiation to RA. With patients 3 and 6 there was a response at 10 nM RA, a concentration close to the reported normal plasma level for RA.[43]

Because of the synergy of combinations of RA with PGE$_2$ or DIA on differentiation of HL-60 (see above), we examined the effects of these combinations on fresh human APL cells. PGE$_2$ (10 nM) alone had no effect on differentiation (patient 3) and the combination of 10 nM PGE$_2$ and 100 μM RA resulted in levels of differentiation that were slightly higher than those observed with 100 nM RA alone (Table 7, patient 2 and patient 3, day 7). While these results are suggestive that combinations of RA and PGE$_2$ synergistically induce differentiation of fresh APL cells, a definitive determination must await further experimentation.

In contrast to the results with PGE$_2$, the combination of DIA and RA appears to be clearly

Table 7
INDUCTION OF DIFFERENTIATION OF FRESH CELLS FROM PATIENTS WITH ACUTE PROMYELOCYTIC LEUKEMIA (APL)

Patient identification	Treatment				Differentiation, % NBT at day			
	RA (nM)	PGE$_2$ (nM)	DIA	Other	3	5	6	7
1. PV	0				0	0		
pb	100				35	79		
221080	1000				37	85		
	0		+		0	2		
	100		+		92	100		
	1000		+			98		
2. PV	0					3.5		
bm	100					66		
101280	1000					80		
	100	10				77		
	100		+			96		
3. PV	0				7	4		2
bm	10				4	12		38
220481	100				7	22		46
	1000				10	26		71
	0	10			5	4		4
	100	10			2	24		59
	0		+		4	5		5
	100		+		19	98		99
4. GS	0				8	11		
	100				10	56		
230481	1000				14	69		
5. MS	0					2.5		
bm	100					37		
101280	1000					41		
	0		+			7		
	100		+			72		
	1000		+			81		
6. MR	0				1	2		
pb	10				65	88		
220682	300				68	92		
	1000				75	93		
	0		+		0	2		
	10		+		77	93		
	300		+		81	90		
	0			DMSO, 180 mM	1			
	0			Ro 22-9343, 10 nM	5	9		
	0		+	Ro 22-9343, 10 nM	5	4		

synergistic in inducing differentiation of fresh APL cells (Table 7). The concentrations of DIA employed in these experiments had no effect alone on differentiation (Table 7, patients 1, 3, 5, and 6). However, with a combination of DIA and RA the rate and/or extent of differentiation was markedly greater than what was observed with RA alone. This promotion of differentiation by DIA was observed in all cases except for patient 6 whose cells, because they were very responsive to RA alone, probably masked a greater DIA effect than that observed.

Two other inducers of HL-60 differentiation were tested on the cells of patient 6 (Table

7). Dimethyl sulfoxide had no effect on differentiation of this patient's cells, even though at this concentration (180 mM) it induces 40% NBT-positivity of HL-60 at day 3 (Figure 6).

Ro 22-9343 is an analog of 1 α,25-dihydroxyvitamin D$_3$ and, on a molar basis, is approximately tenfold more active than 1α,25-dihydroxyvitamin D$_3$ in inducing differentiation of HL-60.[89] In addition, active forms of vitamin D$_3$ have been reported to induce maturation of HL-60 along the granulocytic pathway.[33] However, our own findings, based on morphology, increases in cellular activities of nonspecific esterase and 5'-nucleotidase, and reactivity to monocyte-specific monoclonal antibodies, are that these compounds induce maturation of HL-60 to monocyte/macrophage-like cells. This active derivative of 1α,25-dihydroxyvitamin D$_3$ had essentially no effect, either alone or in combination with DIA, on increasing NBT-positivity of this patient's cells.

X. DIFFERENTIATION OF OTHER MYELOMONOCYTIC CELL LINES BY RA

The monoblast- and monocyte-like cell lines, U-937 and THP-1, grow and are induced to mature by RA in defined medium. In this medium, RA-treated cells, and to a lesser extent untreated cells, adhere to the plastic surface. If, however, 600 μg of bovine serum albumin per milliliter is added, there is essentially no adherence, and the extent of differentiation induced by RA is identical to that obtained in serum-containing medium.[12,90] Combinations of RA and DIA induce differentiation of both of these cell lines synergistically. However, U-937 and THP-1 respond very little, if at all, to DIA alone.[56, 91]

XI. EVIDENCE THAT RA-INDUCED DIFFERENTIATION OF HL-60 DOES NOT REQUIRE CELL GROWTH

When it seemed possible that RA might have clinical utility, it became of interest to examine in vitro the effects of cell-growth-inhibiting chemotherapeutic agents on RA-induced differentiation of HL-60.[92] It was also felt that such studies might yield further insight into the mechanism of RA-induction and, more generally, into granulocytic terminal differentiation.

RA was tested in combination with two chemotherapeutic agents, hydroxyurea and arabinosylcytosine (ara-C). Both of these agents are known to inhibit cell growth by specifically inhibiting DNA synthesis.[93, 94] HL-60 cells were grown at various concentrations of the drug, with and without RA. The concentration of hydroxyurea that inhibited growth by 50% was 100 μM for cultures growing either with or without 1 μM RA (Figure 15). RA alone, as described previously,[30] decreased growth, and increasing concentrations of hydroxyurea decreased the cell number still further. However, hydroxyurea inhibition of cell growth had essentially no effect on the extent of RA-induced differentiation of HL-60 (Figure 16), as measured by the concentration of mature (NBT-positive) cells as a function of the total cell concentration (Figure 16). Thus, in the presence of 1 μM RA, there was essentially a constant value of 0.66 for the mature cells: total cell ratio, with increasing concentration of hydroxurea and decreased proliferation. Growth inhibition by hydroxyurea alone had little if any effect on the extent of HL-60 differentiation.

In a similiar study with various concentrations of ara-C in both the presence and the absence of 0.3 μM RA, the extent of RA-induced differentiation of HL-60 was not markedly reduced by growth-inhibiting concentrations of ara-C (Figures 17 and 18). In addition, ara-C alone appeared to have an inductive effect on HL-60. Thus, at the highest concentration of ara-C, the culture contained approximately 50% NBT-positive cells (0.4 $\times$ 10^5 NBT-positive cells/mℓ/0.8 $\times$ 10^5 total cells/mℓ). However, at the initiation of the experiment, there were 0.2 $\times$ 10^5 NBT-positive cells/mℓ (8% NBT-positive cells $\times$ 2.5 $\times$ 10^5 cells/

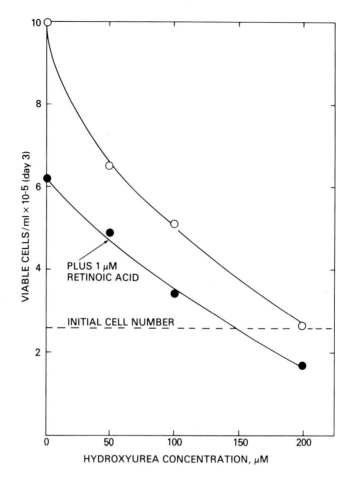

FIGURE 15.   Inhibition of growth of HL-60 cells by various concentrations of hydroxyurea in the presence (●) or absence (○) of 1 μM RA.

mℓ). These nonproliferating mature cells would be resistant to ara-C with the result that ara-C would selectively kill proliferating cells with a consequent enrichment of the population for NBT-positive cells. Thus most if not all of the increase in the percentage of NBT-positive cells in cultures grown with ara-C alone is probably the result of enrichment and not induction. This conclusion is in agreement with the results of others,[18,22] who found little or no morphological maturation of HL-60 at ara-C concentrations lower than 1 μM.

The concentrations at which these drugs were tested are analogous to their plasma levels when they are used as antileukemic agents. RA was used as an inducing agent because of its possible clinical utility, since it has been observed that it induced differentiation of primary cultures of fresh leukemic promyelocytes (see above). Our results indicate that neither hydroxyurea nor ara-C interferes with the differentiative action of RA and that RA does not interfere with their growth-inhibitory activity. Thus, RA and other retinoids can be considered for combination therapy in a program aimed at both inhibiting proliferation and inducing terminal differentiation of promyelocytic and possibly other immature leukemia cells.

XII. ANIMAL MODEL SYSTEMS FOR TREATMENT OF MALIGNANCIES BY INDUCTION OF DIFFERENTIATION

As shown above, some human leukemia cells are induced in vitro to differentiate to nonproliferating end cells with many of the morphological, biochemical, and functional

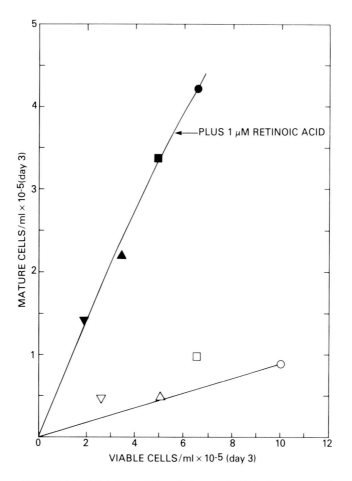

FIGURE 16. RA-induced differentiation of HL-60 in the presence of various concentrations of hydroxyurea. ●, ■, ▲, ▼, with 1 μM RA; ○, □, △, ▽, no RA. Hydroxyurea concentrations: none (○, ●); 50 μM (□, ■); 100 μM (△, ▲); 200 μM (▽, ▼). Mature cells were calculated by the formula: mature cells/mℓ = (% of NBT-positive cells × viable cells/mℓ) × 10^{-2}.

characteristics of normal cells. The question of whether these findings in vitro have applicability in vivo has begun to be explored in the clinic. These studies could be aided greatly if there were animal models for studying differentiation-inducing agents on malignant cells having a close counterpart to human cells. The "perfect" animal model does not exist now; but it can be expected that as the view that malignancy can be treated by inducing differentiation gains acceptance, better animal models will be developed. It has been approximately 25 years since Pierce[95, 96] and Pierce et al.[97] advocated that tumors were a problem of cellular differentiation rather than of proliferation, per se. Only recently has there been strong experimental evidence supporting this advocacy. It can be expected that in the next few years this strategy will be more fully explored, both in the clinic and with animal models. Animal models presently available are outlined below.

A. M1 Leukemia Cells

Induction of differentiation of the murine myeloid leukemia cell line, M1, and its subclones has been studied both in vitro and in vivo (for recent reviews see References 98 and 99). M1 cells are induced to differentiate in vitro into mature granulocytes and/or macrophages by incubation with many agents including bacterial lipopolysaccharides, glucocorticoids,[100]

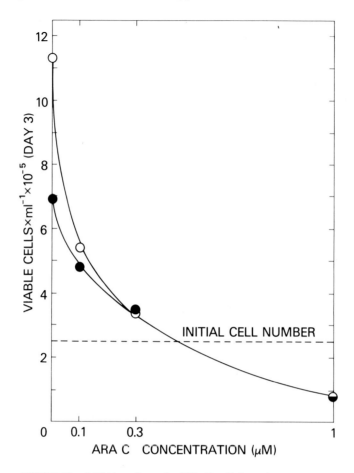

FIGURE 17. Inhibition of growth of HL-60 cells by various concentrations of ara-C in the presence (●) or absence (○) of 0.3 μM RA.

macrophage- and granulocyte-inducing protein(MGI),[101] and 1α,25-dihydroxyvitamin D$_3$.[102] Treatment of syngeneic SL mice or athymic nude mice, previously inoculated with M1 cells, with these agents prolonged their survival time.[100,103,104] This increased life-span could be attributed, at least in part, to an induction of differentiation. An induction of differentiation in vivo was clearly observed when M1 cells were placed in diffusion chambers which were then implanted into SL mice or athymic nude mice and the mice were treated with inducers.[100,103]

B. F9 Embryonal Carcinoma Cells

A murine teratocarcinoma stem cell line, F9, is induced to differentiate in vitro into parietal endoderm by RA.[105] RA-treatment of 129/Sv mice carrying F9 cells significantly retards tumor growth and prolongs the survival time of the mice.[106]

C. HL-60 Cells

HL-60 forms tumors in athymic nude mice.[36] However, tumor formation requires the injection of 3 to 5 × 10^7 cells subcutaneously and appears to be directly related to the passage number of the HL-60. Later passages gave rise to tumors in 3/8 mice while earlier passages gave rise to tumors in only 1/8 mice. In addition, these tumors could not be serially transplanted for more than three generations, either by direct in vivo passaging or by re-establishment of the tumors in tissue culture between inoculations. This system cannot be easily employed for studies on the effects of inducers of differentiation. To our knowledge, diffusion chamber studies have not been conducted.

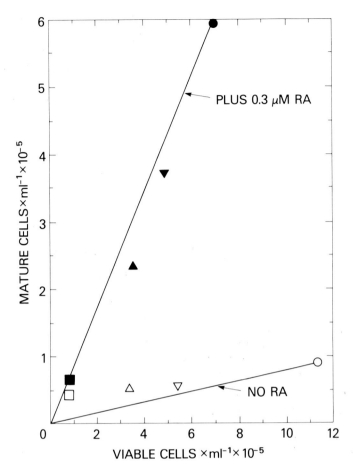

FIGURE 18. RA-induced differentiation of HL-60 in the presence of various concentrations of ara-C: ●, ■, ▲, ▼, with 0.3 μM RA; ○, □, △, ▽, no RA. Ara-C concentrations: none (○, ●); 0.1 μM (▽, ▼); 0.3 μM (△, ▲); 1 μM (□, ■). Mature cells were calculated by the formula: mature cells/mℓ = (% of NBT-positive cells $\times$ viable cells/mℓ) $\times$ 10^{-2}

XIII. CONCLUSION

The availability of tissue-culture cell lines has made it possible to study the regulation of proliferation and differentiation of specific hematopoietic cell types and the effects on these cells of known mediators and modulators. Retinoic acid (RA) is a potent inducer of terminal differentiation of the human promyelocytic cell line, HL-60, and the human monoblast- and monocyte-like cell lines, U-937 and THP-1. RA-induced differentiation occurs as well in serum-free medium or in serum-free medium containing albumin as it does in serum-supplemented medium, indicating that bound RA may be as active as free RA and suggesting that RA may act initially at the cell membrane. The absence of a cytoplasmic RA-binding protein in HL-60 cells and the markedly lower differentiation-inducing activity of two metabolities of RA, 4-hydroxy- and 4-keto-RA, eliminates two other possible mechanisms to explain RA-induction. It is speculated that RA may act after its activation in a reaction with CoA-SH to form retinoyl-CoA, and that an hydroxyl group of a macromolecule is an acceptor for the retinoyl moiety. This retinoylation may be the basis for the chemoprevention, differentiation-inducing, and cytotoxic activities of RA. RA induces differentiation of fresh cells in primary culture of patients with acute promyelocytic leukemia. Combinations of RA and the T-cell lymphokine, differentiation inducing activity (DIA), are synergistic in inducing differentiation of the fresh leukemia cells and the cell lines HL-60, U-937, and THP-1. The combination of RA and agents that increase intracellular cAMP levels (prostaglandin E_2 and cholera toxin) was synergistic in inducing differentiation of HL-60, but had only a small effect on the induction of differentiation of one patient's cells. These results, primarily with HL-60 and fresh APL cells, lends further support to an approach to cancer therapy that attempts to induce differentiation as the primary strategy.

REFERENCES

1. **Lozzio, C. B. and Lozzio, B. B.,** Human chronic myelogenous leukemia cell line with positive Philadelphia chromosome, *Blood,* 45, 321, 1975.
2. **Anderson, L. C., Jokinen, M., and Gahmberg, C. G.,** Induction of erythroid differentiation in the human cell line K-562, *Nature (London),* 278, 364, 1979.
3. **Rutherford, T. R., Clegg, J. B., and Weatherall, D. J.,** K-562 human leukemic cells synthesize embryonic hemoglobin in response to hemin, *Nature (London),* 280, 164, 1979.
4. **Hoffman, R., Murnane, M. J., Benz, E. J., Jr., Prohaska, R., Floyd, V., Dainiak, N., Forget, B. G., and Furthmayr, H.,** Induction of erythropoietic colonies in a human chronic myelogenous leukemia cell line, *Blood,* 54, 1182, 1979.
5. **Lozzio, B. B., Lozzio, C. B., Bamberger, E. G., and Feliu, A. S.,** A multipotential leukemia cell line (K-562) of human origin, *Proc. Soc. Exp. Biol. Med.,* 166, 546, 1981.
6. **Koeffler, H. P. and Golde, D. W.,** Acute myelogenous leukemia: a human cell line responsive to colony-stimulating activity, *Science,* 200, 1153, 1978.
7. **Koeffler, H. P. and Golde, D. W.,** Humoral modulation of human acute myelogenous leukemia cell growth *in vitro, Cancer Res.,* 40, 1858, 1980.
8. **Koeffler, H. P., Bar-Eli, M., and Territo, M. C.,** Phorbol ester effect on differentiation of human myeloid leukemia cell lines blocked at different stages of maturation; *Cancer Res.,* 41, 919, 1981.
9. **Sundstrom, C. and Nilsson, K.,** Establishment and characterization of a human histocytic lymphoma cell line (U937), *Int. J. Cancer,* 17, 565, 1976.
10. **Nilsson, K., Andersson, L. C., Gahmberg, C. G., and Forsbeck, K.,** Differentiation *in vitro* of human leukemia and lymphoma cell lines, *Int. Symp. New Trends in Human Immunology and Cancer Immunotherapy,* Serrou, B. and Rosenfeld, C., Eds., Doin, Paris, 1980, 271.
11. **Koren, H. S., Anderson, S. J., and Larrich, J. W.,** *In vitro* activation of a human macrophage-like cell line, *Nature (London),* 279, 328, 1979.
12. **Olsson, I. L. and Breitman, T. R.,** Induction of differentiation of the human histocytic lymphoma cell line U-937 by retinoic acid and cyclic adenosine 3':5'-monophosphate-inducing agents, *Cancer Res.,* 42, 3924, 1982.
13. **Tsuchiya, S., Yamabe, M., Yamaguchi, Y., Kobayashi, Y., Konno, T., and Tada, K.,** Establishment and characterization of a human acute monocytic leukemia cell line (THP-1), *Int. J. Cancer,* 26, 171, 1980.
14. **Tsuchiya, S., Kobayashi, Y., Goto, Y., Okumura, H., Nakae, S., Konno, T., and Tada, K.,** Induction of maturation in cultured human monocytic leukemia cells by a phorbol diester, *Cancer Res.,* 42, 1530, 1982.
15. **Collins, S. J., Gallo, R. C., and Gallagher, R. E.,** Continuous growth and differentiation of human myeloid leukemic cells in suspension culture, *Nature (London),* 270, 347, 1977.
16. **Collins, S. J., Ruscetti, F. W., Gallagher, R. E., and Gallo, R. C.,** Terminal differentiation of human promyelocytic leukemia cells induced by dimethyl sulfoxide and other polar compounds, *Proc. Natl. Acad. Sci. U.S.A.,* 75, 2458, 1978.
17. **Collins, S. J., Ruscetti, F. W., Gallagher, R. E., and Gallo, R. C.,** Normal functional characteristics of cultured human promyelocytic leukemia cells (HL60) after induction of differentiation by dimethyl sulfoxide, *J. Exp. Med.,* 149, 969, 1979.
18. **Collins, S. J., Bodner, A., Ting, R., and Gallo, R. C.,** Induction of morphological and functional differentiation of human promyelocyte leukemia cells (HL-60) by compounds which induce differentiation of murine leukemia cells, *Int. J. Cancer,* 25, 213, 1980.
19. **Bodner, A. J., Ting, R. C., and Gallo, R. C.,** Induction of differentiation of human promyelocytic leukemia cells (HL-60) by nucleosides and methotrexate, *J. Natl. Cancer. Inst.,* 67, 1025, 1981.
20. **Mendelsohn, N., Michl, J., Gilbert, H. S., Acs, G., and Christman, J. K.,** L-Ethionine as an inducer of differentiation in human promyelocytic leukemia cells (HL-60), *Cancer Res.,* 40, 3206, 1980.

21. **Christman, J. K., Mendelsohn, N., Herzog, D., and Schneiderman, N.,** Effect of 5-azacytidine on differentiation and DNA methylation in human promyelocytic leukemia cells (HL-60), *Cancer Res.,* 43, 763, 1983.

22. **Lotem, J. and Sachs, L.,** Potential pre-screening for therapeutic agents that induce differentiation in human myeloid leukemia cells, *Int. J. Cancer,* 25, 561, 1980.

23. **Lotem J. and Sachs, L.,** Regulation of normal differentiation in mouse and human myeloid leukemic cells by phorbol esters and the mechanism of tumor promotion, *Proc. Natl. Acad. Sci. U.S.A.,* 76, 5158, 1979.

24. **Schwartz, E. L. and Sartorelli, A. C.,** Structure-activity relationships for the induction of differentiation of HL-60 human acute promyelocytic leukemia cells by athracyclines, *Cancer Res.,* 42, 2651, 1982.

25. **Nakayasu, M., Terada, M., Tamura, G., and Sugimura, T.,** Induction of differentiation of human and murine leukemia cells in culture by tunicamycin, *Proc. Natl. Acad. Sci. U.S.A.,* 77, 409, 1980.

26. **Huberman, E. and Callaham, M. F.,** Induction of terminal differentiation in human promyelocytic leukemia cells by tumor-promoting agents, *Proc. Natl. Acad. Sci. U.S.A.,* 76, 1293, 1979.

27. **Rovera, G., Santoli, D., and Damsky, C.,** Human promyelocytic leukemia cells in culture differentiate into macrophage-like cells when treated with a phorbol diester, *Proc. Natl. Acad. Sci. U.S.A.,* 76, 2779, 1979.

28. **Fujiki, H., Mori, M., Nakayasu, M.,Terada, M., and Sugimura, T.,** A possible naturally occurring tumor promoter, Teleocidin B from *Streptomyces, Biochem. Biophys. Res. Commun.,* 90, 976, 1979.

29. **Nakayasu, M., Fujiki, H., Mori, M., Sugimura, T., and Moore, R. E.,** Teleocidin, lyngbyatoxin A and their hydrogenated derivatives, possible tumor promoter, induce terminal differentiation in HL-60 cells, *Cancer Lett.,* 12, 271, 1981.

30. **Breitman, T. R., Selonick, S. E., and Collins, S. J.,** Induction of differentiation of the human promyelocytic leukemia cell line (HL-60) by retinoic acid, *Proc. Natl. Acad. Sci. U.S.A.,* 77, 2936, 1980.

31. **Honma, Y., Takenaga, K., Kasukabe, T., and Hozumi, M.,** Induction of differentiation of cultured human promyelocytic leukemia cells by retinoids, *Biochem. Biophys. Res. Commun.,* 95, 507, 1980.

32. **Breitman, T. R.,** Induction of terminal differentiation of HL-60 and fresh leukemic cells by retinoic acid, in *Expression of Differentiated Functions in Cancer Cells,* Revoltella, R. P., Pontieri, G. M., Basilico, C., Rovera, G., Gallo, R.C., and Subak-Sharpe, J. H., Eds., Raven Press, New York, 1982, 257.

33. **Miyaura, C., Abe, E., Kuribayashi, T., Tanaka, H., Konno, K., Nishii, Y., and Suda, T.,** 1α, 25-Dihydroxyvitamin D_3 induces differentiation of human myeloid leukemia cells, *Biochem. Biophys. Res. Commun.,* 102, 937, 1981.

34. **Breitman, T. R. and Keene, B. R.,** Growth and differentiation of human promyelocytic cell line HL-60 in a defined medium, in *Cold Spring Harbor Conferences on Cell Proliferation,* Vol. 9, Cold Spring Harbor Laboratory, Cold Spring Harbor, New York, 1982, 691.

35. **Newburger, P. E., Chovaniec, M. E., Greenberger, J. S., and Cohen, H. J.,** Functional changes in human leukemia cell line HL-60: A model for myeloid differentiation, *J. Cell Biol.,* 82, 315, 1979.

36. **Gallagher, R., Collins, S., Trujillo, J., McCredie, K., Ahearn, M., Tsai, S., Metzgar, R., Aulakh, G., Ting, R., Ruscetti, F., and Gallo, R.,** Characterization of the continuous, differentiating myeloid cell line (HL-60) from a patient with acute promyelocytic leukemia, *Blood,* 54, 713, 1979.

37. **Fontana, J. A., Wright, D. G., Schiffman, E., Corcoran, B. A., and Deisseroth, A. B.,** Development of chemotactic responsiveness in myeloid prescursor cells: studies with a human leukemia cell line, *Proc. Natl. Acad. Sci. U.S.A.,* 77, 3664, 1980.

38. **Olsson, I. and Olofsson, T.,** Induction of differentiation in a human promyelocytic leukemic cell line (HL-60). Production of granule proteins, *Exp. Cell. Res.,* 131, 225, 1981.

39. **Breitman, T. R., Collins, S. J., and Keene, B. R.,** Replacement of serum by insulin and transferrin supports growth and differentiation of the human promyelocytic cell line, HL-60, *Exp. Cell. Res.,* 126, 494, 1980.

40. **Mather, J. P. and Sato, G. H.,** The growth of mouse melanoma cells in hormone-supplemented, serum-free medium, *Exp. Cell. Res.,* 120, 191, 1979.

41. **Gallo, R., Ruscetti, F., Collins, S., and Gallagher, R.,** Human myeoid leukemia cells: studies on oncornaviral related information and *in vitro* growth and differentiation, in *Hematopoietic Cell Differentiation,* Golde, D. W., Cline, M. J., Metcalf, D., and Fox, C. F., Eds., Academic Press, New York, 1979, 335.

42. **Ruscetti, F. W., Collins, S. J., Woods, A. M., and Gallo, R. C.,** Clonal analysis of the response of human myeloid leukemic cell lines to colony-stimulating activity, *Blood,* 58, 285, 1981.

43. **DeRuyter, M. G., Lambert, W. E., and DeLeenheer, A. P.,** Retinoic acid: an endogenous compound of human blood. Unequivocal demonstration of endogenous retinoic acid in normal physiological conditions, *Anal. Biochem.,* 98, 402, 1979.

44. **Rizzino, A. and Crowley, C.,** Growth and differentiation of embryonal carcinoma cell line F_9 in defined media, *Proc. Natl. Acad. Sci. U.S.A.,* 77, 457, 1980.

45. **Ong, D. E. and Chytil, F.,** Retinoic acid-binding protein in rat tissue. Partial purification and comparison to rat tissue retinol-binding protein, *J. Biol. Chem.,* 250, 6113, 1975.

46. **Breitman, T. R., Collins, S. J., and Keene, B. R.,** Terminal differentiation of human promyelocytic leukemic cells in primary culture in response to retinoic acid, *Blood,* 57, 1000, 1981.

47. **Jetten, A. M. and Breitman, T. R.,** unpublished data, 1981.

48. **Takenaga, K., Honma, Y., and Hozumi, M.,** Cellular retinoid-binding proteins in cultured human and mouse myeloid leukemia cells, *Cancer Lett.,* 13, 1, 1981.

49. **Douer, D. and Koeffler, H. P.,** Retinoic Acid. Inhibition of the clonal growth of human myeloid leukemia cells, *J. Clin. Invest.,* 69, 277, 1982.

50. **Roberts, A. B. and Frolik, C. A.,** Recent advances in the *in vivo* and *in vitro* metabolism of retinoic acid, *Fed. Proc.,* 38, 2524, 1979.

51. **Skubitz, K. M., Zhen, Y., and August, J. T.,** Dexamethasone synergistically induces chemotactic peptide receptor expression in HL-60 cells, *Blood,* 59, 586, 1982.

52. **Brandt, S. J., Barnes, K. C., Glass, D. B., and Kinkade, J. M., Jr.,** Glucocorticoid-stimulated increase in chemotactic peptide receptors on differentiating human myeloid leukemia (HL-60) cells, *Cancer Res.,* 41, 4947, 1981.

53. **Levine, L. and Breitman, T. R.,** manuscript in preparation, 1983.

54. **Hemmi, H., Breitman, T. R., Keene, B. R., and Frank, D. A.,** Comparative functional changes in HL-60 cells induced to differentiate by retinoic acid and dimethylsulfoxide, *Fed. Proc. Fed. Am. Soc. Exp. Biol.,* 41, 683, 1982.

55. **Zakhireh, B. and Root, R. K.,** Development of oxidase activity by human bone marrow granulocytes, *Blood,* 54, 429, 1979.

56. **Olsson, I. L., Breitman, T. R., and Gallo, R. C.,** Priming of human myeloid leukemic cell lines HL-60 and U-937 with retinoic acid for differentiation effects of cyclic adenosine $3':5'$-monophosphate-inducing agents and a T-lymphocyte-derived differentiation factor, *Cancer Res.,* 42, 3928, 1982.

57. **Jaffe, B. M., Behrman, H. R., and Parker, C.W.,** Radioimmunoassay measurement of prostaglandins E, A, and F in human plasma, *J. Clin. Invest.,* 52, 398, 1973.

58. **Berenbaum, M. C., Cope, W. A., and Bundick, R. V.,** Synergistic effect of cortisol and prostaglandin E_2 on the PHA response, *Clin. Exp. Immunol.,* 26, 534, 1976.

59. **Gilman, A. G. and Nirenberg, M.,** Regulation of adenosine $3',5'$-cyclic monophosphate metabolism in cultured neuroblastoma cells, *Nature (London),* 234, 356, 1971.

60. **Kuehl, F. A., Jr. and Humes, J. L.,** Direct evidence for a prostaglandin receptor and its application to prostaglandin measurements, *Proc. Natl. Acad. Sci. U.S.A.,* 69, 480, 1972.

61. **Hittelman, K. J. and Butcher, R. W.,** Cyclic AMP and the mechanism of action of the prostaglandins, in *The Prostaglandins,* Cuthbert, M. F., Ed., J. B. Lippincott, Philadelphia, 1973.

62. **Breitman, T. R. and Keene, B. R.,** unpublished experiments, 1980.

63. **Levine, L. and Ohuchi, K.,** Retinoids as well as tumor promoters enhance deacylation of cellular lipids and prostaglandin production in MDCK cells, *Nature (London),* 276, 274, 1978.

64. **Bonser, R. W., Siegel, M. I., McConnell, R. T. and Cuatrecasas, P.,** The appearance of phospholipase and cyclo-oxygenase activities in human promyelocytic leukemia cell line HL60 during dimethyl sulfoxide-induced differentiation, *Biochem. Biophys. Res. Commun.,* 98, 614, 1981.

65. **Kurland, J. I., Hadden, J. W. and Moore, M. A. S.,** Role of cyclic nucleotides in the proliferation of committed granulocyte-macrophage progenitor cells, *Cancer Res.,* 37, 4534, 1978.

66. **Williams, N.,** Preferential inhibition of murine macrophage colony formation by prostaglandin E., *Blood,* 53, 1089, 1979.

67. **Taetle, R. and Koessler, A.,** Effects of cyclic nucleotides and prostaglandins on normal and abnormal human myeloid progenitor proliferation, *Cancer Res.,* 40, 1223, 1980.

68. **Cavalieri, R. L., Havell, E. A., Vilcek, J., and Pestka, S.,** Induction and decay of human fibroblast interferon mRNA, *Proc. Natl. Acad. Sci. U.S.A.,* 74, 4415, 1977.

69. **Greengard, P.,** Phosphorylated proteins as physiological effectors, *Science,* 199, 146, 1978.

70. **Ludwig, K. W., Lowey, B., and Niles, R. M.,** Retinoic acid increases cyclic AMP-dependent protein kinase activity in murine melanoma cells, *J. Biol. Chem.,* 255, 5999, 1980.

71. **Lotan, R., Giotta, G., Nork, E., and Nicolson, G. L.,** Characterization of the inhibitory effects of retinoids on the *in vitro* growth of two malignant murine melanomas, *J. Natl. Cancer Inst.,* 60, 1035, 1978.

72. **Mastro, A. M. and Rozengurt, E.,** Endogenous protein kinase in outer plasma membrane of cultured 3T3 cells, *J. Biol. Chem.,* 251, 7899, 1976.

73. **Kubler, D., Pyerin, W., and Kinzel, V.,** Protein kinase activity and substrates at the surface of intact HeLa cells, *J. Biol. Chem.,* 257, 322, 1982.

74. **Elias, L., Wogenrich, F. J., Wallace, J. M., and Longmire, J.,** Altered pattern of differentiation and proliferation of HL-60 promyelocytic leukemia cells in the presence of leucocyte conditioned medium, *Leukemia Res.,* 4, 301, 1980.

75. **Chiao, J. W., Freitag, W. F., Steinmetz, J. C., and Andreeff, M.,** Changes of cellular markers during differentiation of HL-60 promyelocytes to macrophages as induced by T lymphocyte conditioned medium, *Leukemia Res.,* 5, 477, 1981.

76. **Todd, R. F., III, Griffin, J. D., Ritz, J., Nadler, L. M., Abrams, T., and Schlossman, S. F.,** Expression of normal monocyte-macrophage differentiation antigens on HL-60 promyelocytes undergoing differentiation induced by leukocyte-conditioned medium or phorbol diester, *Leukemia Res.,* 5, 491, 1981.

77. **Olsson, I., Olofsson, T., and Mauritzon, N.,** Characterization of mononuclear blood cell-derived differentiation inducing factors for the human promyelocytic leukemia cell line HL-60, *J. Natl. Cancer Inst.,* 67, 1225, 1981.

78. **Ferrero, D., Pessano, S., Pagliardi, G. L., and Rovera, G.,** Induction of differentiation of human myeloid leukemias: surface changes probed with monoclonal antibodies, *Blood,* 61, 171, 1983.

79. **Poiesz, B. J., Ruscetti, F. W., Gazdar, A. F., Bunn, P. A., Minna, J. D., and Gallo, R. C.,** Detection and isolation of type C retrovirus particles from fresh and cultured lymphocytes of a patient with cutaneous T-cell lymphoma, *Proc. Natl. Acad. Sci. U.S.A.,* 77, 7415, 1980.

80. **Breitman, T. R. and Olsson, I. L.,** unpublished experiments, 1980.

81. **Tomida, M., Yamamoto, Y., and Hozumi, M.,** Stimulation by interferon of induction of differentiation of human promyelocytic leukemia cells, *Biochem. Biophys. Res. Commun.,* 104, 30, 1982.

82. **Breitman, T. R. and Keene, B. R.,** unpublished experiments, 1983.

83. **Werb, Z. and Cohn, Z. A.,** Plasma membrane synthesis in the macrophage following phagocytosis of polystryrene latex particles, *J. Biol. Chem.,* 247, 2439, 1972.

84. **Driedger, P. E. and Blumberg, P. M.,** Specific binding of phorbol ester tumor promoters, *Proc. Natl. Acad. Sci. U.S.A.,* 77, 567, 1980.

85. **Solanki, V., Slaga, T. J., Callaham, M., and Huberman, E.,** Down regulation of specific binding of [20-^{3}H]phorbol 12,13-dibutyrate and phorbol ester-induced differentiation of human promyelocytic leukemia cells, *Proc. Natl. Acad. Sci. U.S.A.,* 78, 1722, 1981.

86. **Colburn, N. H., Gindhart, T. D., Dalal, B., and Hegamyer, G. A.,** The role of phorbol ester receptor binding in responses to promoters by mouse and human cells, in *Organ and Species Specificity in Chemical Carcinogenesis,* Lagenbach, R., Nesnow, S., and Rice, J. M., Eds., Plenum Press, New York, 1983, 189.

87. **Newburger, P. E., Baker, R. D., Hansen, S. L., Duncan, R. A., and Greenberger, J. S.,** Functionally deficient differentiation of HL-60 promyelocytic leukemia cells induced by phorbol myristate acetate, *Cancer Res.,* 41, 1861, 1981.

88. **Palu', G., Powles, R., Selby, P., Summersgill, B. M., and Alexander, P.,** Patterns of maturation in short-term culture of human acute myeloid leukemic cells, *Br. J. Cancer,* 40, 719, 1979.

89. **Breitman, T. R. and Keene, B. R.,** unpublished experiments, 1981.

90. **Hemmi, H. and Breitman, T. R.,** unpublished results, 1982.

91. **Hemmi, H., Keene, B R., and Breitman, T. R.,** manuscript in preparation, 1983.

92. **Ferrero, D., Tarella, C., Gallo, E., Ruscetti, F. W., and Breitman, T. R.,** Terminal differentiation of the human promyelocytic leukemia cell line, HL-60, in the absence of cell proliferation, *Cancer Res.,* 42, 4421, 1982.

93. **Momparler, R. L.,** A model for the chemotherapy of adult leukemia with 1-β-D-arabinofuranosylcytosine, *Cancer Res.,* 34, 1775, 1974.

94. **Young, C. W. and Hodas, S.** Hydroxyurea: inhibitory effect on DNA metabolism, *Science,* 146, 1172, 1964.

95. **Pierce, G. B.,** Teratocarcinoma: model for a developmental concept of cancer, in *Current Concepts in Developmental Biology,* Moscona, A. A. and Monroy, A., Eds., Academic Press, New York, 1967, 223.

96. **Pierce, G. B.,** The benign cells of malignant tumors, in *Developmental Aspects of Carcinogenesis and Immunity,* King, T. J., Ed., Academic Press, New York, 1974, 3.

97. **Pierce, G. B., Shikes, R., and Fink, L. M.,** *Cancer: A Problem of Developmental Biology,* Prentice-Hall, Engelwood Cliffs, N.J., 1978.

98. **Hozumi, M.,** A new approach to chemotherapy of myeloid leukemia: control of leukemogenicity of myeloid leukemia cells by inducer of normal differentiation, in *Cancer Biology Reviews,* Marchalonis, J. J. and Hanna, M. G., Jr., Eds., Vol. 3, Marcel Dekker, New York, 1982, 153.

99. **Hozumi, M.,** Fundamentals of chemotherapy of myeloid leukemia by induction of leukemia cell differentiation, *Adv. Cancer Res.,* 38, 121, 1983.

100. **Honma, Y., Kasukabe, T., Okabe, J., and Hozumi, M.,** Prolongation of survival time of mice inoculated with myeloid leukemia cells by inducers of normal differentiation, *Cancer Res.,* 39, 3167, 1979.

101. **Lotem, J. and Sachs, L.,** *In vivo* induction of normal differentiation in myeloid leukemia cells, *Proc. Natl. Acad. Sci. U.S.A.,* 75, 3781, 1978.

102. **Abe, E., Miyaura, C., Sakagami, H., Takeda, M., Konno, K., Yamazaki, T., Yoshiki, S., and Suda, T.,** Differentiation of mouse myeloid leukemia cells induced by 1α,25-dihydroxyvitamin D_3, *Proc. Natl. Acad. Sci. U.S.A.,* 78, 4990, 1981.

103. **Lotem, J. and Sachs, L.,** *In vivo* inhibition of the development of myeloid leukemia by injection of macrophage- and granulocyte-inducing protein, *Int. J. Cancer,* 28, 375, 1981.

104. **Honma, Y., Hozumi, M., Abe, E., Konno, K., Fukushima, M., Hata, S., Nishii, Y., DeLuca, H. F., and Suda, T.,** 1α,25-Dihydroxyvitamin D₃ and 1α-hydroxyvitamin D₃ prolong survival time of mice inoculated with myeloid leukemia cells, *Proc. Natl. Acad. Sci. U.S.A.,* 80, 201, 1983.
105. **Strickland, S. and Mahdavi, V.,** The induction of differentiation in teratocarcinoma stem cells by retinoic acid, *Cell,* 15, 393, 1978.
106. **Strickland, S. and Sawey, M. J.,** Studies on the effect of retinoids on the differentiation of teratocarcinoma stem cells *in vitro* and *in vivo, Dev. Biol.,* 78, 76, 1980.

INDEX

A

increased therapeutic activitiy, 104
  levels, 99, 103
  metabolism and properties, 99—102
  phosphorylation, 102
  plasma half-life, 103
  resistance, 102—103
Arabinosylcytosine-CMP, 102
Arabinosylcytosine-CTP, 99—103, 107
Arabinosylcytosine inhibitors, 103—107
Arabinosylcytosine therapy, 99, 105
Arabinosylhypoxanthine, 49
Ara-C, see Arabinosylcytosine
Arachidonic acid, 257
Aspirin, 265
Ataxia telangiectasia (A-T), 198
5-Azacytidine (5-AC), 104—105, 107
5-Azacytidine triphosphate (5-ACTP), 104
6-Azacytidine, 95, 96
8-Azainosine, 122, 123
Azaserine (Aza), 71
8-Azaserine-7-deazaguanine, 50
8-Azaserine-9-deazaguanine, 50
8-Azaserine-7-deazahypoxanthine (allopurinol), 50
8-Azaserine-7-deazainosine (formycin B), 48—51
2'-Azidoinosine (*ara* and *ribo*), 49

B

B16 melanoma, 98, 117
Base methylation, 18
B-cell leukemia, 116
BDF, 126
Benzimidazole, 147
5'-Benzylthioinosine, 49
Biosynthesis, 5—6
Bleomycin, 182, 185
Bovine serum albumin (BSA), 256
Breast cancer, see Mammary cancer
Bredinin, 122, 123, 128
5-Bromo-d-cytidine, 106
5-Bromodeoxyuridine, 252
2'-Bromoguanosine, 49
5'-Bromoinosine, 49
5'-*n*-Butylthioinosine, 49
Butyric acid, 252

C

Carbendazim, 147, 148
Carbocyclic inosine, 49
Carboxylic acid, 125
Carcinogenesis, 215, 216
Carcinoma, Lewis lung, 116, 117
Cardiomyopathy, 166
Cardiotoxicity, of sugar amine-modified anthracy-
  clines, 175—176
CCRF-CEM (T-cell leukemia), 116
CD 8F mammary tumor, 117
Cell

growth and viability, 213, 237—239, 271
  proliferation, inhibition of, 237—239
Cell cycle, 237
Cellular DNA, 182—183
Cellular efflux, 170
Chemical carcinogenesis, 216
Chemical reactions, free-radical, 199
Chemotactic peptide receptor, 256—257
Chemotherapy, combination, 216, 272
C3H/HeJ mammary tumors, 80
5'-Chloroformycin B, 49, 50
2'-Chloroguanosine, 49
5'-Chloroinosine, 49
Chromatin structure, 237, 239
Chromatofocusing, PNP, 40—41
Chromatography, affinity, 40
Clinical studies, 25—26
  on interferons, 217—219
  phase I, 106
CMA, 176
  antitumor activity, 168
  cytocidal activities, 169
  effect on RNA species synthesis, 172—174
  free radical formation and cardiotoxicity, 175
  microsomal metabolism of, 175
Colchicine, 139, 141, 144, 151, 158
  effect on tubulin-dependent GTP hydrolysis,
    145—150
Colon cancer, HCT-8, 80
Colon carcinoma cells, effect of interferons, on, 213
Colon tumor, 117
Colony formation, 195, 249
Combination chemotherapy, 216, 272
Cordycepin, 227, 229—232
Cordycepin analog, 213, 226, 230, 234—235
Cordycepin 5'-triphosphate (3'dATP), 227
C221R osteosarcoma, 80
Cutaneous T-cell leukemia, 116
Cutaneous T-cell lymphoma, 116, 226, 236—237
CX-1 colon tumor, 117
Cyanomorpholinyl group, see CMA
Cyclic adenosine 3',5'-monophosphate (cAMP),
    257—260
d-Cytidilate (dCMP) deaminase, 103, 107
Cytidine, 92, 105
  deamination reaction, of, 95—96
d-Cytidine, 92, 106
Cytidine aminohydrolase, 92
Cytidine deaminase (CDA)
  5-AC as substrate for, 104
  deamination reaction, 96
  diazepin-2-one nucleosides as inhibitors of, 99,
    101
  distribution, 92
  inhibition of, 99—107
  inhibitors, 96—99
  mechanism of reaction, 95—96
  structure-activity relationships, 93
  substrate for, 107
  substrate specificity, 92—95
  tetrahydrouridine inhibition against, 97—98